Life Sciences Research Report 17
Pain and Society

The goal of this Dahlem Workshop is:
To examine strategies in the study of pain and its role in society.

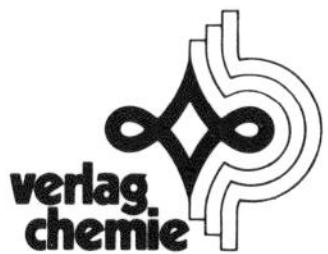

Life Sciences Research Report
Editor: Silke Bernhard

Held and published on behalf of the
Stifterverband für die Deutsche Wissenschaft

Sponsored by:
Stifterverband für die Deutsche Wissenschaft,
Senat der Stadt Berlin, and
Stiftung Deutsche Klassenlotterie Berlin

H. W. Kosterlitz and L.Y. Terenius
Editors

Pain and Society

Report of the Dahlem Workshop on
Pain and Society
Berlin 1979, November 26–30

Rapporteurs:
Harold Merskey · William D. Willis · Berthold B. Wolff ·
Manfred Zimmermann

Program Advisory Committee:
Hans W. Kosterlitz (Chairman) · Jean-Marie R. Besson ·
Albert Herz · Raymond W. Houde · Ainsley Iggo ·
Paolo Procacci · Richard A. Sternbach · Lars Y. Terenius ·
Manfred Zimmermann

Verlag Chemie
Weinheim · Deerfield Beach, Florida · Basel · 1980

Copy editor: M. Cervantes-Waldmann

CIP – Kurztitelaufnahme der Deutschen Bibliothek

Pain and society: *report of the Dahlem Workshop on Pain and Society, Berlin 1979, November 26–30/Dahlem-Konferenzraum. H. W. Kosterlitz and L. Y. Terenius, ed. Rapporteurs: Harold Merskey... – Weinheim, Deerfield Beach (Florida), Basel: Verlag Chemie, 1980.*
(Life sciences research report; 17)
ISBN 3-527-12019-X (Weinheim, Basel)
ISBN 0-89573-099-5 (Deerfield Beach)

NE: Kosterlitz, Hans W. [Hrsg.]; Merskey, Harold [Mitarb.]; Workshop on Pain and Society
<1979, Berlin, West>; Dahlem-Konferenzen

Verlag Chemie GmbH, D-6940 Weinheim

Printed in West Germany

Table of Contents

Central Mechanisms of Pain Control

Recurrent Persistent Pain: Mechanisms and Models

Abbreviations in This Work

5HIAA	serotonin metabolite
5HT	5 hydroxytryptamine, serotonin
5HTP	5 hydroxytryptophan
ACH	acetylcholine
ACTH	adrenocorticotropic hormone
AIB	abnormal illness behavior
βEP	β-Endorphin
βLPH	β-Lipoprotein
BEPs	brain electrical potentials
BK	bradykinin
C1	first cervical segment
CCK	cholecystokinin
CL	centralis lateralis
CNS	central nervous system
CSF	cerebrospinal fluid
DBS	deep brain stimulation
DCS	dorsal column stimulation
DLF	dorsolateral funiculus
DRG	dorsal root ganglion
DRN	dorsal raphe nucleus
ENK	enkephalin
EPSPs	excitatory postsynaptic potentials
GABA	gamma aminobutyric acid
GAD	glutamic acid decarboxylase
HIS	histamine
HRP	horseradish peroxidase
IASP	International Association for the Study of Pain
IPSP	inhibitory postsynaptic potential
KCl	potassium chloride
LSD	D-Lysergic acid diethylamide
NRM	nucleus raphe magnus
OR	opiate receptor
PAG	periaqueductal gray matter
p-CPA	parachlorophenylalanine
PG	prostaglandin
POm	posterior group (medial division)
PT	pain transmission
REM	rapid eye movement
RF	reticular formation
Rmc	nucleus reticularis magnocellularis
SA	slowly-adapting
SCT	spinocervical tract
SES	socioeconomic status
SG	substantia gelatinosa
SGR	substantia gelatinosa of Rolando
S(s)P	substance P
SPA	stimulation producing analgesia
SRT	spinoreticular tract
STT	spinothalamic tract
TENS	transcutaneous electrical nerve stimulation
TNS	transcutaneous nerve stimulation
VIP	vasoactive intestinal peptide
VL	ventralis lateralis
VP	ventralis posterior
VPL	ventralis posterolateralis

Pain and Society, eds. H.W. Kosterlitz and L.Y. Terenius, pp. 1-2.
Dahlem Konferenzen 1980. Weinheim: Verlag Chemie GmbH.

Introduction

H. W. Kosterlitz* and L. Y. Terenius**
*University of Aberdeen, Unit for Research on Addictive Drugs
Marischal College, Aberdeen AB9 1AS, Scotland
**Department of Pharmacology, Uppsala University
Box 573, 751 23 Uppsala, Sweden

Since time immemorial, pain has been the outstanding symptom which persuades the patient to seek the advice of his doctor. Until a few decades ago, the only effective treatment of acute and chronic pain was the administration of analgesic drugs. Since then we have acquired a much better understanding of the anatomical and physiological bases of pain which have made possible a number of new therapeutic approaches to this difficult problem. We are also becoming more aware of the psychological and social factors which influence a person's attitude and reaction to pain whether it be of short or long duration. In the industrialized societies, chronic pain syndromes have considerable economic consequences.

Probably the most significant progress in recent years has been the discovery of the role of certain neuropeptides in the transmission and modulation of the impulses which signal noxious changes and are appreciated as pain. One of these neuropeptides, substance P, seems to facilitate this transmission in the periphery while the opioid peptides, the enkephalins and endorphins, appear to exert an inhibitory modulation, thus limiting the experience of pain to tolerable levels. One of the phenomena which has recently attracted wide attention is acupuncture, and evidence has accumulated that release of enkephalins and endorphins from nerve terminals may be the physiological basis of the pain alleviating effects of acupuncture.

The topic is multidisciplinary in a wide sense. For a long time, philosophers have been engaged in trying to achieve an understanding of the metaphysical meaning of pain. In recent times behavioral scientists have become deeply involved in the problem of pain as they affect the individual and society. Different approaches have been employed by neuroanatomists and neurophysiologists to elucidate the role which different parts of the central nervous system play in the experience and appreciation of different types of pain; neurochemists and particularly neuropharmacologists have aimed at alleviation of pain by analyzing the events at a cellular level and studying their modification by drugs. Finally, neurosurgeons and neurologists have contributed to a great extent to our present-day knowledge of treating pain by electrical stimulation of selected parts of the brain or peripheral nerve.

When the workshop on Pain and Society was planned, it was evident that knowledge in the different areas of research on pain had progressed sufficiently that an attempt could be made to achieve a considerable degree of integration between the various disciplines. We were fortunate in having had the support of outstanding contributors who took part in lively and searching discussions, of which this volume is the record. The panel included anatomists, physiologists, biochemists, pharmacologists, clinicians, psychiatrists, psychologists, sociologists, and, last but not least, philosophers. It is hoped that some of the excitement and friendly controversy of the workshop is mirrored in this book.

Pain and Society, eds. H.W. Kosterlitz and L.Y. Terenius, pp. 3-12.
Dahlem Konferenzen 1980. Weinheim: Verlag Chemie GmbH.

History of the Pain Concept

P. Procacci
Centro di Algologia, Clinica Medica
Università di Firenze, 50134 Florence, Italy

Abstract. The concept of pain follows areas of civilization, philosophical thought, and scientific discoveries. From a first stage, in which pain was considered as a disease due to an "intrusion," we arrive with the great Greek thinkers to the identification of pain as distinctly arising from different sensory modalities. During and after the Renaissance different thinkers, from Leonardo da Vinci to Descartes, tried to explain, according to the scientific knowledge of their times, the origin of different sensations and pain. Great progress in the neurophysiology and psychology of pain has been made in the last one hundred years. A problem which still remains object for discussion is how important are specific nerve-endings and nerves for pain in relation to the input of other nerve-endings and to central integration.

The problem of pain was present at the onset of our civilization. It is strictly related to the concept of sensation and more generally to that of disease. In this short paper, after a brief summary on the primitive civilizations and on the old Mediterranean civilizations, we shall dwell upon the concept of pain in the Western civilization. (For the concept of pain in Eastern civilizations, see Tu, this volume.)

In primitive civilizations lasting until a few decades ago in Australia, New Guinea, and in some islands of Melanesia, pain was referred to as an intrusion upon the human body of objects, magic fluids, or demons (12,13,17). Reference is obviously made to pain caused by an arrow, sword, or spear, which have always been considered objects that allow the magic fluid or the demon to enter the body. This concept is transferred to spontaneous pain, whence the common practice of shamans or sorcerers to make a small artificial wound in the patient to allow the bad fluid or spirit to escape. In some cases the shaman sucks the spirit directly from the wound, taking it in himself and neutralizing it with magic power - a type of therapy which still survives in many countries much more than we think.

This intrusive concept of medicine and consequently of pain remains with some variations in the two great Mediterranean civilizations, the Egyptian and the Assyro-Babylonian (5,8,12,17). Typical of the Semitic peoples is the evolution from the concept of demons and devils to the concept of sin. Pain as a consequence of sin and the typical relationship sin-punishment is found in the Hebraic civilization. This relationship is particularly important because it is largely adopted by the Christian ethic.

Diseases and in particular pain were related to a supernatural cause until the Greek civilization. Alcmaeon of Croton, follower of Pythagoras, defines disease in physical terms: "diseases can be due sometimes to an external cause, as an excess of heat or cold" (13). But the most important contribution to the concept of pain is found in Plato and Aristotle.

Most of Plato's theories on sensations are written in the Timaeus (20). The center of every sensation is the heart. The conversion to the world of ideas seems reserved to the brain but not clearly. Extremely important is the opposition of pain and pleasure. In a well-known passage in Phaedo, the jailor has taken off the ring of the chain from Socrates' leg; the philosopher tells the disciples that he feels pleasure where before he felt pain; consequently, pleasure and pain, though opposed, are strictly tied "as having origin from the same head, while they are two" (19). It is evident that in Plato's thought there is not a clear borderline between psychic and physical basis of pain and pleasure.

Aristotle develops and completes the thought of Plato. Aristotle's concepts on pain are expressed in "De anima" and also developed in other works, e.g., "Ethica Nicomachea" (1,2). He identifies five senses: vision, hearing, taste, smell, and touch. Pain is considered an increased sensitivity of touch. In "De anima" Aristotle also says that "sensations are pleasant when their sensible extremes such as acid and sweet are brought into their proper ratio, whilst in excess they are painful and destructive" (1). For Aristotle the center of the "sensorium commune" remains the heart. The ideas of Aristotle are extremely important because they have been the fundament of medicine for nearly twenty centuries; the "ipse dixit" is the fundament of every scholastic teaching. In Hippocrates' thought pain originates from an imbalance of endogenous humors ("dyscrasia") (10). This idea was followed by all the Hippocratic school and remains parallel to Aristotle's concepts of disease up until the modern age. It may be noted that the recent debate on pain producing substances is philosophically and historically related to this concept.

The most relevant contributions to the physiology of pain in the Greco-Roman times were brought by Galen (9). Galen's importance is based on the fact that he has given a good representation of the central nervous system and studied the effects of nerve and cord sections. Galen thinks that the brain is the center of sensation. Each sense is subserved by a nerve which must be soft in order for the external object to produce its appropriate impression. The soft nerves are sensory and the hard nerves are motor. The brain is softer than any nerve, since it receives all sensations. Galen's knowledge of the cranial and spinal nerves was considerable. He describes how the viscera are supplied by sensory nerves directly from the spinal cord, a really modern concept, and the sympathetic trunks as being "a structure not previously known to anatomists." According to Galen, nature has endowed different organs and tissues with a sensitivity suitable for their physiological functions. Specifically regarding pain, Galen seems to think that the larger nerves are filled with psychic pneuma and are devolved to the finest sensory functions. The smallest nerves subserve the lowest levels of sensitivity consisting of pain alone. As we can see, a relevant group of modern concepts are present in Galen, but he does not elaborate Aristotle's idea of a "sensorium commune" nor does he attempt to locate the soul. This can explain, as Kenneth Keele observes (12), why Aristotle's concepts are more acceptable to the Christian Church and why this part of Galen's work has been neglected.

After Galen, we have a leap of over one thousand years. In the Middle Ages we have important schools of medicine in the Arab countries, in Salerno, and thereafter in the universities of Europe (5,17). But the concept of pain does not show any substantial variation until the Renaissance.

In the Renaissance, under Lorenzo the Magnificent, the famous Academia Platonica was founded in Florence, with Marsilio Ficino, Pico della Mirandola, and other great thinkers. Here the papers of Plato and Aristotle were again commented upon and discussed. We return to the physiology of sensations and of pain with Leonardo da Vinci - also a pupil of the Medici's environment. From a philosophic point of view his concept of pain is similar to the platonic idea of pleasure and pain: in the Codex Atlanticus there is the famous drawing of pleasure and pain represented as a man with two faces (15). In the Windsor manuscripts on anatomy we can see that Leonardo appreciated the function of the spinal cord as a conductor (16). Pain is linked to the sense of touch and passes through the "perforated nerves" to be transmitted to the "sensorium commune," that, according to Leonardo, is located in the third ventricle. Here Leonardo places the site of the soul. Modern anatomy and the physiology of sensation begin with Leonardo.

We cannot describe in detail the thought of other great scientists, such as Vesalius, Varolius, and other Renaissance authors (5,17). The general conclusion is that the center of sensations is in the brain. A tubular system of nerves, described by Leonardo, is generally accepted.

Also, Descartes' studies and conclusions are along the same lines. Very important is his attempt to explain how a sensation arises. For him nerves are not simple hollow tubes, but tubes within which there is a sort of marrow composed of a large number of exceedingly delicate threads starting from the proper substance of the brain. From the porous walls of the cerebral ventricles animal spirit flows in the nerves. Well-known is the figure of the boy published in "L' Homme" (7), in which the paths of heat and burning pain are represented. Pain remains a constituent of touch, according to Aristotle's concept. How Descartes was still tied to the classic views is clear from his opinion that the "res cogitans" and the "res extensa" are connected in the pineal gland.

In the 18th Century, notwithstanding the great progress of anatomy, the physiology of sensation was still tied to the old concepts. Willis, Borelli, Baglivi, and Malpighi - albeit in different manners - always express the fundamental concepts we have already considered (5,17). It is clear that up until the discovery of electrical phenomena in the nerve, the idea of pain and other sensations was necessarily tied to fine threads or to spirits going through the nerves.

Even in modern times discussions on the concepts of pain are still debated. Erasmus Darwin (6), following the Aristotelic idea, thought that pain was a consequence of any excessive stimulation and the result of excessive sensations of touch, heat, sight, taste, or smell. This "intensive" theory of pain was challenged by the idea of receptor specificity formulated by Johannes Müller and incorporated in his well-known doctrine of specific nerve energies (18). The main reason for its success was its simplicity. Indeed, if one adopts the point of view that a given perceptive modality has a definite and specific cellular representation in the brain, the simplest system will be one with a specific receptor apparatus. Furthermore, the obvious specificity of some types of receptors, such as those of vision and hearing, tends to lead one to accept an analogous receptor specificity for other sensory modalities. With regards to the cutaneous end organs, a definite relationship between morphology and function was proposed in the case of Meissner's corpuscles, Merkel's disks, basket endings, and touch, Krause's end bulbs and cold, Ruffini's corpuscles and warmth, and free nerve endings and pain. This theory remained dominant up until recent times.

The first criticism of the theory of specific sensory apparatuses for various sensory modalities was advanced against this strict relationship between ending-structure and function. Careful investigation of sensory function followed by biopsy was performed on a given skin area; the histological examination showed that many of the above-mentioned relations were questionable. Furthermore, various intermediate forms of receptors were found to exist between the known corpuscles, and a difference was observed between nerve-ending structure in glabrous skin and in hairy skin, with no difference in sensibility (21). Recently, however, Iggo (11) has studied in the skin, by both electrophysiological and histological techniques, a sensory ending consisting fundamentally of a corpuscle of Merkel. This "touch corpuscle" shows a high sensitivity to mechanical stimulation and provides a well-documented example of a cutaneous receptor in which a characteristic and distinctive structure is invariably associated with a particular set of functional properties.

Criticism advanced against the attribution of modality specificity to morphological characteristics of end organs does not invalidate a modality-specific physiological theory. It can be maintained that a receptor, whatever its structure, is excited specifically by only one sort of stimulus, thermal, tactile, or painful.

This classical thesis was challenged by Weddell and his group. They proposed that the various cutaneous sensations do not arise from the selective activation of specific receptors, but from a central differentiation between various types of stimuli and that this depends on the spatiotemporal pattern of the excitation of nonspecific sensory endings (14).

In the 1950's, Weddell's thesis gave rise to both agreement and disagreement. In general, agreement came from neurologists and neurosurgeons who found that certain complex clinical states, such as post-herpetic, causalgic, or thalamic pain, could not easily be explained by specific receptors and well-determined pain pathways, while they could be better interpreted by a modification of the spatiotemporal pattern of excitation. Disagreement mainly came from neurophysiologists who, moving from experimental research, tended to favor the specificity of receptors. This point of view is well summarized by Zotterman (22) who concludes that many experimental findings have proved the existence of fibers, and therefore of receptors, highly specific for some sensory modalities.

In the last few years these polemics have been subdued but still remain. It has been shown that a receptor is specific only within a determined range of stimuli. However, the recent discovery of the polymodal receptors (4) has shown that receptors can be excited by different kinds of energy at a given level. The problem today can be identified in these terms: a) Are the high-threshold receptors only nociceptive receptors? b) How important is the discharge of other receptors in coding and integrating the sensation of pain? Another point that is relevant in modern studies of pain is the concept that pain is not an inborn fixed sensation but in humans is in large part a learned sensation, influenced by sociological and ethnological conditions (3). In conclusion, we can say that to date our knowledge of pain is considerable but that there are many aspects which still have to be investigated and discussed; it is this dialectic process which is the most interesting approach to pain.

REFERENCES

(1) Aristotelis de anima libri tres. Ad interpretum Graecorum auctoritatem et codicum fidem recognovit commentariis illustravit Frider. Adolph. Trendelenburg. Berolini, sumptibus W. Weberi, 1877.

(2) Aristotelis Ethica Nicomachea. Edidit et commentario continuo instruxit G. Ramsauer. Lipsiae, in aedibus B. G. Teubneri, 1878.

(3) Benedetti, G. 1969. Neuropsicologia. Milano: Feltrinelli.

(4) Bessou, P., and Perl, E.R. 1969. Response of cutaneous sensory units with unmyelinated fibers to noxious stimuli. J. Neurophysiol. 32: 1025-1043.

(5) Castiglioni, A. 1948. Storia della medicina. Verona: Mondadori.

(6) Darwin, E. 1794. Zoönomia, or the Laws of Organic Life, vol. 1. London: J. Johnson.

(7) Descartes, R. 1644. L' homme. Paris: Angot.

(8) Ebers, P. 1875. Das hermetische Buch über die Arzneimittel der alten Aegypter von Georg Ebers. Leipzig: Engelmann.

(9) Galeni librorum. Venezia: Junta. 1576.

(10) Hippocratis medicorum omnium facile principis opera omnia quae extant. Geneva: Chouet.

(11) Iggo, A. 1965. The peripheral mechanisms of cutaneous sensation. In Studies in Physiology, eds. D.R. Curtis and A.K. McIntyre, pp. 92-100. Berlin: Springer Verlag.

(12) Keele, K.D. 1957. Anatomies of Pain. Oxford: Blackwell.

(13) Keele, K.D. 1962. Some historical concepts of pain. In The Assessment of Pain in Man and Animals, eds. C.A. Keele and R. Smith, pp. 12-27. London: Livingstone.

(14) Lele, P.P.; Weddell, G.; and Williams, C. 1954. The relationship between heat transfer, skin temperature and cutaneous sensibility. J. Physiol. 126: 206-234.

(15) Leonardo da Vinci. Il codice di Leonardo da Vinci della biblioteca del Principe Trevulzio in Milano. Quoted from: The Notebooks of Leonardo da Vinci, translated and edited by Edward MacCurdy, London, 1938.

(16) Leonardo da Vinci. I manoscritti di Leonardo da Vinci della Reale Biblioteca di Windsor. Dell'Anatomia fogli B. Pubblicati da Teodoro Sabachnikoff, trascritti e annotati da Giovanni Piumati. Milano, 1901.

(17) Major, R.H. 1955. A History of Medicine. Springfield: Thomas.

(18) Müller, J. 1840. Handbuch der Physiologie des Menschen für Vorlesungen. Koblenz: Hollscher.

(19) Plato: Phaedo, edited with introduction and notes by W.D. Geddes. London: Macmillan, 1885.

(20) Plato: Timaeus, edited with introduction and notes by R.D. Archer-Hind. London-New York: Macmillan, 1888.

(21) Weddell, G., and Miller, S. 1962. Cutaneous sensibility. Ann. Rev. Physiol. 24: 199-222.

(22) Zotterman, Y. 1962. Nerve fibres mediating pain; a brief review with a discussion on the specificity of cutaneous afferent nerve fibres. In The Assessment of Pain in Man and Animals, eds. C.A. Keele and R. Smith, pp. 60-73. London: Livingstone.

Pain and Society, eds. H.W. Kosterlitz and L.Y. Terenius, pp. 13-26.
Dahlem Konferenzen 1980. Weinheim: Verlag Chemie GmbH.

Phylogenetic Evolution of Pain Expression in Animals

R. Melzack and S. G. Dennis
Department of Psychology, McGill University
Montreal, Quebec H3A 1B1, Canada

Abstract. Throughout the evolution of the vertebrates, the slowly conducting pathways to the brain stem reticular formation continued to evolve and, at the same time, rapidly conducting pathways differentiated and developed, projecting to the ever growing thalamus and cortex. Moreover, descending neural control systems evolved along with the ascending systems. As a result of these evolutionary developments, pain experience and behavior have become less subjected to the push-pull of environmental events and are more variable and dynamic. The growth of the cortex, together with the development of the rapidly conducting transmission systems, allows new dimensions of expression of pain experience and behavior. Flight, fight, and reflex withdrawal are still part of the behavior repertoire, but much more is now possible. The large cortex allows the greater utilization of cognitive activities. Furthermore, increased social cooperation and language provide the basis for the development of complex strategies to cope with pain and suffering. The specialized functions of the parallel conducting systems and the importance of modulating systems (including that of the opioid peptides) are discussed. It is also proposed that the conscious experience of pain in subhuman mammals resembles the pain experienced by man after prefrontal lobotomy; that is, the lack of comprehension of the meaning of death and mutilation preclude the kind of suffering characteristic of some kinds of chronic pain in man.

INTRODUCTION

Pain in man comprises two components - behavior and conscious experience - which can both be measured with appropriate tools. Pain in animals, however, can only be measured by examining overt behavior. The experience of pain is often inferred from the behavior of mammals, and it is not unreasonable to attribute pain experience to birds, amphibia, and fish. Because the nervous systems of all vertebrates are organized in fundamentally the same way, investigators have examined the evolution of new structures, or new forms of neural organization, and have attempted to relate them to the advent of new forms of behavior. Coghill (2), for example, studied the relationships between neural development and behavior in the salamander and drew conclusions that have had an important impact on our understanding of human brain-behavior relationships.

THE COMPLEXITY OF PAIN BEHAVIOR

Pain was long considered to be the function of a reflexive, straight-through input-output system. However, as Melzack and Wall (7) have pointed out, sudden, unexpected damage of the skin usually produces a complex sequence of responses which is similar in most mammals: (a) a startle response, (b) a withdrawal reflex that removes the damaged area from the site of injury, (c) postural readjustment, (d) vocalization, (e) orientation of the head and eyes to examine the injured area, (f) generalized and localized autonomic responses, and (g) a series of behavior patterns such as rubbing the damaged area, flight from the cause of injury, aggression (if the cause is another organism), calling for help, and so forth.

In man, this sequence of behavior is accompanied by conscious experience. It has been proposed (6) that there are three major dimensions to human pain experience: (a) sensory experience which provides information on the location and extent damage as well as the nature of the injury, expressed by such words as crushing, wrenching, burning, stabbing, radiating, and so forth; (b) intensely unpleasant, diffuse affect that colors the entire experience and is associated with motivated behavior of varying complexity, ranging from flight-or-fight to making arrangements for visits to a Pain Clinic; (c) cognitive processes such as thought, evaluation of the meaning of the injury, and making decisions for the most appropriate behavior.

There is also an important temporal factor to pain. Unlike seeing and hearing, which cease when stimulation stops, pain usually persists when tissue has been damaged. If the injury is severe, pain persists for days, weeks, or longer. Normally the pain experience and behavior gradually disappear as healing proceeds. Sometimes, however, pain persists long after healing is completed. Chronic pain such as this is well documented in man but is virtually unknown in animal species. It is evident, then, that there are three temporal sequences: phasic pain, which is usually of short duration, occurs at the onset of injury, and involves a series of complex, rapid adjustments aimed primarily at withdrawal from the source of injury; acute pain, which continues for variable periods of time during rest and protection until healing has proceeded to permit normal behavior; and chronic pain, which persists after healing is completed.

A BRIEF SKETCH OF EVOLUTIONARY PROCESSES

Embryological and anatomical studies of fish, amphibians, and reptiles reveal that, even in the lowest vertebrates, reflexes are modulated by internuncial fibers (the "neuropil") that intervene between sensory and motor transmission (11). During embryological development of these species, behavior becomes increasingly a function of earlier experience (as a result of the engrams it has etched into the neural connections) as well as the ongoing activity of the organism and other inputs occurring at the same time. Behavior, then, is not merely the expression of response to a stimulus, but a dynamic process based on multiple interacting factors. Coghill (2) was first to propound this principle, based on his neuroembryological-behavioral studies of salamanders, which has been substantially confirmed by later investigators (11). Given this fundamental principle - that organisms are not passive receivers manipulated by environmental inputs but act dynamically on those inputs so that behavior becomes variable, unique, and creative - the remainder of evolution becomes comprehensible as a gradual development of mechanisms that make each new species on the evolutionary ladder increasingly independent of the push-and-pull of environmental circumstances.

Studies of the spinal projections of fish, amphibians, and reptiles reveal major spinoreticular components (4,8). These consist of small-diameter, unmyelinated fibers, with many synapses, that conduct slowly to reticular areas in the brain stem. In his studies of reptiles and amphibians after spinal cord hemisection, Ebbesson (4) notes that the lateral funiculus projects primarily to the cerebellum and the medial reticular formation in the brain stem, particularly to the periventricular gray substance. The latter is the most rostral level receiving an input in the frog. Somatic input, then, activates neurons at spinal levels, in cerebellar structures that play a role in coordinated behavior, and in reticular structures. From our present knowledge, it is assumed that the activity in reticular neurons and the limbic structures to which they project is involved in the motivational, driving aspects of behavior.

However, two additional important pathways are seen in amphibians and reptiles. There is a projection to the lateral cervical nucleus and a dorsal column projection to the dorsal column nuclei as well as to vestibular and cerebellar structures. A major clue to the function of the dorsal funiculus is Ebbesson's observation that it is extremely small in the snake but is larger in reptiles and amphibia with well developed limbs. He notes ((4), p. 93) that "the evolution of the dorsal column system indeed appears to be closely related to the evolution of the limbs, and in fact, it appears that the entire dorsal column-medial lemniscus-thalamocortical system has evolved principally in relation to the evolution of the limbs." At the same time, of course, the cortex evolved as selection favored those species with a greater capacity for complex function of the limbs. When the apes left the trees and the forelimbs became free for the manipulation of objects, the development of tools, and related activities, there was a striking growth of both the dorsal column system and the cortex.

All the transmission systems continued to develop during mammalian evolution. The slowly conducting spinoreticular system, as Noback and Schriver ((8), p. 119) point out, is not merely phylogenetically old but has "a long phylogenetic history that is still in progress." That is, its functions are as important as ever, and it has continued to differentiate and evolve. As the thalamus and cortex became increasingly important, the paleospinothalamic tract emerged as a pathway separate from the spinoreticular path. But at the same time, parallel rapidly conducting systems also evolved - the spinocervical tract, the dorsal column system, and the neospinothalamic tract. Indeed; even these systems appear to have undergone evolutionary changes. The spinocervical tract, which is prominent in carnivores, does not exist in a large proportion of humans (9). In contrast, the neospinothalamic tract is relatively small in carnivores and achieves prominence in primates. It is evident, then, that during evolution, the slowly conducting pathways to the reticular formation evolved and, at the same time, faster conducting pathways also differentiated and developed, projecting to the ever growing thalamus and cortex. All these systems act in parallel, although each has specialized functions (3,6).

The growth of the cortex, together with the development of the rapidly conducting systems, allows new dimensions of expression of pain experience and behavior. Flight, fight, and reflex withdrawal are still part of the behavior repertoire, but much more is now possible. The large brain allows the greater utilization of past experience, the evaluation of the meaning of the situation, and the evaluation of strategies to act in pain-producing situations: searching for the most satisfactory place to rest, recuperate and heal; ways of fighting potentially damaging adversaries. Furthermore, animals evolved mechanisms of cooperation and social behavior. Social calls for help after injury occur in the higher mammals such as carnivores and primates. Chimps injured by a fall often call for help and receive physical support from friends as they hobble along. In man, language and the capacity for symbolic expression allow the utilization of language in ways to cope with pain, including the development of the biological and medical sciences as strategies to combat pain and suffering.

So far, we have discussed only the ascending systems, but parallel development occurred in the descending systems from brain stem and cortex. The slowly conducting, multisynaptic "extrapyramidal" pathways were supplemented by the rapidly conducting "pyramidal" paths. In short, along with parallel afferent systems to increasingly complex central processing centers, there developed complex output systems, portions of which projected back to the ascending systems. These thereby allowed feedback loops capable of affecting activity in the more slowly conducting pathways. With all this growth, pain experience and behavior became less subjected to the pull-push of environmental inputs and more variable, plastic, dynamic, and self-determining.

THE EXPRESSION OF PAIN

There are many indices of pain - reflex withdrawal, avoidance behavior, autonomic changes, and, in man, linguistic expression. But not one of these is a certain index of pain experience. When a person says he is in pain, there is usually no reason to question the statement. However, malingerers are a fact of human social life, even though they are rare. Nevertheless, our knowledge of pain mechanisms is still sufficiently inadequate that people who claim to be in pain, even though no lesion or other physical pathology can be found, should be given the benefit of the doubt. It is possible, for example, that they are suffering from referred pain due to the summation of inputs from some minor source of irritation and persistent "memory-like" activity in the central nervous system due to an injury that had healed long before.

Language, generally, is a reliable index of pain, and most languages are rich in words to describe the sensory dimension of pain. The affective dimension is difficult to express - words such as exhausting, sickening, terrifying, cruel, vicious, and killing, come close but are often inadequate descriptors of the affective experience of the pain of cancer or causalgia. These feelings are diffuse and vague; but they drive the organism into activity to stop the pain, sometimes at terrible cost. They may drive people to try anything in their despair, even suicide.

Indices other than language are far less dependable. The damaging stimulus itself is not always a satisfactory index of pain. Visceral tissue can be burned or cut without producing pain, but stretching it usually evokes diffuse, aching pain. Skin, as Bishop (1) reported long ago, is also particularly sensitive to stretch. Wall (10) has recently described the surprising absence of pain during some kinds of injury. These observations suggest that there is a high degree of specialization among receptors. They do not respond to every kind of injury, but to particular kinds. Furthermore, psychological factors such as attention and distraction may also preclude any simple one-to-one relationship between stimulus and response (7).

Nor can reflexes or autonomic responses serve as reliable indices of pain. Spinal animals and paraplegic humans with high total spinal transection show segmental reflexes and appropriate autonomic responses when the skin is damaged but have no pain. Clearly, to infer pain, we must use as many indices as possible and use our best judgment.

PARALLEL CONDUCTION SYSTEMS

It is abundantly clear that pain signals are transmitted to the brain by multiple ascending spinal pathways. Moreover, the phylogenetically old, slowly conducting pathways appear to have maintained their functional importance throughout mammalian evolution. Indeed, the only pathways which seem to have changed in relative importance among mammals are the rapidly conducting spinocervical and neospinothalamic tracts. One of the most surprising recent discoveries is that the dorsal columns - long thought to carry information only about touch and proprioception - also contain fast-conducting pain-signaling fibers. These dorsal column postsynaptic fibers transmit signals evoked by noxious stimuli (damaging pressure and heat) to the dorsal column nuclei and may possibly project to higher areas (3). It is reasonable to assume that all of these pathways play a role in pain processes.

Melzack and Casey (6) noted that information from the spinal cord is projected to the brain along three major ascending systems which contribute to the quality and pattern of pain experience and response. First, there is evidence that the neospinothalamic tract which projects to the somatosensory thalamus and cortex contributes to the sensory-discriminative dimension of pain. Second, the slowly conducting pathways, which project to the medial areas of the brain stem and to the limbic system, are assumed to contribute to the motivational-affective dimension of pain. Third, the most rapidly conducting systems are proposed to comprise a "central control trigger" that activates neocortical or "higher central nervous system" processes, such as evaluation of the input in terms of past experience, which exert control over activity in both the discriminative and motivational systems. It is assumed that these three categories of activity interact with one another to provide (a) perceptual information regarding the location, magnitude and spatiotemporal properties of the noxious stimulus, (b) motivational tendency toward escape, attack, or other action, and (c) cognitive information based on analysis of multimodal information, past experience, and probability of outcome of different response strategies. All three forms of activity, then, influence motor mechanisms responsible for the complex patterns of overt responses that characterize pain.

We now know that the ascending systems are even more complex than Melzack and Casey envisaged. Dennis and Melzack (3) recently reviewed the literature on pain-signaling systems in the spinal cord. Six separate ascending systems (excluding the cerebellar projections) were proposed as having some role in pain-signaling.

The medially coursing systems, it is generally believed, predominantly subserve the affective dimension of pain experience. However, this does not preclude components that might be labeled. as "sensory." For example, the paleospinothalamic tract may be related to the "protopathic" aspects of pain - extremely unpleasant sensations which are poorly localized, diffuse, outlast stimulation, and are difficult to describe. The neospinothalamic tract, in contrast, appears to be predominantly involved in the more localized, discriminable aspects of pain experience. It must be emphasized that these dimensions are not subserved by pathways on a one-to-one basis but are the result of interactions and feedback loops among them.

Yet we are still confronted with a major problem: why are there three rapidly conducting, laterally coursing systems? Dennis and Melzack (3) have suggested that the fast pathways are individually inhibited or facilitated depending on the ongoing behavior or behavioral state of the organism - awake or asleep, fighting or feeding, nest-building or copulating, giving birth or exploring the environment. An important factor which may contribute to this process is the brain's need to obtain light tactile or proprioceptive information from these multimodal systems. None of the three systems is purely nociceptive. Each has a complement of cells responsive only to light tactile stimuli, and, perhaps more importantly, each has a significant population of multimodal cells - units that respond both to light tactile and nociceptive stimuli. Perhaps during a particular behavior pattern, the brain selects one type of information from a system and filters out the other types such as nociceptive inputs. Thus, when a system is functioning in a proprioceptive capacity or monitoring light tactile stimuli, it cannot simultaneously act as a nociceptive system for that part of the body. However, the enormous biological importance of nociception makes it essential that this modality be operative in some form at all times. Therefore, one of the other systems must provide the necessary pain-signaling function for the duration of the behavior. When the ongoing behavior or behavioral state changes, the brain selects other classes of tactile information, perhaps from other systems. When this occurs, a new pattern of differential inhibition and facilitation is imposed on the systems, such that the previously suppressed nociceptive capacity of one system may now be facilitated. In this way, the brain can always extract necessary tactile information from peripheral systems and still maintain vigilance regarding sudden injury or threat of injury.

The medial and lateral systems, in addition to their motivational and perceptual functions, may also provide the substrates for a tonic-phasic distinction in pain-signaling functions (3). The properties of the lateral group ensure speed, security of transmission, and, via thalamocortical relays, rapid integration with all other sensory-motor processes. Such systems would be useful in coding onset or sudden changes in a noxious or potentially noxious stimulus. Responses triggered by such information would have adaptive value in minimizing the damage done by intense stimulation. The medial systems, on the other hand, are generally less rapidly conducting, and synapses are frequent. Their target areas are less indicative of point-to-point relay of information than of global influences on information processing and behavior. Such properties seem more consistent with continuous or tonic information flow. There is less need for directness and speed if the message is to last for hours or days, as would be the case when tissue is damaged. Moreover, once damage is done, there is nothing the animal can do to escape it. Behavior triggered by the message would be better directed toward preventing reinjury and promoting healing. The possibility should also be considered that the medial systems stimulate directly the body's mechanisms for managing trauma, perhaps via hypothalamic mechanisms.

COGNITIVE CONTRIBUTIONS TO PAIN

The most striking feature about pain expression as we ascend that phylogenetic scale is that it becomes increasingly influenced by cognitive activities. Fear, anxiety, attention, and earlier learning have a profound impact on pain in mammals, particularly in primates, and most strikingly in man. Three mechanisms can play a role in this descending control from the brain. First, corticospinal fibers can modulate synaptic transmission at all spinal levels. Second, descending inhibitory influences from the central gray matter and other mesencephalic structures, which produce behavioral analgesia when electrically stimulated, are known to diminish transmission from dorsal horn to spinal afferent cells. Third, painful inputs or other stressing agents and events produce a release of opioid peptides which are capable of diminishing pain. As Hughes and Kosterlitz (5) have pointed out, the opioid peptides, the enkephalins, and endorphins may play a particularly important role in parturition and it is possible that aspects of this system may have evolved in relation to mammalian reproduction activities. Another feature of mammalian reproduction is the fact that sexual behavior often involves pain. Male cats have barbs on their penises and bite into the neck of the female during copulation. Male dogs, after ejaculation, have the penis constricted by specialized vaginal muscle with sufficient force to prevent withdrawal. And some female subhuman primates support the entire weight of much larger males during copulation. It is not surprising, then, that the pituitary produces substances that set a limit on pain. Indeed, all three mechanisms are able to limit the severity of pain, and apart from their possible role in sexual behavior, there are good survival reasons for such effects. Pain, at intense levels, is a disruptive, disorganizing process. Animals, including man, may freeze or become otherwise immobilized by severe pain. By freezing or fainting, animals may be open to even worse injury or loss of life in a dangerous situation. There is obvious survival value, then, in neural and hormonal mechanisms that set a limit on pain.

WHAT DO ANIMALS FEEL?

It is reasonable to assume that mammals below the level of man feel pain as a conscious experience. However, it is equally reasonable to assume that there are experiential differences that relate to differences in neural structure. Man, at the top of the evolutionary ladder, has the largest cortex of all species. And man, more than any other animal, is influenced by the ability to foresee the consequences of events. This fact differentiates between animal and human pain experience. There is no evidence to suggest that animals have any knowledge of death as such, or suffer anticipatory anxiety about becoming lame or disfigured, or have goals of personal fulfillment that can be thwarted by injury or death. These kinds of activities are subserved by the cortex and presumably exert their effects on affective processing by way of the prefrontal cortex (6). It is proposed, therefore, that the primates (probably) and the carnivores (certainly) are comparable to lobotomized people: that they experience the sensory and motivational-emotional components of pain, not the "suffering" or the "big pain" that appear to require a cortex like man's, capable of understanding death and of generating the anxiety that surrounds illness and injury. This is highly speculative, of course, but merits further attention in view of the implications of the ethical issues involved in the experimental study of pain in animals.

Acknowledgements. Supported by Grant A7891 from the Natural Sciences and Engineering Research Council of Canada.

REFERENCES

(1) Bishop, G.H. 1949. Relation of pain sensory threshold to form of mechanical stimulator. J. Neurophysiol. 12: 51-57.

(2) Coghill, G.E. 1929. Anatomy and the Problem of Behaviour. Cambridge: Cambridge University Press.

(3) Dennis, S.G., and Melzack, R. 1977. Pain-signalling systems in the dorsal and ventral spinal cord. Pain 4: 97-132.

(4) Ebbesson, S.O.E. 1969. Brain stem afferents from the spinal cord in a sample of reptilian and amphibian species. Annals N.Y. Acad. Sci. 167: 80-101.

(5) Hughes, J., and Kosterlitz, H.W. 1977. Opioid peptides. Br. Med. Bull. 33: 157-161.

(6) Melzack, R., and Casey, K.L. 1968. Sensory, motivational, and central control determinants of pain: a new conceptual model. In The Skin Senses, ed. D. Kenshalo, pp. 423-443. Springfield: C.C. Thomas.

(7) Melzack, R., and Wall, P.D. Pain mechanisms: a new theory. Science 150: 971-979.

(8) Noback, C.R., and Schriver, J.E. 1969. Encephalization and the lemniscal systems during phylogeny. Annals N.Y. Acad. Sci. 167: 118-128.

(9) Truex, R.C.; Taylor, M.J.; Smythe, M.Q.; and Gildenberg, P.L. 1970. The lateral cervical nucleus of cat, dog, and man. J. comp. Neurol. 139: 93-104.

(10) Wall, P.D. 1979. On the relation of injury to pain. Pain 6: 253-264.

(11) Whiting, H.P. 1955. Functional development in the nervous system. In Biochemistry of the Developing Nervous System, ed. H. Waelsch, pp. 85-102. New York: Academic Press.

Pain and Society, eds. H.W. Kosterlitz and L.Y. Terenius, pp. 27-36.
Dahlem Konferenzen 1980. Weinheim: Verlag Chemie GmbH.

The Existence of Pain in Animals

G. Carli
Istituto di Fisiologia Umana
53100 Siena, Italy

Abstract. Most of our knowledge of pain responses comes from laboratory experiments where artificial stimuli elicit a constant set of responses. Nociceptive stimuli, however, may also induce eating, copulation, or other responses which are difficult to interpret. Two main approaches to determine the existence of pain in animals are discussed. The first one consists of studying animal behavior while there is a continuous nociceptive stimulus, as, for instance, in some pathological conditions or following mechanically produced body lesions. The second approach involves the recording of animal responses during damaging fights with members of the same species (i.e., conspecifics). The nature of the response, however, varies according to the different functions of aggressive behavior and to animal interactions. It is suggested that in normal life and in social interactions, animals avoid, as much as possible, exposure to nociceptive stimuli.

INTRODUCTION

It is commonly assumed that receptors which selectively respond to noxious stimuli are present in all mammals, although they have been adequately studied in only a few animal species (rats, cats, monkeys). This supposition comes mainly from the observation that all animals respond to nociceptive stimuli. In most of the behavioral studies performed in the laboratory, experimental procedures are required to keep most of the parameters of the stimulus constant: for instance, identical stimuli are applied over and over again to determine the regularity of the response. The low variability of the environmental conditions has several advantages, e.g., confidence in the results, constancy in the nature of the response, higher speed of learning, etc. The difficulties in interpreting behavioral experiments performed by using artificial stimuli are easily illustrated by the effects of electric shocks and tail pinches on rats. If two seemingly friendly rats are subject to painful electric shocks, they begin to fight. The number of attacks depends on such things as shock intensity, size of the chamber, length of the session, and age of the animals (6). Even if another rat is not present, attacks may be directed to inanimate objects. Electric shock may also induce copulatory behavior, depending on stimulus conditions. Tail pinch induces eating behavior, similar to normal eating patterns, when food pellets are available. This behavior is elicited by pinches of different intensities not necessarily nociceptive. But tail pinch may also induce both drinking of palatable fluids and maternal behavior according to the objects available in the environment.

To understand the pain experience on the whole, it is appropriate also to study animal behavior in more natural conditions, e.g., where a subject is exposed to noxious stimuli of various nature and, in different circumstances, may select the most suitable response. In the present review, the existence of pain will be inferred by the animal response to nociceptive stimuli. Moreover, it will be shown that the pain response may be modified by several parameters besides the stimulus intensity. Attention will be focused on two main topics: a) the evaluation of symptoms which may lead the experimenter to diagnose a condition of persistent pain, and b) the interactions among animals which may elicit a pain experience.

SIGNS OF PERSISTANT PAIN

Conditions which would ordinarily lead to intense pain in humans sometimes produce less overt behavioral changes in animals who may exhibit immobility. Even in the absence of superficial lesions, veterinarians can assess a state of continuous pain by careful clinical examination. For small mammals, the limbs, trunk, vertebral column, and abdomen are palpated and watched for signs such as resistance to movement and tensing of the muscles. In the dog, a very useful localizing sign of dermal hyperesthesia is the contraction of the cutaneous muscle (panniculus) following a gentle prick with a needle. In normal areas the skin twitch is absent and no behavioral response is recorded (5). Sometimes, examination is impossible, because even touching the hair of the hyperesthetic area elicits vocalization and aggressive or fearful behavior. In limping horses, the source of pain may be identified by the fact that local anesthesia of the affected area will restore normal movements. In a horse with intestinal distension, a condition of severe abdominal pain may be inferred from persistent pawing, wallowing, and "cold sweat." Dogs may display persistent abnormal postures. For instance, in cervical disk protrusion, the head and neck are held low and rigid, while in low thoracic and lumbar disk lesions, arching of the back is recorded. Also, the dog occasionally wimpers and whines for no apparent reasons and may awake and cry during the night. Tendon reflexes are found exaggerated and respiration increased. Spontaneous or surgical removal of the compression abolish all manifestations. Although interpretation of behavioral signs in the absence of body lesions may be sometimes very difficult, central pain phenomena are reported in veterinary medicine. McGrow describes a Boston terrier that whined and cried continuously, as if in pain: a brain tumor was found in the left thalamus upon necroscopy (5).

With limb muscle rupture, which may occur in racing dogs and horses, local symptoms (hematoma) and functional disturbances (lameness) may suggest a condition of severe suffering. With bone fractures and traumatic injuries to joints, or infections, local metabolic and electromyographic modifications have been described. Hnik et al. (4) have shown that following the fracture of metatarsal bones in rats, an injection of turpentine into the paw induces muscle atrophy. This atrophy, although transient in character, progresses more rapidly than denervation atrophy; it is reduced by long-lasting anesthesia and is called reflex atrophy since it is prevented by dorsal rhizotomy. The chronic nociceptive stimulus also produces local modifications of the electromyographic activity (contraction of flexor and relaxation of extensor muscles) and a sharp increase of up to twelve-fold in corticosteroid plasma levels.

The amount or the depth of body lesions, the inflammatory reactions of tissues, and the presence of bleeding cannot be indicative of pain when behavioral responses are absent. Licking, scratching, biting of the affected region, and in limb injuries, limping during locomotion leave no doubt about the animal's distress. Licking is an excellent protective response; it cleans the damaged tissues, stimulates local blood circulation, and triggers, by activating large myelinated afferent fibers, central mechanisms that reduce the noxious input. Scratching usually indicates the release of local substances; persistent scratching up to self-mutilation may be due to damage of the superficial surface due to contact with irritants, photosensitization to ingestion of some plants, or skin invasion by certain types of parasites. In experimental pain, injections of irritants such as formalin in unrestrained rats and cats lead to behavioral reactions which can easily be monitored, and the pain intensity can be quantified according to a rate scale. The volume and the concentration of formalin determine the amount of tissue damage and the duration of behavioral manifestations. In cats, we have observed that high dosages (2ml of 37% formalin), causes absolute insomnia for 1-6 hours and suppression of REM sleep for 9-29 hours. In the rabbit, formalin injection may either decrease or increase the duration of hypnosis (tonic immobility) according to the intensity of the stimulus.

Summing up, a careful examination of animal behavior may lead to the diagnosis of a sustained pain condition.

INTERACTIONS AMONG ANIMALS WHICH MAY ELICIT A PAIN EXPERIENCE

Weapon-like Structures and Defense Organs

Weapon-like structures and defense organs limit the number of strategies of attack and defense of a given animal species: their absence or presence determines their use. During development, for instance, escape behavior may change to defensive fighting. In the newborn mouse, a tail pinch is followed by a succession of squeaks and a few walking movements. At the time of the appearance of the first teeth (9 days of age), the young mouse reacts to the same stimulus by biting the forceps or the experimenter's fingers (8).

Weapon-like structures may be used for a) deep body penetration (caused, e.g., by long horns which maximize the chances of killing an opponent), b) large body surface damage (caused by, e.g., claws, teeth, tusks, short horns), and c) trauma (mainly caused by hooves). Weapon-like structures that maximize surface damage can be rapidly used and withdrawn in instantaneous violent attacks. On the other hand, a weapon-like structure achieving deep penetration places the aggressor in danger: withdrawal is more difficult and the weapon may cause its owner a neck or skull fracture as the victim struggles violently to disengage itself (2). All kinds of weapon-like structures may produce pain reactions.

Defense organs are most suitable to neutralize attacks of conspecifics: dermal shields, for instance, are located where weapons are most likely to make contact. Fighting mountain goats whirl around each other and each has his head closest to the opponent's rear, the dermal shield being thickest in the rump. The importance of strategies is illustrated by the following example. In bighorn sheep, rams have double-layered skulls, interconnected with bone, that allow them to absorb the tremendous impact of head butting without injury to the head or the brain. After one attack, the two contenders, seeming to ignore each other, maneuver for the best position of the next charge. Some are adept at getting uphill of their opponent since a downhill charge is more effective, others adopt the strategy of the "sneak attack," in which the opponent is charged from the side or behind when he least expects it. Such encounters are most effective because they may produce deep wounds and bone or rib fractures. According to Geist (2), weapon-like structures and defenses in mammals are arranged in certain patterns. Short, sharp tusks and horns in medium-sized and large mammals (wild boar, mountain goat, giraffe, Indian rhinoceros, and hippopotamus) are paired with thick, often large, dermal armors on the body. In ungulates, antlers have a dual function as weapon and shield: the primary function of the points, twists, and surface texture of the antlers is to allow a grip on the opponent's antler. In very small ungulates and in most carnivores, we find weapon-like structures capable of inflicting serious injury, but there is no structural defense against them.

Thus, natural selection leads to weapon-like structures that inflict the highest degree of trauma and pain, and for defense, to organs and strategies that protect the regions most exposed to the weapons of conspecifics.

Responses to Injuring Attacks

In simple experimental conditions, the intensity of the response is related to the intensity of the stimulus. Nociceptive stimuli may elicit responses ranging from a withdrawal response to flight reactions, vocalization, and fainting. In natural habitat, the behavior of fighting animals may be analyzed in the light of three main hypotheses: a) animals are under a state of analgesia or hypoalgesia, and the fight stops for reasons independent of pain; b) animals do not feel pain during the combat but know from previous experience that injuries will hurt them later on, and they behave accordingly; c) animals do feel pain and their response is related to the stimulus. There is no need of implicating an analgesic state in the fights which terminate before any physical contact or damaging lesion has occurred. When body injuries are produced, either hypothesis b) or c) is acceptable: in both instances, a pain experience is involved and the response is somehow related to the stimulus.

In this connection it has to be stressed that, even in long-lasting fights, the physical contact between competitors is usually of short duration and immediately followed by behavioral changes. Intensity and duration of a damaging attack also depend upon either the strength of the releasing stimuli or the responses of the contenders. One of the responses to mild painful stimuli is retaliation which contributes to the continuation of the fight. The risk of a counterattack is perhaps the main parameter limiting the use of dangerous weapons. Challenge gestures during a fight may either increase the power of the damaging actions or stop them. Three main responses may stop a combat: submission signals, absence of counterattacks, or flight reactions. Injuring fights may erupt for a variety of reasons, such as territorial possession, dominance, sexual conflicts, parental discipline, defense from predators, etc. (9). The myth that conspecifics have evolved "bloodless" combats in which participants do not seek to harm each other despite their ability to do so is now devoid of evidence. The annals of extreme violence among mammals are beginning to lengthen: repetitive attacks of previously wounded animals unable to defend themselves efficiently, group aggression, and warfare and killing are being found far more common and "normal" with the increase in time devoted to the observation of animals in their habitat.

Functions of Aggressive Behavior

Aggressive behavior is a result of circumstances and serves very different functions. In territorial conflict, aggressive behavior has a geographic aspect: animals defend particular areas. The territorial defender first uses the most dramatic signaling (weapon, rush, or scare threats) to repulse the intruders. Physical aggression is usually employed as a last resort and terminates when the losing contender leaves the field. Submission signals may help to interrupt the fight, but they are not very critical. Jane Goodal (3), a pioneer observer of Africa's chimpanzees, noted that males of a community, in groups of three or four, patrol the boundaries searching for clues to locate strangers. If they meet a group from another community, they are likely to withdraw after exchanging threats; but if a single chimpanzee is encountered, or a mother and a child, then patrol males usually chase and, if they can, severely beat the stranger.

The purpose of dominance aggression is to exclude subordinates from desired objects and to prevent them from performing actions to which the dominant animal claims priority. Social rank may be established through combats or threats of force. Submission and appeasement signals are the main responses preventing and interrupting a losing fight (7). The dominant animal enjoys some impunity, since subordinates do not usually retaliate when he attacks. An attack on a previously defeated animal consolidates dominance and reduces its fighting capacities. Dominance combats should not be mistaken for sparring and other forms of harmless clashes, through which males learn the proper orientations and actions where fighting is a test of strength. Moreover, during sparring, juveniles are exposed to stimuli of different intensities (heavy pressure, fortuitus painful pressure, and blows) which they learn to evaluate carefully. In mountain sheep, the rule is that, although the dominant may solicit the sparring, it is the subordinate who starts and ends it. Dominance attacks may start quite early in life: suckling pigs use their temporary but short, sharp, canine teeth in encounters that determine which position each will occupy along the row of maternal teats. The further forward a piglet can establish itself, the better will be the milk supply and its growth, and the smaller will be the chances of being trampled by the mother's hind legs.

Possessing an established territory or maintaining high social rank permits a better selection of mates and a more favorable breeding ground. Therefore it is not surprising that in many mammals aggression is intense only during the mating season. The seasonal rise in the androgen titer of males is generally associated with an increase in aggressiveness. In male rhesus monkeys, plasma testosterone levels are correlated with aggressiveness, while the correlation with rank in the dominant order is less precise. Geist (1) has discovered that sexual and aggressive behavior are closely linked in the mountain sheep: a) they mature in parallel during development, b) rams are stimulated to sexual acts after fighting, and c) females use aggressive behavior on exhausted males to stimulate them to copulate. Other interesting sexual relationships are present in goats. Males are potentially very dangerous but, outside the rut, are less aggressive and subdominant to females. In animals with sexual monopolies, such as wolves and camels, the dominant tries to prevent competitors from mating. However, the dominant may be attacked by subordinates during mating, hit hard, and displaced. During intense courtship, the mountain goats approach females rapidly from the rear and deliver a hard kick with the front leg between or along their haunches. Some kicks are strong enough to push the female forward. Noxious attacks by males on females may be related to mating behavior: the male cat bites the skin of the female's neck and holds this neck grip as long as he is mounting. In amadryas baboons, the male recruits young females to build up a harem and harasses them throughout their lives to prevent them from straying. Attacks may also be delivered for appeasing reasons: in monkeys the dominant male may punish subordinates or juveniles to break up fights.

In more general terms, it should be stressed that even the most aggressive animal species engage only rarely in damaging combats. This sporadic experience is associated with changes in the arousal and in the vegetative systems, most typical of intense emotional states. Finally, animals may self-induce body lesions to gain freedom, for instance, they may bite or stretch a trapped paw until it separates from the body. In monkeys, one of the offense-defense gestures is the biting off of one's own hand.

CONCLUSION

Animals, as humans, are exposed to nociceptive stimuli from early infancy. The pain experience becomes associated with intense emotional states. Among conspecifics, producing body lesions is perhaps the most extreme form of communication of the animal repertoire. In normal life and in social interactions, animals avoid the risk of body lesions as much as possible.

Acknowledgement. I wish to thank S. Lovari for his suggestions during the preparation of the manuscript.

REFERENCES

(1) Geist, V. 1965. On the rutting behavior of mountain goat. J. Mammal. 45: 551-568.

(2) Geist, V. 1978. On weapons, combat and ecology. In Aggression, Dominance and Individual Spacing, eds. L. Krames, P. Pliner and T. Alloway, pp. 1-30. New York: Plenum Publishing Corporation.

(3) Goodal, J. 1979. Life and death at Gombe. National Geogr. 155: 592-621.

(4) Hnik, P.; Holas, M.; and Payne, R. 1977. Reflex muscle atrophy induced by chronic peripheral nociceptive stimulation. J. Physiol. (Paris) 73: 241-250.

(5) Horlein, B.F. 1978. Canine Neurology. Philadelphia: W.B. Saunders Company.

(6) Johnson, R.N. 1972. Aggression in Man and Animals. Philadelphia: W.B. Saunders Company.

(7) Jolly, A. 1972. The Evolution of Primate Behavior. New York: The McMillan Company.

(8) Scott, J.P. 1967. Discussion of the paper of Leakey L.S.B. In Aggression and Defense, eds. C.C. Clemente and D.B. Lindsley, pp. 47. Berkeley: University of California Press.

(9) Wilson, O.E. 1975. Sociobiology. The New Synthesis. Cambridge: The Belknap Press of Harvard University Press.

Pain and Society, eds. H.W. Kosterlitz and L.Y. Terenius, pp. 37-52.
Dahlem Konferenzen 1980. Weinheim: Verlag Chemie GmbH.

Ontogenetic and Cultural Influences on the Expression of Pain in Man

K. D. Craig
Department of Psychology, University of British Columbia
Vancouver, B. C. V6T 1W5, Canada

Abstract. The individual differences in pain expression are the consequence of variations in the genetic endowment, the natural environment, and socialization influences. A transition from innate patterns released by noxious events to complex cognitive, affective, and behavioral reactions can be observed during the course of development. The family and community influence sensitivity to noxious external and interoceptive events, memories of prior pain experiences, the nature of the emotional reaction, conceptual information used to explain and cope with situational demands, the mode of expressing distress, and the execution of skills designed to minimize further injury and enhance recovery. Family interaction patterns provide for the transmission of societal concepts, standards, and normative practices. Parental role-modeling and precedents, children's propensities to attend to and emulate others' actions, and the use of strong controls to ensure conformity to expected roles, yield pain behavior that is determined by social realities as well as tissue insult. Substantial cultural variations in pain expression can be traced to family interaction patterns.

INTRODUCTION

Individual differences in pain expression are striking phenomena. Some people bear pain with surprising equanimity, whereas others react to the same tissue insult with intense suffering. These differences are attributed commonly to variable genetic endowments and unique life histories, but there are lamentable deficiencies in our knowledge of the specific origins. Adopting the ontogenetic perspective permits a description of the unfolding patterns of pain expression during different periods of the life span from birth to old age. Fundamental characteristics of the neurophysiological systems involving pain, that have important bearing on socialization of pain expressions, are their potential for adaptation to environmental demands and capacity to mediate changed behavior as dictated by learning experiences. Considered alone, the biological endowment gives rise across children and adults to the progressive maturation of discriminable patterns of pain response, as well as individual variations in pain behavior. But, this only represents a partial description of the formative influences. Transactions between the individual and his or her physical and social environments lead to the development of patterns of expression that systematically reflect unique characteristics of those environments. The inherent plasticity of the systems mediating pain experience and behavior, and their sensitivity to family, community, and cultural influences, necessitate socio-psychological analyses.

The behavioral expression of pain as affected by social antecedents and consequent conditions, rather than pain experience, was of primary interest for several reasons. First, the scientific study of pain can only infer subjective experience from overt expressions. Second, while the personal, subjective experience of pain represents its most important component, the public manifestations strongly affect other people. These lead to complex interactions between suffering individuals and others in the social environment. Pain behavior usually represents the hurt person's best possible solution to situational demands, as dictated by prior experience, awareness of the situation, and the trauma of the tissue insult. The experience is not static and its social sequelae have an impact on ensuing experiences. Expressions of pain symbolize a need for help and most people respond promptly with sympathy and efforts at compassionate caretaking. However, empathic distress and personal threat may lead to defensive avoidance of people in pain. Fortunately, cultural norms and expectations to engage in helping others in pain are observable throughout the life cycle.

During the course of development, the family and community influence the structure and functions of perceptions, memory, cognitive representational activities, problem-solving, and behavioral skills (1). Social influences determine the sensitivity to noxious external and interoceptive events, the memories of prior pain experiences, the nature and severity of emotional reactions, the conceptual information used to explain what happened and its future implications, and finally, at the behavioral level, the mode of expressing distress and the execution of skills designed to minimize further injury and enhance recovery.

DEVELOPMENTAL SEQUENCES

At the beginning, it is worth noting that a substantive body of knowledge on pain in children does not exist. The lack of systematic research has serious implications since supposition dictates assessment and treatment of children's pain. Eland and Anderson (7) described the unfortunate consequences for children of the following prevalent beliefs, amongst others: children do not experience pain with the same intensity as adults, children recover quickly, and children cannot tell you where it hurts.

Measuring Pain in Children

The measurement issues in the study of pain in children are of major importance. While adult verbal pain reports have limitations (6), they provide a sensitive and reliable index of subjective experience, and adults at least have recourse to this means of influencing others. Very young children do not have language available as a medium of communication, and a facility for using speech to describe the subtleties of subjective distress emerges only slowly. Concerned observers are compelled to interpret other forms of expression. Children are capable of engaging in vigorous reactions to painful events and considerable information is available in nonlinguistic vocalizations, withdrawal and avoidance behavior, facial expressions, gesticulations, and postural adjustments. Nevertheless, there are very few studies that examine the convergence of these behavioral events on subjective distress; moreoever, the extent to which observers interpret these actions as signifying pain and react to them as such, is unknown.

Problems in interpreting the most prominent expression of pain in children, crying, illustrate the difficulties. Parents successfully discriminate their own child's pain cries from other forms of crying and tend to react with affective distress and concern (13). However, other adults do not differentiate pain as a source of crying as readily and are relatively less distressed. Furthermore, the vocal cues signaling that painful events have elicited crying are most salient at the beginning when the sudden, intense vocal ejaculation and the breathing pattern is particularly meaningful. Within minutes the crying begins to resemble that instigated by hunger or fatigue.

The absence of a satisfactory metric for pain appears to have contributed to controversies on the extent to which children suffer from surgical procedures during early infancy. Preoperative procedures, such as endotrachial intubation, and surgery are undertaken in children with minimal anesthetic more often than in adults. In part, this reflects the risks of deleterious effects of anesthetics on homeostatic mechanisms. Nevertheless, disagreement exists on the extent to which young children suffer. One would expect systematic behavioral observation to be undertaken with painful procedures, but there is a paucity of data and even routine procedures such as circumcision lead to discrepant accounts as to the severity of pain expressed (11,15). This measurement problem also contributes to the absence of evidence on the long-term effects of pain experienced during early infancy. Immaturity in the central nervous system suggests that the capacity for sustained memory may be limited. Nevertheless, young children's electrophysiological reactions to noxious events resemble those of adults, and capabilities for complex perceptual and cognitive processing are increasingly recognized at very early ages (16).

Difficulties in interpreting the psychological significance of children's unique expressions of pain should also engender caution in inferences about children's experiences of pain. Adults' conception of pain and suffering may be imposed inappropriately, as young children's experiences probably do not correspond to those of adults. Elaboration of the experience of pain along evaluative, affective, and sensory dimensions requires substantial socialization and experience. The risk of misinterpretation may be of considerable importance considering strong tendencies for parents and other adults to react energetically with compassionate caretaking when children are assumed to be in pain. Adults generally react conservatively when engaged in decision making about activities and events that pose risks of physical harm for children. When combined with children's tendencies to react intensely to injuries, the risks of misattributing nuances and intensities of pain appear considerable. Parents' perceptions and expectations determine the manner in which they treat their children and are predictive of the course of the children's development.

Potentials of Infants to Experience Pain

Neonates and infants are responsive to noxious stimuli. Strong stimuli generate efforts to withdraw from contact, and screams, cries and considerable nonverbal signs of agitation and distress. Few systematic studies have examined changes in sensitivity throughout childhood, but there is evidence that the neonate experiences relatively little pain during the first few days of life, with sensitivity increasing rapidly thereafter (11). Pain reactions evoked by the initial prick for blood samples in neonates are distinguished readily from other patterns of crying by their sudden loud onset, without preliminary moaning, and an initial long cry followed by an extended period of breath-holding in expiration. This is followed by a conventional rhythmic pattern of crying (13). Infants' cries encode stimulus intensity since they react with lustier cries to more noxious events.

The newborn's reaction to noxious stimuli tends to produce a total motor response, suggesting that expressive mechanisms have not become differentiated or that the locus of stimulation is not readily identified. Between 3-12 months the reaction to a pinprick begins to include withdrawal of the touched extremity (15). Individual differences in pain reactivity appear early in life, as do other temperamental differences which ultimately may relate to individual pain behavior. During infancy, ranges of individual differences resemble those that are so problematic in adults.

The data in the literature on sex differences in pain reactivity tends to be inconsistent, but there is evidence that at an early age females react more intensely to noxious stimuli than males (10). Apparently, the tendency for men to present themselves as forebearing has its basis in biological predispositions as well as in socialization to sex-appropriate roles.

LEARNING EXPERIENCES

The usual course of growing up provides innumerable misfortunes that permit intense learning about pain and its source. Painful experience may emerge from normal events, such as teething, or from disorders, such as colic. Various medical and dental procedures also inflict painful discomfort. Growing up only gradually corrects the skill deficits, inexperience, and lack of coordination that create hazards for children, and they inevitably sustain numerous cuts, scrapes, bruises, and bites. Finally, intensive learning experiences result from the pain inflicted by others in the form of corporal punishment and during childhood games. Serious and protracted pain disorders in children frequently lead to major life adjustments and stressful changes in patterns of family interaction.

A capacity to anticipate pain and to perceive the environment as potentially harmful soon emerges. Levy's (9) study of infants' reactions to inoculations indicated that, under the age of about 6 months, children did not cry prior to the needle puncture. Thereafter, the children began to recall signal qualities of the inoculation situation and responded fearfully to such cues as the needle, white coats, and restraint. The infant's growing awareness of circumstances relating to pain is also evident in nonverbal emotional expressions (8). Using anatomically-based criteria for recognizing discrete facial expressions of affect in infants 1-9 months old, observers successfully identified a characteristic expressive response to pain that could be distinguished readily from other emotional expressions, including the positive affects and sadness, anger, and fear. The development of a sequence of emotional expressions that indicate an emerging capacity to recognize, anticipate, and respond to events leading to pain was observed in the seventh or eighth month of life. There was a transition from a spontaneous pattern of expression suggesting unanticipated pain, to a sequence suggesting fear of the inoculation needle, pain as a reaction to the actual event, and anger following the event. Pain appears to become embedded in a complex network of thoughts and feelings at a very early age.

SOCIALIZATION OF PAIN EXPRESSION

Two principal sets of factors lead to the transformation of pain from an innate pattern released by noxious events to a complex affective experience influenced by past history and contextual events: a) the developing capacities of the child to encode and process information and to interact with the environment, and b) the social consequences of pain, best indicated by the compelling impact of expressions of physical distress upon others. With rare, but unfortunate, exceptions, the urgency signaled by expressions of pain provokes caretaking and intimate interactions with others. An involvement of adults inevitably must reflect their preconceptions of the nature and meaning of pain, injuries, and diseases, and how one should deal with them.

Social Modeling of Pain Experience

Opportunities to observe others' experiences with pain and physical danger are major sources of socialization influence on pain expression (5). The capacity to benefit from others' experiences with pain provides for the prevention of injury or disease and related pain states and, should injury become inevitable, skill in minimizing the stress and the physical and psychological trauma associated with it. To witness suffering in others leads to an awareness of the kinds of events that are potentially harmful, how one is likely to feel in similar unfortunate circumstances, and how one should behave to minimize the immediate or long-term consequences of personal injuries leading to suffering.

Vicarious emotional sensitivity tends to be particularly pronounced when others express distress in settings posing physical danger or react fearfully to creatures that are potentially harmful. Affective reactions to stimulus events signaling these risks are readily conditioned, whether the individual is exposed personally or vicariously to harm. The ready capacity to associate neutral cues with risky events in one's own or others' experiences may reflect the evolutionary development of biological predispositions to learn to fear events threatening physical danger or the force of early direct and vicarious learning experiences with pain.

It is noteworthy that vicariously acquired emotional reactions, may be unrelated to the actual threat posed by an event. Children frequently are unable to cognize the rationale justifying adult behavior. In these circumstances they emulate qualities of the behavior of their parents and other adults without comprehending its purposes or consequences. In this manner, familial and ethnocultural styles in expressing pain may be transmitted from generation to generation.

Gradually, children acquire skills that promote personal well-being and minimize risks of painful encounters. The general sequence in the acquisition of personal and social skills tends to be one of initial observational learning of requisite information, followed by tentative trial and exploratory behavior, and finally, corrective feedback from the environment that either promotes further adaptive changes or maintains the skill (1). Information derived from personal and vicarious encounters with pain becomes organized in the form of knowledge concerning the probable relationships among various antecedent events, experiences and behavior, and consequent events. The individual then can maximize personal benefits by acting in accordance with rules.

As with all skill acquisition, the consequences of behavior assume a crucial role in either maintaining the behavior or leading to further refinement. The operant approach to therapeutic management of chronic pain disorders has demonstrated convincingly the reinforcing effects of numerous socially delivered consequences that can be contingent upon pain behavior. These may well delay recovery and lead to entrapment in the role of an invalid, rather than promote health.

Adults exert considerable influence on the behavior of young children to ensure conformity to their expectations of how one should behave when at risk of harm or when suffering. Children complain frequently about pain, partly as a result of the inevitable crises of childhood, and partly because such complaints constitute powerful controls over adult behavior. As with other patterns of maladaptive interpersonal relationships, pain behavior and sick roles may be used to coerce others to comply with demands. Seeing others suffering, particularly loved ones, tends to be highly aversive. Providing care can terminate empathic distress, which may constitute positive reinforcement for pain behavior, while the negative reinforcement for caretaking behavior provided by termination of the pain complaints can entrap both the suffering party and the caretaker in their respective roles.

The Acquisition of Pain Language

The advent of language permits novel access to subjective experiences. The observer no longer must witness the child at the time of injury or during the painful trauma in order to assess the nature of the experience but can rely increasingly upon verbal report. Crying is at first exclusively expressive and indiscriminate, but toward the end of the first year it becomes "goal-directed" and is used with the intent to influence others (13). Gradually verbal repertoires for expressing painful distress come to include expressions that range from the nondifferentiated cries of young children to the articulated language that adults use to describe their present and past experiences.

The transition from reflexive crying to dispassionate descriptions of personal suffering tends to be slow and gradual. Studies of early language acquisition in one and two year olds indicate that words for pain are among the first learned (14). However, young children have relatively few words available to describe personal emotional states in their early vocabularies, in contrast to words referring to objects. Given that children acquire vocabularies by naming objects exhibiting salient properties of change, and that pain generates highly intrusive changes in experience, pain language would be expected to assume some priority.

Ultimately, skill in using a complex vocabulary to describe pain emerges, and differential diagnoses can be made on the strength of subtle differences in word usage. Because an articulate language for interoceptive experience has not evolved, expressions prevail that describe properties of the external environment and how pain may have been caused. Thus, people refer to pain as stabbing, shooting, burning, or bursting. Recent studies of pain language suggest a broader range of descriptive terms that fall into sensory, affective, and evaluative categories.

Developmental trends in children's concepts of illness are instructive, given the role of pain in most illness states. Campbell (2) interviewed children and their mothers to determine their definitions of illness. Content analyses indicated that youngsters of different ages shared a consensus with the definitions changing to conform increasingly to those of the typical adult. Younger children characterized illness in terms of vague, nonlocalized feelings ("Feeling bad", "Not right"), whereas older children gave more attention to specific diseases or diagnoses ("Appendicitis," "Chicken pox") and to disruptions in conventional role behavior ("Dont't go to school," "Stay home from school"). Mothers displayed more conceptual sophistication by including non-obvious symptoms of illness, changes in mood and motivational states, and increases in sick role behavior. In addition, children were more knowledgeable if they had been hospitalized or their mothers had been particularly concerned about the child's health and reported increased nurturing when the child was sick.

The development of language skills serves more than to allow the child to describe experiences that exist independent of the linguistic system or to effect some control over the social environment. Language clarifies ambiguity, attaches meaning to events, and provides for conceptual structure. Because the social environment assumes a primary role in the acquisition of language, the prevailing conceptual system would also be expected to influence children's pain concepts.

FAMILY DETERMINANTS

Patterns of family interaction provide the basis for the transmission of societal practices as well as patterns of behavior unique to the particular family. Consistent with the formulation that observational learning and corrective feedback assume primary roles in the shaping of children's patterns of pain expression, parents exert two basic forms of influence. First, they model those forms of pain complaint that represent their personal resolution to the problem of painful injuries and diseases. Second, they exert strong sanctions to conform to their personal expectations of how their children should react to somatic events and behave when ill. The emotionally stressful nature of children's painful cries and complaints, young children's vulnerability to physical harm, and societal expectations that parents will assume responsibility for the safety of children, combine to ensure parental involvement when the well-being of their children is in question. Under these circumstances, parents use their best intervention techniques to exact control. These may include strict surveillance, explicit verbal instructions, modeling demonstrations, physical guidance, and corporal punishment for failure to abide by rules. The presence of parental precedents, children's propensities to attend to and emulate others' actions, and the use of strong controls to ensure conformity to expected roles, combine to yield pain behavior that is as much determined by social realities as the objective characteristics of noxious events.

Compliance with parental expectations and standards leads to mutually gratifying experiences for parents and children. The parents react generously, with praise and expressions of satisfaction over the children's actions that appear to sustain health, and the parents experience relief that their children have avoided physical danger. Given that parental role-modeling and reinforcement practices are constrained by societal norms, the patterns of behavior learned by children are likely to be consistent with community standards and would receive further support from extra-familial sources. Only with the development of cognitive and behavioral skills, do parents become less directive and rely upon verbal guidance and self-control.

The impact of the family on pain behavior is most evident when children have witnessed in others pain due to illness that is exceptionally intense, affect-ridden, prolonged, or frequent. Under these circumstances, children become predisposed to unusual patterns of pain complaint themselves (5). For example, children who display uncooperative behavior and distress reactions during dental treatment tend to have family members who have had unfavorable dental experiences and displayed adverse attitudes themselves. In addition, when children complain of recurring abdominal pain unrelated to organic pathology, the probability is high that other family members will have had a history of pain syndromes of similar severity (3,5). Empathic communication of parental distress, instruction in identifying somatic states and symptoms, and skill in engaging clinicians appear to be important sources of the children's problems. Other psychosocial problems occur frequently in these families, including emotional problems, marital distress, and school and work absenteeism. While these contribute to patients' problems, findings that the family histories are replete with illnesses and somatic complaints and family members preoccupied with health concerns suggest that observational learning effects are crucial. Overreaction to pain in these families may reflect a general failure to use adaptive coping skills. For example, tendencies to exaggerate the severity of painful experiences can provoke substantial anxiety and distress. Imagining painful experiences leads to the patterns of physiological arousal that are ordinarily associated with the painful experiences themselves (4).

Christensen and Mortensen (3) present evidence that it is the parents' current attitudes toward pain rather than past histories that affect their children's recurrent pain behavior. The incidence of parents' abdominal disorders during childhood was unrelated to their children's complaints, but concurrent problems were. Distant members of families of pain patients may also show a greater prevalence of pain problems. Mohammed, Weisz, and Waring (12) found that a group of chronic pain patients who were also depressed had a greater prevalence of pain problems among their spouses, their own family, and their spouses' families in contrast to a control group of depressed people. The study suggests either intrafamilial facilitation of pain complaints or that chronic pain patients select spouses with similar problems.

The existence of "pain prone families" also suggests that ill health encourages tendencies to attribute health problems to others. This could lead to entrapment of others in sick roles. We have observed that patients with chronic back pain, who did not benefit from surgical care, tended to attribute greater ill health to both their children and themselves than control parents. Illness attribution has been found to promote action relevant for health. Mothers, in particular, ensure that children receive medical attention. In addition, parents treat children who are ill, or are misperceived as being ill, differently from children of good health. The differences may reflect the child's real needs, but the special treatment also may be the consequence of parental anxiety and over protectiveness and be unrelated to genuine ill health.

Other family factors less directly related to parental instruction have been associated with variations in pain behavior. Chronic pain has been reported to be more prevalent in large families, in younger children from large families, in members of lower socio-economic classes, and where there is parental abuse and neglect. Perhaps there is inadequate training in skills of health care, or conditions foster acquisition of dramatic pain complaints in the life styles of these families.

Changes in pain sensitivity and expressive patterns have been reported through the adult age-range (18). The research does not make it clear whether the differences reflect maturation of the neural systems mediating pain, general biological aging influencing the capacity to engage in potentially painful work, or changes in social roles influencing the appropriateness of expressions about pain.

CULTURAL VARIATION

Cultural variations highlight the role of social learning experiences as determinants of pain expression. Ethnocultural differences in the manner of expressing pain have been demonstrated frequently. In the classic study, Zborowski (20) interviewed and observed groups of Irish, Jewish, Italian, and "Old-American" surgical patients in pain, along with their families, to determine their attitudes toward pain and pain expression. In brief, the Jewish and Italian patients had a low tolerance for pain and were quite emotional in their responses. The Jewish tended to be pessimistic and attempted to mobilize others to give them the best possible care. In contrast, the Italians did not try to enlist help from others. Those Americans of Anglo-Saxon origin tended to bear pain with a minimum of outward expression. Irish patients also were reluctant to admit pain and withdrew from family and friends. Tursky and Sternbach (17) related similar attitudinal differences among subcultures in the United States to psychophysical and psychophysiological reaction patterns to experimental pain, indicating the attitudes were associated with differences in pain experience as well as in modes of expression. Weisenberg (18) reported similar findings and proposed that the ambiguity of the pain experience necessitated the use of others' experiences and behavior to determine what reactions are appropriate.

It is important to note that differences between groups have been small in contrast to the variability within groups, and there is considerable overlap across groups. Research in this area suffers major limitations, including poor group definition, limited sample sizes, questionable assessment of the intensities or types of clinical or experimental pain, failures to replicate, contradictory data, and overgeneralization (19). Furthermore, group differences are deemed to reflect stable traits with the impact of situational variables neglected. Pain expression is more flexible and situation-specific than has commonly been believed.

Acknowledgement. Supported in part by Canada Council research grants and a Social Sciences and Humanities Research Council of Canada Leave Fellowship.

REFERENCES

(1) Bandura, A. 1977. Social Learning Theory. Englewood Cliffs, N.J.: Prentice-Hall.

(2) Campbell, J.D. 1975. Illness is a point of view: The development of children's concepts of illness. Child Devel. 46: 92-100.

(3) Christensen, M.F., and Mortensen, O. 1975. Long-term prognosis in children with recurrent abdominal pain. Arch. Dis. Child. 50: 110-114.

(4) Craig, K.D. 1968. Physiological arousal as a function of imagined, vicarious and direct stress experiences. J. Abnorm. Psychol. 73: 513-520.

(5) Craig, K.D. 1978. Social modeling influences on pain. In The Psychology of Pain, ed. R.A. Sternbach, pp. 73-110. New York: Raven Press.

(6) Craig, K.D., and Prkachin, K.M. 1978. Social modeling influences on sensory decision theory and psychophysiological indexes of pain. J. Pers. Soc. Psychol. 36: 805-815.

(7) Eland, J.M., and Anderson, J.E. 1977. The experience of pain in children. In Pain: A Source Book for Nurses and Other Health Professionals, ed. A.K. Jacox, pp. 453-476. Boston: Little, Brown and Company.

(8) Izard, C.E.; Huebner, R.R.; Rissner, D.; McGinnes, G.; and Dougherty, L. 1980. The young infant's ability to produce discrete emotional expressions. Devel. Psychol., in press.

(9) Levy, D.M. 1960. The infant's earliest memory of inoculation. J. Genet. Psychol. 96, 3-46.

(10) Maccoby, E.E., and Jacklin, C.N. 1974. The Psychology of Sex Differences. Stanford: Stanford University Press.

(11) Merskey, H. 1975. Pain, learning and memory. J. Psychosom. Res. 19: 319-324.

(12) Mohamed, S.N.; Weisz, G.M.; and Waring, E.M. 1978. The relationship of chronic pain to depression, marital adjustment, and family dynamics. Pain 5: 285-292.

(13) Murray, A.D. 1979. Infant crying as an elicitor of parental behavior. Psychol. Bull. 86: 191-215.

(14) Nelson, K. 1973. Structure and strategy in learning to talk. Monog. Soc. Res. Child. Devel. 38: Whole No. 149.

(15) Poznanski, E.O. 1976. Children's reactions to pain. Clin. Ped. 15: 1114-1119.

(16) Stone, L.J.; Smith, H.T.; and Murphy, L.B., eds. 1978. The Infants First Year. New York: Basic Books.

(17) Tursky, B., and Sternbach, R.A. 1967. Further physiological correlates of ethnic differences in responses to shock. Psychophysiol. 4: 67-74.

(18) Weisenberg, M. 1977. Pain and pain control. Psych. Bull. 84, 1008-1044.

(19) Wolff, B.B., and Langley, S. 1968. Cultural factors and the response to pain: A review. Amer. Anthropol. 70: 494-501.

(20) Zborowski, M. 1969. People in Pain. San Francisco: Jossey-Bass.

Pain and Society, eds. H.W. Kosterlitz and L.Y. Terenius, pp. 53-62.
Dahlem Konferenzen 1980. Weinheim: Verlag Chemie GmbH.

The Suffering of Severe Intractable Pain

M. R. Bond
University Department of Psychological Medicine
Southern General Hospital, Glasgow G51 4TF, Scotland

Abstract. Suffering severe pain involves the whole being and for most ill people this means enduring greater physical distress than pain alone. The powers of endurance of each individual are based upon their physical and mental constitution and strongly moulded during the years of childhood and adolescence by culturally determined attitudes to pain and suffering in their peers and elders. In Western civilization strong emphasis has been placed upon the enobling effects of enduring the suffering of pain - an attitude which has its roots in pre-Christian philosophy and in Christian theology. Although this view of suffering pain remains pre-eminent amongst British hospital patients, there are signs of a change towards a less tolerant attitude towards being in pain and it is suggested that the change may bring increased rather than reduced suffering for a person with pain. The sources of this change are a matter for debate and possible contributors include increased but false expectations about the power of modern medicine to abolish pain, a weakening in the influence of religion and the appearance of a philosophy of materialistic individualism in society.

SOCIAL DEVELOPMENT OF ATTITUDES TO THE SUFFERING OF PAIN

The suggested title of this paper directs thought towards the precise nature of suffering and to what it means to an individual to have to endure severe intractable pain. This subject is seldom discussed in the scientific literature of pain but is a frequent source of interest and inspiration to novelists, poets, and writers of religious works. In order to gain insight into what it means to suffer severe intractable pain, and in preparing this paper, the author has specifically talked to many patients enduring it. In general these conversations have reinforced a long-held personal view that suffering accompanying severe intractable pain is an emotional experience which arises from the totality of each sufferer's being, both present and past, and his or her social heritage. In other words, although pain is a trial of the moment, the suffering aroused by it is rooted in each person's cultural background and history, and his or her personal growth and experience of pain through life. It has become very clear that understanding the influence of cultural values upon suffering and pain is of considerable importance to those who attempt to analyze the feelings and behavior of a person in pain, and yet it is a subject that is generally overlooked in the education of most doctors and nurses. For this reason the historical background to our attitudes to pain sufferers and their own to the pain they suffer is considered before examination of the mental and behavioral elements of suffering.

Any observant visitor to a hospital ward in Britain will become aware, sooner or later, that ability to endure pain with little or no complaint is admired and regarded as highly desirable behavior. Most patients in pain, especially men, learn this even more quickly! Stoicism in a pain sufferer is rewarded with admiration, sympathy, and more material expressions of approval, notably administration of pain relieving medicines. In contrast complaints of pain, especially if regarded as excessive or unnecessary are punished by expressions of disapproval, both verbal and practical, in the form of withholding analgesics or the administration of placebo substances. The attitude that suffering and pain should be borne with patience and fortitude has been expressed in many ways in prose and poetry, for example,

'Know how sublime a thing it is
to suffer and be strong.'

(Henry Wadsworth Longfellow 1807-1882, The Light of Stars)

and again,

'There is nothing the body suffers
the soul may not profit by.'
(George Meredith 1828-1909, Diana of The Crossways).
These are not merely sentiments confined to 19th century American and British poets. Recently Steven Brena writing about pain and religion (2) dedicated his book to,
'All those who have learned to suffer
in silence and understanding.'

The high value placed upon endurance of pain and suffering can be traced back in Hebrew history and to the Greek civilization of the 6th century B.C. - in particular to the intellectual and mystic philosopher, Pythagoras, who founded his school at Croton in Magna Graecia, now Southern Italy. His moral philosophy has had a surprisingly lasting effect upon attitudes to suffering in Western Civilization. He praised moral purity and in particular regarded the endurance of pain as one of the most salutory ways of gaining self-discipline and demonstrating self-control. At a much later time, Christianity in the Middle Ages, which had absorbed many of the teachings of Plato, Aristotle, and Pythagoras, viewed human suffering of pain as evidence of sin or punishment for trespass against religious dogma and as a beneficial form of preparation in life for salvation after death. It is obvious that such beliefs have played an important role in giving meaning to suffering and to the enduring of pain. Returning to the words pain and punishment etymological studies reveal a longstanding link between them because the origins of the word pain in Greek and Latin are 'poine' (suffering) and 'poena' (penalty), but it seems that whereas in early times pain was seen to be the cause of punishment, later it came to be regarded as the effect of it, and this was especially obvious in medieval theology (6). Some of our own patients enduring severe pain comment angrily that they feel unjustly punished (by God) when others, whom they regard as having been greater sinners than themselves, remain healthy. Therefore, despite the gradual loss of power and influence of theologians from the time of the Renaissance onwards and despite the rapid advances of science, there are many sufferers of severe pain today whose sentiments would be familiar to their medieval forefathers. However the view that to endure pain as well as one is able and for as long as possible, though prominent amongst pain sufferers, shows signs of weakening - a process which is to be viewed with some concern. A small but increasing number of pain sufferers in Britain expresses dissatisfaction with medical treatments for pain and with doctors and nurses unable to provide total or substantial pain relief which is regarded as both possible and each person's 'right.' There are several factors which may contribute to this attitude which has the potential for increasing rather than reducing suffering, as the frustrations, anger, and anxiety generated by failure to obtain expected relief heightens pain and lowers endurance, especially when the pain seems 'purposeless' as in advanced cancer. This attitude may be related to the general public's impression, gained from newspapers, magazines, radio, and television, that medicine has reached an advanced level of scientific sophistication where total pain relief ought to be possible, though clearly this is not the case. Medicine is indeed highly technical and becomes increasingly so year by year, but, one suspects, without more than a superficial interest amongst many doctors in improving their power to deal with individual human suffering by means other than the use of physical methods. However this deficiency is not new to society, having been recognized in general terms 150 years ago by Thomas Carlyle who wrote critically of it in Signs of the Times:

'Not the external and physical alone is now managed by machinery, but the spiritual also..... For the same habit regulates not our modes of action alone, but our modes of thought and feeling. Men are grown mechanical in head and heart, as well as in hand' (7).

Other factors which may play a part in the breakdown of attitudes towards enduring pain include lessened demands from society for self-control in speech and behavior evident in films, on television, and in the streets, the benumbing effects of almost ceaseless exposure to the pain and suffering of others worldwide through the media and increased social mobility with the loss for many of the traditional supporting role of the family. Last and perhaps most significant of all is the demystification of the Christian religion for many by scientists and theologians who have mistakenly applied scientific analytic methods to their creed.

MENTAL AND BEHAVIORAL ASPECTS OF THE SUFFERING OF PAIN

Severe chronic pain is experienced in a number of benign and malignant disorders. At times it is the only symptom (as in post-herpetic neuralgia), but more often it accompanies other symptoms of which several, especially breathlessness, diarrhea, or vomiting, may be less endurable than pain, thereby contributing more to suffering than pain alone. The total burden imposed on the sufferer may be increased by the side effects of treatment. Therefore a balance must be struck between the latter and a desirable level of symptom relief. For example, considerable suffering may occur during treatment with cytotoxic drugs or irradiation therapy. Analgesics in quantity produce unpleasant gastrointestinal disturbances, and those of the narcotic group have the power to alter consciousness to such an extent that some patients would rather retain their senses by taking less potent medicines and suffer some pain. At times the unknown element in treatment adds to suffering. Fear of surgery, especially of mutilation, for example, by mastectomy, and the need for devices like colostomies, often produce additional anxiety. However, experience shows that explanations about the nature of an illness, its likely outcome, the nature of treatment required, and any possible discomforts reduce anxiety in most patients and thus reduce suffering (1).

Severe pain, whether acute or chronic, leads to increased self concern, withdrawal from social contacts, and to reduction in tolerance for external stimuli such as light or sound.

In acute severe pain states, fear and anxiety are the predominant emotions and are most marked where the outcome of the patient's plight is unknown, and amongst those who, under normal circumstances, have the greatest liability to emotional breakdown when under stress. There has been debate about the extent to which severe and persistent pain alters personality, and to summarize the literature on this issue, it seems that most authors accept that certain premorbid characteristics become more evident, especially tendencies to anxiousness, depression, or preoccupation with health (9). Relief of pain brings about a reversal of the change, the extent of which depends upon whether the patient is cured or merely relieved of a major symptom but not of the underlying illness or disability. When pain is severe and intractable without clear prospects of relief, a different range of emotions is arounsed. Anger and resentment about failure to gain relief are common, especially amongst those who regard their pain as 'meaningless.' In some, especially those who find difficulty in expressing emotion, especially anger, depression of mood develops. This is especially obvious where the sufferer feels helpless in the grip of events beyond his or her control and hopeless, as it seems others have also lost control over the disease process and its treatment leaving no comfort for the future. These feelings are generally attributed to psychological causes but could as easily be regarded as the product of an increasingly secular society and as an expression of 'Godlessness.' Therefore it seems that the lack of firm spiritual beliefs enhances the bleakness of a life of suffering, a life in which the future may either remain unknown or be filled with the prospect of continued and increasing suffering ending in death which is in itself often feared as a painful and final event. When pain becomes chronic, an interesting phenomenological change may be observed. Patients begin to talk of pain as alien, as unwelcome though often commanding total attention, as invasive, malign, almost tangible, and coming from without the self. To speculate, this may be an essential part of the process of gaining control over an unavoidable experience which is potentially destructive to emotional integrity and which as a result becomes a major preoccupation in life. In fact, the daily battle with pain may become essential for preservation of life! This statement is based on the observation that, at times, sudden and total relief of severe chronic pain in patients with advanced cancer is followed by a state of complete calm lasting only days and ending in death.

In contrast to those with a very obvious physical cause for severe pain, are two groups of patients present at clinics complaining of severe intractable pain for which a satisfactory explanation cannot be found in physical terms. The larger of the two groups consists of individuals who appear emotionally depressed to a variable extent and who have severe pain which is presented as the leading symptom and which is often experienced in the region of the face (5). Both depression and pain disappear on treatment with antidepressant drugs, and it is clear that the total suffering is a consequence of mental rather than physical illness in patients who may have a history of similar illnesses in the past and often a good premorbid personality. Patients in the smaller group usually have a very long history of pain. They complain vociferously about the intensity of suffering and pain but outwardly fail to show the behavior and appearance of those with severe pain of known physical origin. Trained primarily to cope with the latter, many doctors find it difficult or impossible to believe that these patients have pain and this, coupled with a long history of negative investigations for possible physical causes, tends to arouse hostility and rejection. However, twenty years ago independent and germinal papers by George Engel (3) and Thomas Szasz (10) demonstrated that complaining of pain for this group is a genuine expression of anguish, of suffering, of the feeling of being a 'painful person.' The existence of the 'pain prone' and 'painful person' is beyond doubt, and such individuals exhibit an abnormality of personality development in which being in pain and suffering plays a major role in stabilizing psychic life and in the manipulation of interpersonal relations (8, 9). Therefore this form of suffering, which is undoubtedly extreme at times, serves a purpose other than as an indicator of physical damage to the body. But, it is an essential component of mental life and it is not seen as alien to the self in contradistinction to the severe pain of chronic physical illness. Thus, rather than being destructive, paradoxically it protects mental and social integrity. The need for pain and suffering is so strong and so much a part of the person that all but a few of those with it reject any form of treatment ultimately, whether physical or psychological, and yet continue to attend one clinic after another ostensibly seeking investigation and cure - a form of behavior which validates their occupancy of the sick role status. In recent years behavioral psychologists have investigated this group very thoroughly and proposed that its members have a learned disorder beginning either with experiences of painful illness in childhood or later in adult life, and they claim modest success in treatment using operant conditioning techniques designed to eliminate old behaviors and to teach new ones (4). To conclude, it is clear that there are several conceptual frameworks within which pain problems and the suffering associated with them may be analyzed and treated, namely, the neurobiological, psychodynamic, behavioral, and ethico-religious paradigms. This observation is central to the understanding of pain and suffering and one which has only recently begun to filter into the minds of those who care for individuals in pain.

CONCLUSION

The main objective of this working paper is the formulation of questions designed to provoke discussion about the suffering of severe pain. Three issues identifiable in the text merit consideration and they are:

1) Is the attitude that severe pain should be borne with fortitude advantageous to pain sufferers in the present age?

2) Are attitudes changing towards a reduction in tolerance for suffering? If so, what is their implication for those who seek but cannot find relief for pain?

3) In the face of inability completely to relieve and prevent severe intractable pain by traditional medical methods, what alternative ways of reducing suffering should be investigated and/or promoted by the medical and other professions involved in caring for those with pain?

REFERENCES

(1) Bond, M.R. 1976. Psychological and psychiatric aspects of pain. In Modern Perspectives in Psychiatric Aspects of Surgery, ed. J.G. Howells, pp. 109-139. New York: Brunner/Mazel.

(2) Brena, S. 1972. Pain and Religion. Springfield, IL: Charles C. Thomas.

(3) Engel, G.L. 1959. Psychogenic pain and the pain prone person. Am. J. Med. 26: 899-918.

(4) Fordyce, W.E. 1976. Behavior Methods in Chronic Pain and Illness. St. Louis: C.V. Mosby Co.

(5) Lascelles, R.G. 1966. Atypical facial pain and depression. Br. J. Psychiat. 112: 651-659.

(6) Merskey, H., and Spear, F.G. 1967. Pain: Psychological and Psychiatric Aspects, pp. 15. London: Bailliere, Tindall and Cassell.

(7) Phelps, G. 1979. A Short History of English Literature, pp. 171. London: The Folio Press.

(8) Pilowsky, I. 1978. Psychodynamic aspects of the pain experience. In The Psychology of Pain, ed. R.A. Sternbach, pp. 203-218. New York: Raven Press.

(9) Sternbach, R.A. 1974. Pain Patients: Traits and Treatments. New York and London: Academic Press.

(10) Szasz, T.S. 1957. Pain and Pleasure: A Study of Bodily Feelings. New York: Basic Books.

Pain and Society, eds. H.W. Kosterlitz and L.Y. Terenius, pp. 63-78.
Dahlem Konferenzen 1980. Weinheim: Verlag Chemie GmbH.

A Religiophilosophical Perspective on Pain

W. Tu
Department of History, University of California
Berkeley, CA 94720, USA

Abstract. Pain experience involves a complex interaction of physical, mental and spiritual factors. The symbolizations of pain in Christian, Buddhist, and Confucian traditions, while seemingly irrelevant to current scientific investigations of pain, provide a cultural-social milieu in which a significantly large population of the human community learn to articulate pain in a way meaningful to them. Panpsychism, as a religiophilosophical perspective on the mind-body problem, seems particularly suited to accommodate various new advances in pain research without losing sight of the important historical perceptions on the subject. If panpsychism as an interpretive position is tenable, the Taoist approach, on which much of Chinese medical theory is based, may provide a fruitful means to explore further the physiology and psychology of pain.

If we take pain to be a complex phenomenon, involving sensation, emotion, cognition, motivation, and, in the perception of Chinese medical theory, energy (2,6,12), an intriguing problem in the understanding of pain is to determine the level of sophistication on which it is articulated. Recent advances in what may be called the science of pain have yielded so many concrete results (7,8,9,13) that the promise of a precise definition of pain, as a solvable problem, seems near at hand. It is likely, some more optimistic researchers of this common human experience are ready to propose, that as our knowledge of the neurophysiological or biochemical processes of pain further develops, it will bring about the long overdue solution to most, if not all, of the puzzling problems of pain. The increasing currency of concepts such as "pain control" and "pain management" suggests that the alleged pain epidemic is at last controllable and manageable (12).

As a layman in pain research, I must defer to the experts to comment on the truth-value of the various claims currently put forth in professional scientific journals. However, I am under the impression, admittedly based on very limited exposure to the vast literature on the subject, that the word "pain" has already assumed so many layers of meaning in its technical usage that to an expert, no matter how broadly he or she conceives of it, the senses of pain in ordinary language are relegated to the background. To be sure, it makes sense to note the difference between acute pain and chronic pain; and it seems helpful to distinguish a painful sensation as a mental awareness and the total subjective pain experience. But to characterize "life in the working-class family" as "worlds of pain" (15) is, in the view of the experts, irrelevant to their overall concern. Indeed, the nature of a scientific inquiry demands that the object of study be defined in precise terms. If _life_ is characterized as painful, it is an attitude, a belief, or a world view, hardly the subject for a research project that could lead to clearly observable conclusions.

Yet, undeniably, pain as a human experience involves a complex interaction of physical, mental, and spiritual processes (6). Even if we can explain objectively the genetic reasons for the occurrence of a painful sensation, the actual experience of pain is not reducible to them. In fact, the kinds of pain that are easily identifiable as physical and thus controllable and manageable by pharmacologic approaches constitute the least problematical aspects of the pain experience (9). A much more difficult issue is the pain that seems to have been conditioned by psychological, social, and cultural factors as well (17). Perhaps the implicit dichotomy between physical and non-physical pain is misleading. So long as pain experience is intensely personal, it is necessarily shaped, as it were, by the forms of life of those who care to articulate it.

The articulation of pain entails self-description which, in turn, reveals attitude, belief, and world view (11). Of course it is highly desirable that we pinpoint scientifically what pain is (allowing for different but complementary explanations). In fact, it can significantly enhance our knowledge of the nervous system and even the structure and function of the brain. But, so long as pain experience remains universally present and yet must be individually interpreted, it raises profound questions of meaning. These questions can never be fully answered; they will continue to challenge us. Pain, in this view, is not a problem to be solved but a deceptively simple code. We need to examine, among other things, a variety of symbolic structures in which it manifests itself, in order to have it properly deciphered.

In an attempt to decipher the message of pain from a Christian theological perspective, C. S. Lewis observes in his thought-provoking The Problem of Pain written almost four decades ago:

> But the truth is that the word Pain has two senses which must now be distinguished. a. A particular kind of sensation, probably conveyed by specialised nerve fibers and, recognisable by the patient as that kind of sensation whether he dislikes it or not (e.g., the faint ache in my limbs would be recognised as an ache even if I didn't object to it). b. Any experience, whether physical or mental, which the patient dislikes. It will be noticed that all Pains in sense a become Pains in sense b if they are raised above a certain very low level of intensity, but that Pains in the b sense need not be Pains in the a sense. Pain in the b sense, in fact, is synonymous with "suffering," "anguish," "tribulation," "adversity," or "trouble," and it is about it that the problem of pain arises ((6), p. 90).

In the light of recent studies on pain, we may want to refine our conceptions to a much greater degree of precision. We may want to suggest, for example, that chronic pain rather than acute pain seems to raise more problems for the researcher. However, his underlying thesis that human suffering is pain experience laden with ethicoreligious implications still poses perennial perceptual questions (14).

I do not intend to argue that a critical examination of theological views on pain necessarily increases our understanding of the pain experience in the Christian West. While I am aware that such an examination may provide some clue to a comparative analysis of the intriguing issues such as pain threshold, pain tolerance, and the pain sensitivity range (13,17), my purpose is simply to note some of the salient features of this particular perspective on pain. To begin, it is vitally important that we treat enduring religious insights not as superstitious or pseudoscientific opinions but as symbolizations of reality formulated by some of the most subtle and influential minds in a given cultural tradition (14).

It is misleading to say that the Christians glorify pain as a purifying experience, but the view that pain (and for that matter death) is the means of redemption and sanctification is widely held among those who do not deny Christ. Theologians may disagree with Pope Pius XII when he flatly pronounced: "In the garden of humanity, ever since it ceased to be called the earthly paradise, there has ripened, and will always ripen one of the bitter fruits of original sin: pain." Historically, however, martyrdom as "the supreme enacting and perfection of Christianity" embraces pain as an integral part of "Trial" or "Sacrifice." Through the agonizing experience of pain, the Christian doctrine suggests, one can be made whole. Thus, the full acting out of the believer's surrender to God demands pain: "this action, to be perfect, must be done from the pure will to obey, in the absence, or in the teeth, of inclination" (6). The vivid image of Crucifixion, heightened by the graphic portrayal of the skilled artists, speaks directly to this experience commonly shared in Christian communities (14).

In the Christian perception, it should be further stated, pain unlike error or sin is unmasked, unmistakable, and therefore immediately recognizable evil. Since pain in itself has no tendency to proliferate, the knowledge that there is something wrong when one is being hurt does not require any "undoing." By contrast, after an error or a sin is committed, we need to remove not only the causes but also correct or repent what we have already done. This is the reason for Lewis to characterize pain as "sterilised or disinfected evil" (6). Yet, theologically, it is this evil as a form of "retributive punishment" that awakens us to the possibility of a primarily remedial or corrective good because man is by nature fallen but redeemable: "God whispers to us in our pleasures, speaks in our conscience, but shouts in our pains" (6).

If the Christians believe that pain is inherent in the very existence of a world where people must be roused to respond to God's calling, the Buddhists accept "pain" (<u>dukkha</u>, also rendered as ill, sorrow, turmoil, suffering) as a defining characteristic of human life. Understandably the experience of pain is pregnant with spiritual meanings in Buddhism. Indeed, it is the point of departure of the most sacred doctrine in all of Buddha's teachings. The so-called Four Noble Truths, which the Buddha is alleged to have first preached at Benares immediately after his enlightenment, are essential to all schools in the Buddhist tradition:

> 1. What then is the Noble Truth of Pain? Birth is pain, decay is pain, sickness is pain, death is pain. To be conjoined with what one dislikes means suffering. To be disjoined from what one likes means

> suffering. Not to get what one wants, also that means suffering. In short, all grasping at (any of) the five skandhas (components of a person) involves suffering.
> 2. What then is the Noble Truth of the Origination of Pain? It is that craving which leads to rebirth, accompanied by delight and greed, seeking its delight now here, now there, i.e., craving for sensuous experience, craving to perpetuate oneself, craving for extinction.
> 3. What then is the Noble Truth of the Stopping of Pain? It is the complete stopping of that craving, the withdrawal from it, the renouncing of it, throwing it back, liberation from it, non-attachment to it.
> 4. What then is the Noble Truth of the steps which lead to the stopping of Pain? It is this Noble Eightfold Path, which consists of: Right views, right intentions, right speech, right conduct, right livelihood, right effort, right mindfulness, right concentration ((3), p. 43).

The Four Noble Truths thus contain the characterization of all existence as pain, the observation that this pain arises from craving for objects which are figments of distorted human minds, the insistence that there is liberation from pain, and the advocacy of the Middle Path, which consists of eight modes of spiritual discipline, as the authentic method for attaining this liberation (3). Pain, as Buddha's teaching has it, is a view of life as well as a physical-emotional-mental complex which defines the nature of human existence.

This Buddhist interpretation of pain is predicated on a highly sophisticated notion about the meaning of spiritual insight: a human being has no enduring substance (ātman) and is only an ever-changing conglomerate of material, affectional, and psychic agents (dharma). The world we experience in our everyday living results from numerous patterns of continuous interaction among these agents. The objects of our perceptions are thus without independent bases of existence. As Frederick J. Streng explains:

> The "arising of existence," which generally is also the arising of turmoil [pain], comes about through interdependent and reciprocal forces of the factors [agents]—forces which find their roots in man's ignorant clinging to the objects that "he" unwittingly is fabricating! For "the arising of existence" to cease, the fabricating ignorance must cease; and the quelling of ignorance requires spiritual insight (prajñā). When fabricating ignorance is overcome and the residue of the fabricating force has dissipated, then there is nirvāṇa—the "dying out" of the flame of desire for illusory objects ((16), p. 30).

Pain so conceived does not at all resemble the "primitive" view that as a disease, it is caused by the intrusion of an alien element into the body. Nor does it resemble the Hebraic idea of retributive punishment as a result of sin. Even though it seems compatible with the Platonic interpretation of pain as sensation, it goes beyond the conceptual category of the unpleasant as opposed to the pleasant feelings. For its purpose is to establish a general thesis about human suffering. On the Buddhist view, pain as a pervasive human experience is not merely obvious suffering engendered by some psychosomatic disorder. Rather, as hidden suffering, it underlies human existence as a whole. Thus, pleasant feelings themselves are by no means a sign of well-being or even a clear indication of painless relief. For they may involve the suffering of others, they are likely tied up with anxiety for fear that the experienced pleasure cannot last, they can bind us still further to conditions that will lead to a great deal of suffering, and they often fail to satisfy the inmost longings of our hearts (3). The implicit message is that pain features prominently in all modalities of human life: birth, aging, sickness, and death. Sensory pleasures are short-lived, riddled with anxiety and hardly satisfying to our inner cravings. The only way to transcend pain and to experience a lasting spiritual bliss is through enlightenment: the art and joy of the destruction of craving.

Inherent in the Buddhist ethicoreligious perspective on pain is a suggestive paradox. The cultivation of sensory pleasures may lead to more agonizing pain. The right path to relieve pain is not to seek pleasurable feelings but to develop a disinterested attitude toward it. This spirit of detachment, far from being an artificially adopted attitude, is a manifestation of an intensely religious form of life. While worldly pleasures are shifting, trivial, superficial, and insignificant, experiences of pain properly understood can strengthen our body, purify our soul and deepen our spirit. This view is articulated not only in Christian theology and Buddhist religiophilosophy but also in Confucian ethical thought:

> When Heaven is about to confer a great responsibility on any man, it will exercise his mind with suffering, subject his sinews and bones to hard work, expose his body to hunger, put him to poverty, place obstacles in the paths of his deeds, so as to stimulate his mind, harden his nature, and improve wherever he is incompetent. [Mencius, 6A:15]

It may not be farfetched to note that pain experience as a "trial" for great historical personalities and thus for sharpening our own ethicoreligious awareness is also commonly shared by Greek philosophers, by the Church fathers in the middle ages and by Hindu ascetics. Indeed, the Neo-Confucians take pain as a heightened experience, disturbing in itself but significant for human communion. It is through the ability to share the pains of others that one becomes a sensitive and responsible participant of society. The person who can heartlessly bear the sufferings of those around him is seriously deficient in basic humanity.

With this background understanding, we can now proceed to a preliminary description of a religiophilosophical perspective on pain which, for lack of a better designation, will be referred to as a form of "panpsychism." In an attempt to formulate an essay on the subject, Thomas Nagel specifies four premises as necessary conditions for establishing the philosophical doctrine of panpsychism. The first premise is material composition. Since "any living organism, including a human being, is a complex material system," "anything whatever, if broken down far enough and rearranged, could be incorporated into a living organism" (10). An obvious implication of this for us is that pain as a sensation is based on a multidimensional structure of physical properties. If studied and analyzed with sufficient sophistication, it can be broken down to perceptible or decipherable material units and processes, such as afferent fibers, neurons, nociceptors, theomoreceptors, various pathways, possibly "gates" and so forth.

The second premise is nonreductionism, which means "ordinary mental states like thought, feeling, emotion, sensation, or desire are not physical properties of the organism—behavioral, physiological, or otherwise—and they are not implied by physical properties alone" (10). On this view, pain as a sensation, not to mention the more complex notion of pain experience, is not reducible to neurophysiological or biochemical explanations, no matter how comprehensive they are. The third premise is realism, which maintains that mental states are properties of the organism. Even relational properties such as belief and perception are no exception, for they also involve some nonrelational aspect. This premise further maintains that mental states are no less real than behavior, physical stimuli, and physiological processes (10).

Thus, to deny that mental properties can be entailed by physical properties is not to cast doubt about the "reality" of mental properties. The premise that physical interpretation of human activities does not explain the mental is based on the assumption that such an interpretation cannot account for the self-awareness of any conscious mental state of the possessor. The problem of pain is a case in point. Since self-ascriptions of pain experience require no evidential grounds, analysis of the objective neural system, or for that matter the cerebral cortex, can never by itself imply anything that is nonobjectifiable. Yet the multiple possibilities of sensation are real as physical phenomena. To be sure, mental states often depend on what is going on in the physiology of the body and are intimately connected with nerve and brain processes. However, despite their belonging to the organism, they are neither reducible to nor explainable by it. This leads us to the fourth premise, <u>nonemergence</u>.

This premise assumes that "all properties of a complex system that are not relations between it and something else derive from the properties of its constituents and their effects on each other when so combined." In other words, it rejects the proposition that "an observed feature of the system cannot be derived from the properties currently attributed to its constituents." Of course, it is quite conceivable that our obtained knowledge about a complex system fails to recognize further vital constituents that it possesses or our understanding of already identified and analyzed constituents lacks the sophistication of knowing further properties and functions that they have (10). To say that there are no truly emergent properties of complex systems, however, is to deny that mental states can be totally independent of the biology and physiology of the organism. Pain as a sensation, in this sense, is not an emergent property which does not derive from the structures and functions of the constituents of the body. In fact, it is the result of their effects on each other.

With these four premises, the so-called mind-body problem assumes a different shape of meaning. Indeed, the whole procedure of trying to establish causal connections between mental and physical processes will have to be fundamentally revised. If we accept panpsychism so defined, dualism may still be used as a heuristic device, but we must declare that it is epistemologically untenable. The practice of reducing mental processes to physical processes is rejected because it seems to be an easy way out of the mind-body problem; it may explain the problem away without offering plausible answers. However, admitting the reality of mental occurrences is not to deny that mental states have causal explanation. Even though we do not ascribe them to either organisms or for that matter souls as subjects, we believe that they are necessitated by something inherent in the complex system itself (10).

This panpsychist viewpoint enables us to see the religious insights on pain in a new light. On the surface, the conception of a living organism as a complex material system is diametrically opposed to a theological or religious interpretation of human existence. However, by maintaining that the mental states are nonreducible and real, there is no reason to doubt that a living organism has symbolic significance laden with deep religious import. Leaving aside the issue of genesis, which of course can be taken as a deceptively simple encoding of a complex message, panpsychism impels us to appreciate what is normally taken as "the proto-mental properties of dead matter" with a sense of awe. Precisely because it is difficult to imagine how a chain of explanatory inference could ever get from the mental states of whole animals back to their material compositions, thought, feeling, emotion, sensation, or desire requires much more complex symbolization to make it sensible as a common human experience.

Panpsychism as a religiophilosophical perspective allows a fruitful exploration of the relevance of well-articulated religious insights to our understanding of basic human experiences such as pain. For one thing, the symbolizations of pain in major religious systems have become so much an integral part of our subjective mental states, it is ill-advised to relegate them to the background as outmoded opinions on a technical subject. Recent studies in psychology clearly show that the transition from a reflective response to pain sensation to a disinterested description of a pain experience involves a long and gradual process in human development (2). By analogy, we may very well take symbolizations of pain in major religious systems as highly integrated insights on a perennial human concern from various civilizational perspectives. Needless to say, the evolution of these insights into complex symbolic systems has been agonizingly slow. This is at least part of the reason that hermeneutics as philosophy of interpretation remains one of the most difficult disciplines in the humanities (14).

The Christian idea of pain as both an indication of human fallibility and an authentic possibility for self-purification may not have much to do with neurophysiological analysis of pain, but as an enduring feature in experiencing and articulating pain among those who are confirmed Christians, it seems to have exerted a profound influence on the dualistic conception of pain in Western literature. By contrast, since the Buddhists perceive pain as a defining characteristic of human existence, they seem to be willing to endure pain experience as a matter of fact. While the Confucians share the Christian theology of suffering as "trial," they do not have any notion of original sin. To them, it is both desirable and necessary to cure pain, if one intends to preserve one's well-being. It is true that the Neo-Confucians take pain experience as evocative of sympathy and thus valuable for social solidarity. Their purpose of life, nevertheless, is to improve the human condition through moral education so that pain and suffering can be controlled and reduced. Since they do not entertain the possibility of a Buddhist Western Paradise where ultimate joy prevails, they devote themselves to the transformation of the secular world.

Admittedly, if we take panpsychism seriously as a religio-philosophical perspective on pain, we cannot accept the Christian idea of soul as an independent cause for the emergence of mental states. Nor can we uncritically subscribe to the Buddhist claim that no causal interpretation is possible in respect to either external things or inner experiences. Furthermore, it prompts us to probe the possibility that an alternative model for human physiology, such as the idea of "energy fields" in Chinese medicine, may turn out to be a more satisfying overall conceptualization of the interaction between physical and mental processes. Recent studies on the effect of auriculo-acupuncture on pain (5), for example, should provoke us to examine closely the Yin-Yang model of Taosim (4,12). It is plausible that the Taoist organismic theory with emphasis on a dynamic interplay between bipolar and yet complementary forces is just such an alternative model.

The Yin-Yang model, in the words of Manfred Porkert, signifies several interconnected "systems of correspondence" (12). These systems are not material structures but energy fields. The interior of the body thus conceived consists of dynamic interplays of various energetic spheres in which the physical organs function as material substrata. This conception of human physiology is significantly different from the anatomical approach which takes the organism as a combination of related parts. As Nathan Sivin observes, in the classical Chinese medical theory, each energetic sphere "is defined, not by physical properties, but by its specific role in the processing, storage, and distribution of vital energy and thus in the maintenance of life." While modern Western medicine "deals with material structures and tissues which are able to perform certain functions, Chinese medicine deals with functions to which physically demonstrable organs happen to be attached" (12). It is thus conceivable, from the Chinese viewpoint, that a functional system of energetic sphere may exist and perform a vital role in the organism without being attached to any specific organ, as in the case of the *san-chiao* (12).

Furthermore, according to this explanatory model, energy is distributed throughout the body, from the inmost spheres to the tips of the fingers, by a series of "conduits" ("sin-arteries" or "meridians"). The so-called acupuncture points are actually hundreds of sensitive "foramina" (*hsüeh*) locatable near the periphery of the body as parts of the overall system (12). The workability of auriculo-acupuncture on pains of distant locations of the body seems to suggest a particular modality of the interconnectedness of the energetic spheres (1,5). Acupuncture or moxibustion treatment of pain can thus be interpreted as doctor's intervention with a view to "restoring proper phasing of the energetic flow, restoring to that dynamic balance in the order of time which for Chinese defines health." Understandably, "a remarkable variety of investigative methods, ranging from electrical measurement of skin potentials to the microscopic search for special subcutaneous structures" (12) have not yet brought about anticipated results. A more fruitful line of inquiry is perhaps to conduct a comprehensive examination of the idea of "energetics" (or "the forms of energy") in Chinese medical literature. For instance, if we have a better sense of how *ch'i* ("energetic configuration") is functionally defined in Chinese internal medicine, we can then proceed to a more focused investigation of one of its salient features. This of course requires a deeper commitment than simply the desire to learn a practical technique. It may also, in Lewis' words, "raise almost intolerable intellectual problems" for those of us who have never questioned the validity of the conceptual scheme in which the human body has been scientifically studied.

REFERENCES

(1) Andersson, S. A., and Holmgren, E. 1975. On acupuncture analgesia and the mechanism of pain. American Journal of Chinese Medicine 3 (4): 311-334.

(2) Bresler, D., and Trubo, R. 1979. Free Yourself from Pain. New York: Simon and Schuster.

(3) Conze, E. 1951. Buddhism: Its Essence and Development. Oxford: Bruno Cassirer Limited.

(4) Kao, J. 1977. Chinese alchemy: confluence and transformation. American Journal of Chinese Medicine 5 (3-4): 233-240.

(5) Leung, C. Y., and Spoerel, W. E. 1974. Effect of auriculo-acupuncture on pain. American Journal of Chinese Medicine 2 (3): 247-260.

(6) Lewis, C. S. 1962. The Problem of Pain. New York: Macmillan.

(7) Melzack, R., and Wall, P. D. 1965. Pain mechanisms: a new theory. Science 150: 971-979.

(8) Melzack, R., and Wall, P. D. 1970. Psychophysiology of pain. International Anesthesiology Clinics: Anesthesiology and Neurophysiology 8 (1): 3.

(9) Merskey, H., and Spear, F. G. 1967. Pain: Psychological and Psychiatric Aspects. London: Bailliere, Tindall & Cassell.

(10) Nagle, T. 1979. Panpsychism. In Mortal Questions, pp. 181-195. Cambridge: Cambridge University Press.

(11) Polanyi, M. 1958. Personal Knowledge: Towards a Post-critical Philosophy. New York: Harper & Row.

(12) Porkert, M. 1974. The Theoretical Foundations of Chinese Medicine: Systems of Correspondence. Cambridge, Mass.: MIT Press.

(13) Procacci, P.; Corte, M. D.; Zoppi, M.; and Maresca, M. 1974. Rhythmic changes of the cutaneous pain threshold in man. Chronobiologia 1: 77-96.

(14) Ricoeur, P. 1976. The Symbolism of Evil. Boston: Beacon Press.

(15) Rubin, L. B. 1976. Worlds of Pain: Life in the Working-class Family. New York: Basic Books.

(16) Streng, F. J. 1967. Emptiness: A Study in Religious Meaning. Nashville, Tenn.: Abingdon Press.

(17) Wolff, B. B., and Langley, S. 1968. Cultural factors and the response to pain: a review. American Anthropology 70: 494-501.

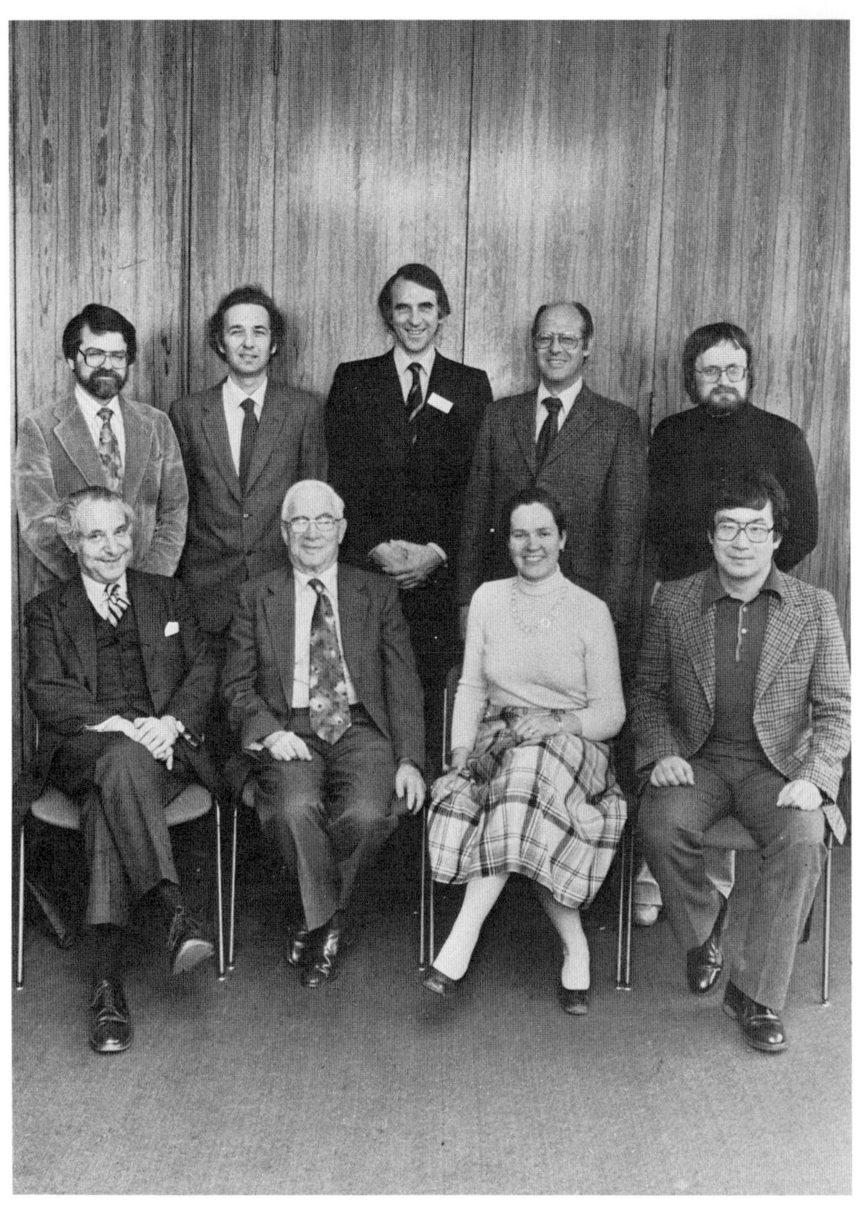

Group on <u>Evolution of Expression of Pain (Acute and Chronic)</u>
Seated, left to right: Bert Wolff, Hans Kosterlitz, Jane Dum, Wei-ming Tu. Standing: Ken Craig, Giancarlo Carli, Michael Bond, Ron Melzack, Hartmut Brinkhus.

Pain and Society, eds. H.W. Kosterlitz and L.Y. Terenius, pp. 81-92.
Dahlem Konferenzen 1980. Weinheim: Verlag Chemie GmbH.

Evolution of Expression of Pain (Acute and Chronic) Group Report

B. B. Wolff, Rapporteur
M. R. Bond, H. Brinkhus, G. Carli, K. D. Craig,
J. E. Dum, H. W. Kosterlitz, R. Melzack, W. Tu

INTRODUCTION

In Western civilization the concept of pain as a specific sensation is of relatively recent origin, having been developed during the last centennium (3). Views of pain have progressed from religious-hedonistic notions to the idea of pain as a sensory modality to that of pain as a personal experience associated with complex behavior patterns, influenced by many psychological and sociocultural variables (see Procacci, this volume). In contrast, the modern consideration of pain from a philosophical and religious perspective is presented by Tu (this volume). It is recognized that the distinction should be made between the mind-body and good-evil dualism in Western philosophical and religious thought (6) and the Eastern concept of a dynamic interaction by energy fields, e.g., the Yin-Yang model, for constructing explanatory and interpretative systems (10,11).

A second concern relates to the existence of pain in animals. Melzack and Dennis (this volume) outline the evolution of new ascending pathways allowing greater plasticity of expression, especially in the higher vertebrates and man, while Carli (this volume) presents evidence from behavioral studies and observations to support the view that animals can and do feel pain.

The development of pain expression and experience from innate reflexes to a complex learned behavior sequence, modulated by cognitive, affective, and sociocultural factors, is discussed by Craig (this volume). Bond (this volume) further develops the concept of suffering in Western civilization in association with pain.

No attempt will be made to discuss or summarize these six papers as they are published in detail in these Proceedings. However, they serve as a trigger for the discussion leading to the following questions and statements presented in full in this report.

Major concerns exist with regard to terminology, definitions, and conceptual studies needed to understand pain. It is recognized that pain is a unique and individual experience, which is composed of several dimensions. It is suggested that a phylogenetic approach is helpful. The concept of a three-tiered system (8) with sensory-discriminative, motivational-affective, and cognitive-evaluative factors as the three determinants of pain appears to be most convenient (Fig. 1).

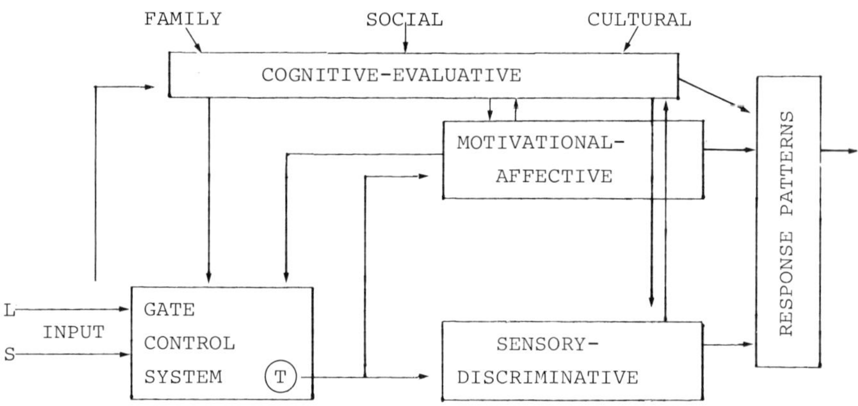

FIG. 1.

There is a basic sensory-discriminative level, shown by all animals and man, in which there is some kind of pain-related response (e.g., withdrawal) following a noxious stimulus, which does not require higher level involvement. These sensory level responses seem to serve a useful purpose in our study of pain, although it may be questioned as to whether or not they ought to be labeled "pain."

The second, motivational-affective level is generally accepted as an important component of the pain experience and is related to motivational aspects of behavior, although it may not always be easy to relate it to the triggering stimulus.

The third, cognitive-evaluative level is highly complex, influenced by many extrinsic variables, such as the family, social milieu, and cultural group. This cognitive level in turn interacts with both the motivational-affective and the basic sensory-discriminative levels, which in turn can influence each other. In addition, processing already occurs at the first synaptic level as shown in Fig. 1 and discussed in the gate theory (9).

It is suggested that the proposed three-tiered system may be useful in the analysis of acute and chronic pain. The existence of automatic or innate behavior patterns is accepted. These patterns, in turn, may be related to the first sensory level. It is thus possible that acute pain may be heavily weighted by such innate behavior patterns. As thought or cognition developed in higher animals and humans, a graded plasticity of response became possible. Chronic pain, in contrast to acute pain, may be an outcome of such cognitive modulation of the pain-related response. Therefore, it is recommended that the strategies in the study of pain and its role in society must include both genetic and environmental (i.e., learned) factors and observations.

In terms of phylogenetic development, it is suggested that in the higher animals, pain or the expression of pain may in fact be related to the highest levels of functioning, probably involving both the motivational-affective and cognitive-evaluative levels.

Finally, the group agreed that in both higher animals and man, pain is a private datum - not directly measurable (5). Because different individuals have undergone unique past experiences and have been subject to varying social and cultural influences, it is to be expected that they perceive pain in different fashions. However, in spite of this problem, it is agreed that pain can be evaluated and measured from several different perspectives.

Nine fundamental questions were developed for detailed discussion.

1. PAIN EXPERIENCE IN ANIMALS

Question: Given the evolutionary evidence, what can we infer about the nature of the pain experience in animals?
Statement A: Pain is an individual subjective experience. We can only infer its existence in animals and humans.

The reiteration of this statement serves as a starting point for this topic. It is emphasized that there is not only a developmental evolution of the newer ascending and descending neural systems (pathways) in higher animals and man, but that the older systems also continued to evolve. Thus, it is implicit that mammals below the level of man can also feel pain similar to man but with fewer of the cognitive attributes (5). The possibility of comparing pain in animals with that of lobotomized patients was discussed, but it was decided that it is anthropomorphic and risky to make analogies from human to animal behavior. Furthermore, pain perception in lobotomized patients is not as simple as was once thought. Similarly, one should be aware of the limitations of drawing analogies between animals and man, and therefore, one should not extrapolate from humans to animals and vice versa.

An important strategy for studying pain is to carry out observations in the natural habitat. Experimental behavioral studies of the total intact animal in the laboratory should be designed to reflect the total behavior patterns related to the day-to-day activity of animals in their natural habitat.

Statement B: Based on our knowledge of the evolution of pain expression in man, and because pain is an individual subjective experience, we conclude that it is only possible to infer the qualities or nature of pain perceived by animals, children, or other people.

2. ETHICAL CONSTRAINTS ON EXPERIMENTAL PAIN STUDIES

Question: What are the ethical constraints on experiments which inflict pain in humans and animals?

It was indicated that while a scientist may have the most expert knowledge about a given experiment, he has biases which may impede his evaluation of the ethical implications of his own or similar experiments by others. Similar conflicts of interest may diminish the effectiveness of the peer review system. Society increasingly demands more and better control of such research, including veto power.

The "Golden Rule" states "...Therefore all things whatsoever ye would that men should do to you, do ye even so to them: For this is the law and the prophets..." (14). The "Golden Rule" was discussed at length and criticized for possibly attempting to impose a code of ethics or sets of morals on individuals or groups not willing to accept such criteria. This problem was already recognized by George Bernard Shaw (13), who stated, "...Do not do unto others as you would they should do unto you. Their tastes may not be the same..." Therefore, the following modification of the "Golden Rule" was suggested. "Do not do unto others what you would not have done to yourself, and do not do unto others what they would not have done unto themselves."

Statement C: In view of the inadequacy of our knowledge, we believe that ethical decisions related to research on pain should be made by the broadest representation possible, involving a multidisciplinary group with "outside" lay representation.

The following strategies were proposed:

a) To develop a code of ethical guidelines for pain research.

b) In humans, to use the subject as a collaborator OR to have an advocate or ombudsman for the subject.

c) To improve methods of pain measurement.
d) To perform only experiments that can be justified in humane as well as scientific terms.
e) To ensure human care for man (Standard Hospital Care) and animals (Veterinary Guidelines).

3. PAIN AND SUFFERING

Question: What is the relationship between pain and suffering?

It was observed that usually "pain and suffering" are associated, although they may be considered separately. It was agreed that both pain and suffering are psychological states and that, therefore, the language of psychology and not of physiology should be applied to them. It follows that the term "analgesic" is appropriate for human studies, but should be avoided for animal experiments, where the term "antinociceptive" seems more reasonable.

Masochism was discussed. It was proposed that masochists do not so much seek out pain and noxious states per se, but that such states provide a "means to an end," especially the need for humiliation and sexual arousal.

It was suggested that pain may frequently be associated with "secondary gain," such as in compensation cases, avoidance of work, sympathy, etc. However, some participants objected to this view of "secondary gain."

The group was unable to recommend strategies for the study of the relationship between pain and suffering, except to emphasize their psychological nature.

4. CROSS-CULTURAL MEASUREMENT OF PAIN

Question: What advantages could be gained from cross-cultural measurement of pain and how could this be accomplished?

In a lengthy discussion it was pointed out that there is a dearth of controlled anthropological and cross-cultural studies in the field of pain (16). While we are aware of cultural diversity, there is no consensus as to how this is related to the individual. The concept of cultural or ethnic sterotypes (17) was severely criticized. While there appear to be substantial differences in the expression of pain between different cultures, there is no definitive evidence on the reasons for these and physiological differences.

Statement D: Although pain expressions are highly divergent among different cultural groups, there is no evidence to indicate that any such group is deficient in any aspect of the pain experience.

The participants suggested that there exists an important need to develop strategies for cross-cultural studies.

5. DEVELOPMENTAL CHANGES IN PAIN EXPERIENCE

Question: Are there significant changes in pain experience throughout the human lifespan? How shall they be measured?

There seems to be little information about the perception of pain in children. Many pediatricians believe that children are relatively insensitive to pain. Therefore, children may be prescribed inadequate doses of analgesics. In contrast, the public takes the attitude that the elderly are expected to suffer more pain, and hence there is frequently a compliance with such notions by the elderly. Yet, there is some experimental evidence that thresholds of pain may increase with age (12,15). Furthermore, it is considered that there are as yet no specific nonverbal pain tests for young children. The importance of close interpersonal contact between infant and parent and of imprinting in animals was discussed. Absence of such contact may lead to abnormal behavior patterns, known as the "Isolation Syndrome" (1). Abnormal behavior has also been observed in animals reared in partial isolation (2,7).

Statement E: The following procedures and studies are suggested in order to acquire knowledge in this area.

a) Develop specific, nonverbal tests of pain for children.

b) Compare and study groups of retarded as well as of emotionally and socially deprived children.

c) Compare the differential effect of the mother and father on pain in the young infant.
d) Evaluate the role of crying in young children.
e) Carry out further studies of pain in the elderly.

6. STUDY OF PAIN IN NATURAL SETTINGS

Question: What are the benefits and methods for studying pain in natural settings in man and animals?

It is important to investigate pain in both man and animals in their natural habitat. The laboratory obscures the plasticity of the nervous system. It is noted that in the normal habitat, animals do not seek pain. However, during natural fighting (e.g., mating rivalry), there are signs of pain-related behavior, although appropriate experiments have never been performed. The apparent lack of pain sensations during sport activities in man were also noted. There is no real evidence that there are differences in pain sensation among women of different cultures during childbirth.

Statement F: There is need for studies of pathology in animals and man, e.g., dental pain, low back pain, labor and postpartum pain, etc.

7. MOOD AND PAIN

Question: Is there a correlation between mood and pain, and what is the basis of it?

A considerable discussion ensued on the relation of anxiety and/or depression to pain. Pain may be felt at the site of a previous injury. Mood changes may precede or follow pain (e.g., migraine, dysmenorrhea), suggesting a two-way system: Changes in mood may result in pain, and vice versa, changes in pain may cause alterations in mood. Anxiety may reduce an individual's threshold of pain, while chronic pain is usually associated with depressive behavior (4). The role of reserpine and the catecholamines was discussed in depression and hypertension. The importance of the opiate system for both analgesia and hyperanalgesia was emphasized. The reciprocal relationship of such chemical mediators was stressed.

In animals, maternal deprivation may play a role in the eliciting of pain. Continuous stressful stimulation may produce changes in the observable pain behavior.

Statement G: There is much evidence that pain and mood are related and that there may exist a chemical basis for this reciprocal relationship.

8. ROLE OF EARLY EXPERIENCES

Question: What is the impact of early experience - in the family, society, culture - on pain perception and response? What are the implications for early intervention, prevention, and treatment?

Early experience is not important, but one must not forget or overlook genetic factors. The relationship of the parent and child in early life is very significant in the socialization process. Intense, prolonged pain in a close family member has an impact on the child. The child's expression of pain often reflects the influence of the parent and of other family members, i.e., "pain-prone" family. Yet, in some cultures, sick parents may actually encourage early familial intervention in the health care of the very young.

Statement H: Little is known about early intervention and treatment of pain in young children.

9. AVOIDANCE OF PAIN AND SUFFERING

Question: To what extent should pain and suffering be avoided? What are the positive functions of pain to the individual and society? Is society fostering invalidism?

Pain may be of benefit to either the individual or society. If one is hurt and vocalizes, the cry may serve as communication and hence it is social. On the other hand, an individual may need his pain - there is then an individual asset. Religion plays an important part - some regard pain as "sin" for which one may atone (6). "Pain" may be "credited" for future pleasure.

In some Oriental cultures it is idiomatic to chastize an individual for failing to feel pain - it is human to feel pain.

Modern concepts have changed. Now frequently the patient demands and does not plead for help for his pain. Pain may thus facilitate aggressiveness. Similarly, therapists or institutions may tout a specific treatment by implying that it can cure.

The predominant attitude of society is to help the suffering patient. Yet, unwittingly, certain components or requirements of health care, e.g., welfare, may potentiate invalidism. Society, while utilizing altruism, exerts a paradoxical dual influence on the patient - rehabilitation and dependence.

REFERENCES

(1) Clancy, H., and McBride, G. 1975. Isolation syndrome in childhood. Dev. Med. Child Neurol. 17: 198-219.

(2) Cross, H.A., and Harlow, H.F. 1965. Prolonged and progressive effects of partial isolation on the behavior of Macaque monkeys. J. Exp. Res. Person. 1: 39-49.

(3) Dallenbach, K.M. 1939. Pain: History and present status. Am. J. Psychol. 52: 331-347.

(4) Davidson, P.O., ed. 1976. The Behavioral Management of Anxiety, Depression and Pain. New York: Brunner/Mazel.

(5) Keele, C.A., and Smith, R. 1962. The Assessment of Pain in Man and Animals. The Universities Federation for Animal Welfare. London: E. & S. Livingstone, Ltd.

(6) Lewis, C.S. 1940. The Problem of Pain. London: Geoffrey Bles: The Centenary Press.

(7) Lichstein, L., and Sackett, G.P. 1971. Reactions by differentially raised Rhesus monkeys to noxious stimulation. Dev. Psychobio. 4: 339-352.

(8) Melzack, R., and Casey, K.L. 1968. Sensory motivational, and central control determinants of pain: a new conceptual model. In The Skin Senses, ed. D. Kenshalo. Springfield, IL: C.C. Thomas.

(9) Melzack, R., and Wall, P.D. 1965. Pain mechanisms: A new theory. Science 150: 971-979.

(10) Needham, J. 1954. Science and Civilization in China. Cambridge: University Press.

(11) Porkert, M. 1974. The Theoretical Foundations of Chinese Medicine: Systems of Correspondence. Cambridge: MIT Press.

(12) Schludermann, E., and Zubek, J.P. 1962. Effect of age on pain sensitivity. Percep. Motor Skills 14: 295-301.

(13) Shaw, G.B. 1903. Maxims for revolutionists. In Man and Superman, pp. 225-244. London: Archibald Constable & Co., Ltd.

(14) St. Matthew, Ch. 7:12, King James version.

(15) Wolff, B.B., and Jarvik, M.E. 1965. Quantitative measures of deep somatic pain: Further studies with hypertonic saline. Clin. Sci. 28: 43-56.

(16) Wolff, B.B., and Langley, S. 1968. Cultural factors and the response to pain: A review. Am. Anthrop. 70: 494-501.

(17) Zborowski, M. 1952. Cultural components in response to pain. J. Soc. Issues 8: 16-30.

RECOMMENDED FURTHER READING

(1) Bonica, J.J., ed. 1980. Pain Research Publications: Association for Research in Nervous and Mental Disease, vol. 58. New York: Raven Press.

(2) Bonica, J.J.; Liebeskind, J.C.; and Albe-Fessard, D.G., eds. 1979. Advances in Pain Research and Therapy, vol. 3. Proceedings of the Second World Congress on Pain. New York: Raven Press.

(3) Melzack, R. 1973. The Puzzle of Pain. New York: Basic Books.

(4) Sternbach, R.A., ed. 1978. The Psychology of Pain. New York: Raven Press.

(5) Weisenberg, M., ed. 1975. Pain: Clinical and Experimental Perspectives. St. Louis, IL: C.V. Mosby Co.

(6) Zborowski, M. 1969. People in Pain. San Francisco: Jossey-Bass.

Pain and Society, eds. H.W. Kosterlitz and L.Y. Terenius, pp. 93-122.
Dahlem Konferenzen 1980. Weinheim: Verlag Chemie GmbH.

The Anatomy of Pain and Pain Modulation

A. I. Basbaum
Department of Anatomy, University of California
San Francisco, CA 94143, USA

Abstract. A review of studies on the anatomy of pain demonstrates that most of our knowledge centers on the organization of and input to the superficial dorsal horn of the spinal cord. There is new information on the origin of pain transmission pathways, but the thalamic and cortical areas involved in pain are largely unknown. Most anatomical studies of pain modulation have concentrated on the descending systems which control spinal pain transmission neurons. Recent analyses of aminergic-peptidergic interactions in the dorsal horn are an important first step in resolving the local circuitry underlying pain modulation.

THE ANATOMY OF PAIN

It is somewhat surprising that anatomical studies have provided some of the most recent and important advances in our understanding of pain mechanisms. These anatomical studies are the result of new tracing techniques based on axoplasmic transport procedures (autoradiographic tritiated amino acid and retrograde horseradish peroxidase studies), the morphological analysis of functionally identified neurons (by intracellular filling with horseradish peroxidase), and perhaps most significantly, the localization of peptides by highly sensitive immunohistochemical techniques. This report will review the anatomical observations in peripheral and central nervous system which bare on aspects of pain generation and pain modulation. Some major points of disagreement will be highlighted and some critical questions which remain unanswered will be raised. A brief review of the distribution of several neuropeptides will be included insofar as the distribution implies a role in pain or pain modulation. With a view to minimizing the numbers of citations, many excellent papers have not been included. Other comprehensive reviews of this problem should be examined (7,16,22,26,46,48). The discussion will begin at the sensory receptor and move centrally, towards thalamus and cortex, at which point the deficiencies in our understanding become glaringly apparent.

The Peripheral Apparatus

Although there is now general agreement that there are specialized nerve endings which respond to different somatic stimuli, our knowledge of the receptor morphology for primary afferent fibers responding to noxious stimuli is almost non-existent. Neither the Aδ high threshold mechanoreceptor nor the C polymodal nociceptor has been associated with specialized endings. The long held view that there are unspecialized, "free nerve endings" is still taught. Kruger et al. (50) reported some initial electron microscopic observations of receptors for high threshold mechanoreceptors. They found characteristic unmyelinated terminals which contain dense core vesicles. Each ending is surrounded by Schwann cell processes. Their observations were limited but are hopefully a first start towards resolving this important problem.

As to the nature of the afferent fibers responding to noxious stimuli, it is clear that they are exclusively of small caliber. Not all fine fibers, however, are nociceptors. The proportion of C fibers responding to non-noxious stimuli is much greater in the cat than in the primate (40% vs 10%), but the significance of this difference is not known.

Although our knowledge of peripheral "pain" receptors is limited, there have been several interesting observations relating to the peripheral afferent fiber. Two of these have drastically revised what may be considered long-standing biological dogma. In the first case, Coggeshall and his collaborators (20) have observed that in several mammalian and submammalian species, up to 30% of ventral root axons are unmyelinated. Moreover, a proportion of these unmyelinated ventral root fibers are afferent fibers; their cell bodies are located in the dorsal root ganglion. This observation goes counter to the Bell-Magendie Law, i.e., that only afferent fibers course in dorsal roots and only efferent fibers course in ventral roots. Physiological studies demonstrated that many of these ventral root afferents are responsive to noxious stimulation. More recently, by incubating cut ventral roots with horseradish peroxidase, the central projection of these afferents has been studied. Of particular interest to the anatomy of pain mechanisms is the observation that the finest fibers in the ventral root, on entering the ventral horn, course dorsally and terminate in the superficial dorsal horn, i.e., they merge with small diameter primary afferent fibers which enter over the dorsal roots (54). Thus, a considerable number of nociceptive afferent fibers have apparently been overlooked and must be considered in future evaluations of pain mechanisms. It has, in fact, been suggested that the return of pain after dorsal rhizotomy may reflect preserved afferent input over ventral root fibers. Some neurosurgeons have taken this suggestion to heart and advocate dorsal root ganglionectomy (to sever afferents in dorsal and ventral roots) in preference to dorsal rhizotomy for the relief of peripheral pain.

Equally surprising is the recent observation that section of primary afferents distal to the dorsal root ganglion produces considerable degeneration of central terminals. Previous studies, of course, implied that central degeneration only results from dorsal rhizotomy or ganglionectomy. The new observation was first described by Grant (36) and has subsequently been used to evaluate the central termination of putative "pain" transmission primary afferent fibers, specifically those innervating tooth pulp (35). For example, removal of tooth pulp produces terminal degeneration in spinal trigeminal nucleus caudalis and interpolaris. Some degeneration has even been reported contralateral to the tooth pulp removal. Section of primary afferents distal to the ganglion has also been used to map the differential central termination of Aδ and C fibers (see below).

Organization of the Spinal Dorsal Horn: Cytoarchitecture

Until very recently there has been considerable confusion concerning the nomenclature of the superficial dorsal horn. Some studies refer to lamina II only as the substantia gelatinosa; others include lamina III. For a short time, Gobel reintroduced the original Rolando terminology, i.e., all superficial layers I, II, and III are part of the substantia gelatinosa. Fortunately, there is now a revised nomenclature which is agreed upon and which seems to hold for primate (69) as well as for the cat. Interestingly, it is quite consistent with the original description by Rexed.

The superficial lamina I, the marginal layer, contains both large and small neurons. Many of these project into the contralateral anterolateral fasciculus. The substantia gelatinosa, ventral to the marginal layer, contains small neurons. It can be subdivided into an outer half (IIo or IIa) with few myelinated fibers and an inner half (IIi or IIb) which contains a characteristic population of small myelinated fibers. The distinction between IIo and IIi is also characterized by the presence of substance P immunoreactivity, in I and IIo but not IIi (40, 41). Ventral to IIb is the nucleus proprius - it is not certain whether distinguishing a lamina III from lamina IV is valid or necessary.

In two recent papers, Gobel (33,34) has provided a comprehensive Golgi analysis of the marginal zone and substantia gelatinosa. Using sections cut tangential to the marginal zone, Gobel recognized at least four classes of marginal neurons. What is important for this report is his conclusion that the dendrites of marginal neurons are restricted to the marginal zone. Thus, marginal neurons must receive their input from axons which arborize in the marginal zone. Although Beal (10) has described marginal neurons with dendrites penetrating the substantia gelatinosa, Gobel feels that these are, in fact, within the substantia gelatinosa and are probably stalk cells (see below). Although this appears to be a semantic argument, it is relevant to the question as to which neurons are the neurons transmitting nociceptive inputs. Since no local axonal arborization was detectable in Golgi preparations of the marginal neurons, Gobel concluded that all marginal neurons are projection neurons. He, of course, could not distinguish between marginal neurons at the origin of the spinothalamic tract versus, for example, those with long ascending or descending propriospinal axons.

Gobel also described several classes of substantia gelatinosa neurons. Of these, two have been particularly well characterized - the stalk cell and the islet cell. The stalk cell, located at the I-II border, has a large dendritic tree which is concentrated in the substantia gelatinosa. Its axon arborizes in the marginal zone. Gobel has suggested that the stalk cell is an excitatory interneuron which feeds on to marginal neurons. As such it forms part of the ascending pain transmission pathway. His conclusion is based on the observation that marginal neurons have "wide dynamic range responses." Since his data argue that large fibers terminate deep in the marginal zone and since marginal neurons do not have dendrites below lamina I, he postulated that the stalk cell provided the "non-nociceptive" large diameter fiber input.

The islet cell is a bipolar neuron with long dendrites that arborize along a rostral caudal axis entirely within the substantia gelatinosa. Its axon also arborizes within the substantia gelatinosa. There is also a prominent glomerulus in the substantia gelatinosa; its characteristic feature is a large scalloped primary afferent terminal surrounded by pre- and postsynaptic dendrites (32). It has been suggested that many of the dendrites surrounding the central or "C" terminal derive from islet cells. Recent ultrastructural studies of single islet cells filled iontophoretically with horseradish peroxidase have confirmed this hypothesis (11). Since immunohistochemical studies have described glutamic acid decarboxylase immunoreactive dendrites in the glomerus (4), it has been suggested that the islet cell dendrites are GABAergic.

Light et al. (57), however, also using intracellular recording from and labelling of dorsal horn neurons, reported that there are far more than two classes of substantia gelatinosa neurons. They concluded that no recognizable correlation between soma morphology and physiological function could be discerned. They further concluded that what is important is the location of the dendrites, not the location or the morphological identity of the soma. According to these authors, those cells with dendrites in the marginal zone will have predominant Aδ input; those in the substantia gelatinosa will have unmyelinated C fiber input. A cell in lamina V with dendrites in the substantia gelatinosa would thus also have a C fiber input.

Contrary to Gobel's view that stalk cells are excitatory is Narotsky and Kerr's (62) observation that lesions of the Lissauer tract produce degeneration of boutons on proximal marginal dendrites; the same synapses do not degenerate after dorsal rhizotomy. The proximity of the boutons to the soma led to the suggestion that they derive from substantia gelatinosa interneurons which inhibit marginal pain transmission neurons. Clearly, the functional role of single substantia gelatinosa neurons cannot be discerned by anatomical analyses alone. Hopefully, further studies of the physiology of the substantia gelatinosa will shed some new light on this region.

Organization of the Spinal Dorsal Horn: The Afferent Input

Following on some 19th century observations which Lissauer reported, Ranson (71) using pyrimidine silver techniques which stain normal axons, reported that, in cat, the dorsal root is divisible into a medial, large caliber fiber population and a lateral, small caliber fiber population. On the assumption that small fibers transmit nociceptive information, section of the lateral division was recommended and used in animals for "selective" block of pain. Over the years, subsequent studies questioned the validity of the initial anatomical observation. Snyder (74), however, using electron microscopic, serial reconstruction of the dorsal root entry zone concluded that a segregation of large and small diameter fibers in the root can, in fact, be recognized in the primate although it was not demonstrable in the cat. Kerr (46), however, reported that a distinction can also be seen in the cat. At the dorsal root entry zone, however, in both cat and monkey, there is a marked lateral segregation of small diameter fibers. Many of these are clustered in the Lissauer tract. The medial division contains the larger diameter axons which course through the dorsal horn to terminate in the nucleus proprius and ventral horns.

By dipping cut dorsal roots in horseradish peroxidase, it is possible to fill primary afferent axons and terminals in the dorsal horn. There have been several beautiful demonstrations of the primary afferent input into the dorsal horn with this technique. Combining this procedure with selective section of medial and lateral divisions of the root has also revealed the differential termination of large and small diameter fibers. Light and Perl (55) demonstrated a preferential small caliber fiber termination in the superficial dorsal horn. More recently, intracellular recordings from identified primary afferent fibers and subsequent injection of horseradish peroxidase into these axons have provided a detailed picture of the central termination of single afferent fibers. Single high threshold (Aδ) mechanoreceptors terminate in lamina I, outer II, and V; non-nociceptors terminate in inner II, III, and IV (56). Hopefully, improvements in the technique will permit successful impalement of unmyelinated fibers and thus provide greater detail concerning the terminal pattern within the superficial dorsal horn.

The preferential termination of small diameter fibers in I and outer II (SGo) is further supported by a host of anatomical studies, e.g., acid phosphatase staining is densest in lamina I and II; in the dorsal root ganglion it is most concentrated in small diameter cell bodies. Similarly, the dense substance

P and somatostatin immunoreactivity in the superficial dorsal horn (59) probably derives from small diameter fibers, since the corresponding immunoreactivity of the dorsal root ganglion is also found exclusively in small somata.

Although it is agreed that small fibers terminate superficially, there is considerable controversy over the differential termination of Aδ and C fibers. Based on differential degeneration patterns at different times after dorsal root section, attributable to large and small fibers, La Motte (51) concluded that unmyelinated axons terminate in the substantia gelatinosa while Aδ fibers terminate more superficially in lamina I. Ralston (69) has reported a similar organization for primary afferent input in the superficial dorsal horn of the primate. His studies used ultrastructural observation of degenerating terminals as well as autoradiographic localization of labelled primary afferent terminals. He found three types of degeneration after dorsal root section. The different degeneration patterns occurred at different times after root section and in different dorsal horn lamina. The earliest degeneration was found in lamina II and III and was concurrent with myelinated fiber degeneration in the Lissauer tract. The latest degeneration occurs in the SGo and SGi and occurs concomitantly with the first signs of degeneration of unmyelinated fibers in the tract of Lissauer. On physiological grounds, Perl and his colleagues (57) arrived at a similar conclusion. Marginal neurons in lamina I were driven primarily by Aδ input and substantia gelatinosa neurons by C input.

In contrast, Gobel (33,34) maintains that C fibers terminate in the marginal zone, Aδ fibers in lamina II. His evidence is based on the fact that section of trigeminal nerve, distal to the Gasserion ganglion, produces degeneration first in the substantia gelatinosa and this is preceeded by degeneration of small diameter myelinated axons in the descending tract of lamina V. Subsequently, terminal degeneration was observed in the marginal zone and this occurred in temporal contiguity with the appearance of degenerating unmyelinated fibers in the descending tract.

Interestingly, Dubner and his colleagues (12) concluded that the recorded Aδ input to the marginal neuron is secondary to activation of substantia gelatinosa interneurons. This conclusion derived from recordings of pairs of substantia gelatinosa and marginal neurons. The substantia gelatinosa neurons were always driven first by the Aδ input. One must always keep in mind that physiological studies can rarely determine whether the input to a given neuron is mono- or disynaptic, particularly when longer conduction times over small myelinated and unmyelinated fibers are being examined.

Central "Pain" Pathways

Although there have been numerous advances in our understanding of the anatomical and functional organization of spinal cord mechanisms of pain transmission, our knowledge of the relevant ascending pathways and their brain stem and thalamic termination is very limited. The emphasis is still placed on the spinothalamic tract (STT), although it is recognized that the STT is not a pure "pain tract" but carries non-nociceptive information as well. Consistent with a variety of modalities being represented in the spinothalamic tract are the recent observations on the cells of origin of spinothalamic tract neurons using the horseradish peroxidase technique. In the primate, Albe-Fessard et al. (2) used retrograde transport of this enzyme and demonstrated that marginal neurons project both to the intralaminar nuclei and lateral thalamus. Cells in lamina IV and V project laterally. Carstens and Trevino (18) reported that neurons of lamina I, IV, V, VII, and VIII of the spinal cord are labelled after large thalamic injections of horseradish peroxidase. Interestingly, the greatest number of non-marginal spinothalamic tract neurons in lumbar cord of the cat are in lamina VII and VIII; in cervical enlargement they are found in lamina V. In primate, however, this difference was not present. More recently, these authors made smaller thalamic injection of horseradish peroxidase and demonstrated differential cells of origin of axons projecting to medial and lateral thalamus. Neurons of lamina I project primarily to lateral thalamus; VII and VIII projects primarily medially. The posterior thalamus receives a predominant input from lamina IV and V. Giesler et al. (29) found a similar organization in the rat.

Although most studies emphasize that the substantia gelatinosa consists of interneurons, there is some recent evidence that a small population of SG neurons in primate (79) and rat (28) project. Whether these are displaced marginal neurons or whether they constitute a separate spinothalamic tract cell population remains to be determined.

The course and termination of ascending fibers of the anterolateral quadrant has been reinvestigated in both cat and primate. A major revision in the thalamic distribution of spinothalamic tract fibers in the cat was revealed. Although it was previously reported that these terminate in the ventroposterolateral thalamus (VPL), Boivie (14) clearly demonstrated this to be incorrect. In fact, the fibers of the spinothalamic tract terminate more rostrally, in a small region which serves as a transition zone between the caudal VPL and the rostral ventrolateral nucleus. This same region receives cerebellothalamic projections (13). Apparently previous descriptions of the spinothalamic tract input to the VPL resulted from high cervical cordotomies which concomitantly destroyed fibers of the cervicothalamic tract.

In general, the results from primate are more consistent with early observations (15). The spinothalamic tract terminates in various thalamic sites including the posterior (POm), intralaminar (centralis lateralis) and ventral thalamus, and in the zona incerta. Unlike the cat, the VPL receives an input from the spinothalamic tract, but it is less dense than previously described. As in the cat there is also a projection to the transition zone between VPL and the ventralis lateralis (VL). Kerr (47) has also reexamined spinothalamic and spinoreticular projections, with emphasis on distinguishing the ventral from the lateral spinothalamic tracts. By making isolated ventral funiculus lesions (sparing the ventrolateral funiculus), he demonstrated an ascending system which shares many features with that of lateral spinothalamic tract, but with a few differences. The projection to the reticular core of the brain stem was entirely ipsilateral; in the thalamus there were bilateral projections to the intralaminar and ventral thalamic nuclei. Only the ventral spinothalamic tract was shown to project to the periventricular gray and to the nucleus of Darkschewitsch. Because of the minimal differences in terminal patterns of the ventral and lateral spinothalamic tracts, however, Boivie (15) concluded that there is no reason to distinguish the two.

Since a lesion of the anterolateral quadrant severs numerous ascending systems in addition to the spinothalamic tract, it has often been suggested that other pathways transmit ascending "pain" information. The most often cited is the spinoreticular system. Certainly neurons of the reticular formation respond to noxious stimuli, have large receptive fields, often bilateral, and therefore could be involved in pain transmission. Lippmann and Kerr (58), however, concluded that spinoreticular pathways are unlikely to be important. They made midline myelotomies to sever crossing fibers of the spinal cord. Since they found no degeneration in the reticular formation (and since pain is associated with crossed fiber systems), they concluded that spinoreticular fibers are predominantly ipsilateral and thus are not important for pain transmission. Nevertheless, since the collaterals of crossed spinothalamic tract fibers also terminate in the reticular formation, the role of the reticular nuclei should not be overlooked.

The Thalamus and Cortex

Despite the anatomical evidence for a spinothalamic projection system, it is not known which thalamic terminal region is relevant for pain transmission. Three regions have received the most attention: the posterior thalamus, particularly POm, the VPL-VL transition zone, and the intralaminar nuclei, particularly centralis lateralis. Although the earliest studies emphasized that posterior thalamic neurons have a predominant nociceptive input (68), this may be largely related to the depth of anesthesia (19). The intralaminar nuclei have long been associated with pain transmission (49), however, the precise region from which recordings were made has never been adequately delineated. Nevertheless, unlike POm and VPL, there appears to be a predominant nociceptive input to this region. Importantly, the properties of these neurons are more similar to spinoreticular and brain stem reticular neurons, suggesting the importance of a spinoreticular-reticulomedial thalamic pain transmission system.

The "pain" responsiveness of the VPL-VL transition zone is not known. An interesting hypothesis was raised by Boivie (15). He suggested that the direct spinothalamic projection to VPL in the primate corresponds functionally to the cervicothalamic projection in cat; while the projection to the transition zone in primate is functionally similar to the same projection in cat. This reasoning appears to downplay the role of VPL in pain transmission. Hopefully, physiological studies of the transition zone will shed light on its role.

Although our knowledge of the anatomy and physiology of the thalamic role in pain transmission is limited, our understanding is even more deficient when it comes to the cortex. If we examine the cortical projection areas of the three thalamic regions which receive spinothalamic tract projections, attention is focused on a wide area, including SI, SII, motor cortex, and retroinsular cortex. The VPL, of course, projects to the SI cortex; more anterior parts of the SI cortex are innervated by more anterior parts of VPL. The cortical projection of the transition zone would thus lie in rostral SI, i.e., in cortical area 3a. Since 3a contains units responding primarily to innocuous inputs, its role and that of the VPL-VL transition zone in pain transmission are still unresolved.

Although early studies implied that the intralaminar nuclei do not project to the cortex, it is now clear that CL projects to the parietal cortex, including SI, and to the motor cortex (75). Assuming that the large cerebellar input to the intralaminar nuclei dominates the CL to motor cortex projection, it is possible that the spinothalamic tract has access to SI via CL. Again, we are faced with inadequate physiological data. Few neurons with noxious inputs have been demonstrated in SI or in more posterior parts of the parietal cortex.

Finally, the cortical projection of the POm region should be considered. Burton and Jones (17) emphasized that POm projects selectively to the retroinsular field, just caudal to SII. Their data argue that cortical pain responsiveness would be found in the retroinsular cortex, not in caudal SII as had been reported. Again physiological studies are required to answer that question.

It is clear that inadequate physiological studies make it difficult to determine which spinothalamic tract projection sites are important for pain transmission and which subserve other roles. Although anatomical studies can demonstrate terminal fields of the spinothalamic tract, their functional significance remains unknown. It is particularly important to determine the terminal projection of identified spinothalamic tract neurons. Because of interference from anesthesia and perhaps because of convergent input from inhibitory nonnociceptive spinal systems and from cerebellothalamic inputs, it is impossible to find pure "pain" responsive thalamic units. Microantidromic stimulation of spinothalamic cells, a technique presently used in Willis' laboratory, is tedious but is a necessary approach.

Neuropeptides and Pain

It is difficult to review the anatomical literature relating to pain and pain control without discussing the neuropeptides (for reviews, see (24,38,66)). One is constantly struck by the variety of peptides in the superficial dorsal horn, specifically lamina I and the substantia gelatinosa. Demonstrating their presence, however, is far easier than determining their function. Fortunately, the functional properties of many of the elements within this region are known; thus the presence of a peptide in a particular cell type or axon terminal is, in some cases, indicative of a particular function.

The list of peptides in the superficial dorsal horn is long, but without question, it is substance P which is most often associated with nociception. Substance P is localized in small dorsal root ganglion cells (39); these cells are the predominant source of the dense SP immunoreactivity in lamina I and IIa of the dorsal horn. Since iontophoresis of substance P excites central nociceptors (37), and since substance P is found in synaptic vesicles (5,67) and is released by electrical stimulation of small diameter peripheral axons (45), it has been suggested that substance P is a neurotransmitter for "pain." As described above, however, not all small fibers are nociceptors. Thus, it is possible that substance P is also released by a population of non-nociceptors. The presence of substance P in tooth pulp afferents (63), however, strongly suggests that some primary afferent nociceptors contain substance P. Whether it is a neurotransmitter or neuromodulator remains to be determined. Its mode of action would be better understood if we knew the content of the remaining, small, agranular vesicles in terminals containing substance P.

A second population of small dorsal root ganglion cells contains the peptide somatostatin (39). This peptide is also found in the superficial dorsal horn and is released into the CSF by peripheral nerve stimulation (45). The populations of dorsal root ganglion cells containing substance P or somatostatin do not overlap; this implies a different functional role. Physiological studies are not conclusive, but a possible inhibitory action of somatostatin on nociceptors is suggested (70).

The number of dorsal horn peptides which originate from primary afferent fibers continues to grow. It now includes cholecystokinin (CCK) and angiotensin (38,44,53). The central action of these peptides is not known. Of particular interest to pain studies, however, is the octapeptide, CCK. Not only is CCK found in the superficial dorsal horn (44,53), but it is also densely concentrated in cell bodies of the midbrain dorsal raphe (44). The latter region is a major locus from which analgesia is produced by electrical brain stimulation (64).

More recently, Hökfelt (personal communication) and his colleagues demonstrated vasoactive intestinal polypeptide (VIP) and CCK in dorsal root ganglion cells. Although substance P and somatostatin are exclusively located in small dorsal root ganglion cells, a population of large cells was VIP or CCK immunoreactive. Since only a few large diameter nociceptive fibers have been reported, it is likely that CCK and VIP are associated with nonnociceptors.

Not all peptides in the superficial dorsal horn derive from primary afferents; this fact argues against the possibility that the presence of multiple peptides is artifactual, reflecting failure of a given antibody to distinguish between the various peptides. Of particular importance are two peptides which probably derive from spinal interneurons, enkephalin and neurotensin. Enkephalin-containing cell bodies are found in some interneurons of the substantia gelatinosa (41). More recently, a population of marginal, enkephalin-containing neurons was reported ((30), and see below). Enkephalin immunoreactivity is concentrated in lamina I and II (a and b). In the cat, lamina IIa has somewhat less enkephalin staining (31). Additional staining is found in lamina V and VII and densely around the central canal. The mechanism of enkephalin action is not clear; both pre- and postsynaptic inhibitory actions have been postulated (Zieglgänsberger, this volume). Although a significant proportion of spinal cord opiate receptors is located on primary afferent fibers (52), axo-axonic synapses in which enkephalin-immunoreactive terminals are presynaptic have not been seen (43). This indicates a possible "non-synaptic" action of ENK on primary afferents.

Neurotensin cell bodies are also found in the substantia gelatinosa (77). In contrast to enkephalin, however, the densest, non-cellular immunoreactivity is found in lamina II; much less is seen in the marginal layer. Since marginal neuron dendrites rarely penetrate the substantia gelatinosa, it would appear that these neurons are influenced less by neurotensin than by enkephalin or substance P. In contrast, oxytocin immunoreactivity is found primarily in the marginal layer of the dorsal horn (76). The staining probably derives from oxytocin-containing hypothalamic neurons. Although the functional significance of this pathway is unknown, the restricted distribution to lamina I suggests postsynaptic modulation of central nociceptors. Other studies have described glutamic acid decarboxylase (GAD) immunoreactivity in substantia gelatinosa cells and terminals (4). This may underly a GABA-mediated presynaptic inhibition of primary afferents. It is important to establish whether GAD-containing perikarya and/or terminals also contain one of the peptides of the substantia gelatinosa.

Determining the origin of superficial dorsal horn peptides is complicated by the presence of bulbospinal peptide-containing axons. For example, some serotonin-containing raphe spinal axons contain substance P (40). Since some raphe spinal axons inhibit central nociceptors, it is particularly confusing to label substance P a "pain" or nociception transmitter. For the same reason, one must exert caution in interpreting CSF changes in substance P levels produced by noxious stimulation. An increase in substance P, for example, might reflect activation of a descending inhibitory system by a noxious stimulus (7). Evidence for a descending enkephalinergic pathway has also been reported (42). These neurons are located in regions of medulla from which antinociception can be obtained by electrical stimulation. It is not known whether the terminals of this descending pathway make synaptic contacts similar to those made by local enkephalin interneurons. Clearly ultrastructural studies demonstrating the synaptic relationship of the many dorsal horn peptides are necessary. Despite the difficulties inherent in immunohistochemical studies at the electron microscopic level, the next few years should produce significant progress in our understanding of the synaptic organization of peptides and the functional role of the many neuropeptides in the superficial dorsal horn.

THE ANATOMY OF PAIN MODULATION

Despite the controversy over which spinal cord neurons contribute to pain perception, which spinal pathways conduct nociceptive information, and what the relevant thalamic and cortical receiving areas are, there has been much less difficulty in the analysis of pain modulatory systems. Perhaps this is because behavioral studies have successfully demonstrated multiple modes and sources of pain modulation. Moreover, with restricted lesions, it has been possible to antagonize the effects produced by these modulatory systems. Thus some relevant modulatory systems have been delineated. Quite the opposite, of course, is true for the generation of pain. Barring complete spinal transection, lesion studies have consistently failed to eliminate pain for an extended period of time. Certainly the unsatisfactory results after anterolateral cordotomy or spinal tractotomy for the relief of intractable pain in humans has raised questions concerning the existence of "pain pathways."

Since the pioneering studies of Hagbarth, Magoun, and Lundberg and their colleagues (which followed upon the early studies of Sherrington), it was known that the brain stem exerts strong control over spinal cord neurons. For some reason the relationship of these descending modulatory systems to the control of pain was not recognized or at least was not emphasized until the late 60s. At that time, Reynolds (72) and subsequently Mayer and Liebeskind (60) and their colleagues demonstrated that potent analgesia could be produced by electrical brain stimulation in freely moving animals. Most of the early studies focused on the midbrain periaqueductal gray (PAG) from which stimulation-produced analgesia (SPA) was best elicited.

A directional anatomical analysis of these pain modulatory systems, however, did not begin until it was also demonstrated that stimulation of the serotonin (5-HT)-containing, medullary nucleus raphe magnus (NRM) also produced potent analgesia (64) and that a lesion of the spinal dorsolateral funiculus (DLF) antagonizes the analgesic action of opiates and electrical brain stimulation from the PAG (7). In a series of anatomical studies (6,8), our laboratory demonstrated that the NRM projects via the spinal DLF and terminates densely in the marginal layer and in the substantia gelatinosa of the spinal dorsal horn and in analogous regions of the medulla, i.e., in the trigeminal nucleus caudalis. There is also a projection to lamina V, VI, and VII.

Since the region of dorsal horn to which NRM projects contains pain transmission neurons, it was subsequently demonstrated in both the cat (26) and the primate (78) that raphe stimulation profoundly inhibits pain transmission neurons of the spinal dorsal horn. Since the PAG projects minimally to the spinal cord and since a PAG-raphe projection was demonstrated (1,27), it was proposed that the raphe-spinal projection was the critical link in the analgesia produced by PAG stimulation, PAG opiate injection, or systemic injection of narcotics.

In addition to the raphe-spinal projection, it was shown that the part of the reticular formation located just lateral to NRM, i.e., the magnocellular reticular formation also projects to the same regions of the dorsal horn, via the DLF. Some authors considered that Rmc is merely a lateral extension of the raphe; others assume that the two are independent. The issue is relevant to whether 5-HT is essential for the modulation. It has, for example, been proposed that NRM and Rmc are at the origin of parallel descending modulatory systems, one serotonergic and the second nonserotonergic (7). Certainly not all NRM neurons are serotonergic. Furthermore, the recent evidence that some NRM neurons contain both serotonin and substance P (40) raises additional possibilities for the anatomical substrate for descending control. As Willis and his colleagues (78) have appropriately pointed out, to assume that the raphe-spinal pathway is exclusively designed for pain modulation is almost certainly wrong.

There is already evidence that visceral systems are modulated; there may also be modulation of cells with non-nociceptive input.

The data reviewed above demonstrate that the PAG-NRM-spinal cord system is a possible neural substrate for the analgesic action of electrical brain stimulation and opiates. The mechanism of exogenous opiate action, however, and the role of NRM in that action, rather than becoming clearer, are exceptionally obscure and are areas which require much further study. There is a serious lack of agreement concerning the primary locus of opiate action. Early studies pointed to the PAG; the subsequent discovery of moderate concentrations of opiate receptors in the PAG (3) was consistent with this view. With the exception of Feldberg (25), who demonstrated opiate responsiveness on the ventral surface of the medulla, most investigators considered that raphe neurons are not opiate sensitive but are indirectly activated from the PAG.

More recently, the story has become exceptionally complicated. First Satoh and Takagi and their collaborators (73) demonstrated that in rat microinjection of nanogram quantities of opiates into the paragigantocellular reticular formation (Pgl), located just lateral to the NRM, produced potent, naloxone-reversible analgesia. Injections into NRM or into the more dorsal reticular formation were much less effective. Although Hökfelt has demonstrated enkephalin immunoreactivity in NRM (41), because of the paucity of opiate receptors in that region (3), the site and mechanism of action of local injection of opiates is difficult to explain. It is unlikely that diffusion of the peptide accounts for the action, since the effective sites were so restricted. More recently, Besson and his colleagues (23) reported that in the rat the NRM not the Pgl was most sensitive to microinjection of opiates. Clearly their data are in direct contradiction to those of Satoh and Takagi.

Besson's laboratory has also demonstrated that the analgesic action of NRM stimulation is reversed by the opiate antagonist naloxone (65). This observation has been difficult to account for, since in other laboratories the inhibitory action of NRM stimulation on spinal pain transmission neurons was not naloxone-reversible. The question, of course, concerns the site of the naloxone action. Interestingly, in the cat, the NRM contains few enkephalin cell bodies and no terminals (30). Assuming that the absence of enkephalin-immunoreactivity in the terminals implies a paucity of opiate receptors, it would appear that opiates do not act at the level of the raphe. If this were true, then the reversibility of raphe stimulation by naloxone must take place elsewhere, for example, at the opiate receptors in the spinal cord (52). Hopefully, techniques based on combined transport of retrograde markers and peptide immunoreactivity will make it possible to determine the axonal projection of individual peptide-containing neurons of the medulla. Alternatively, studies designed to increase the sensitivity of the localization of opiate receptors may establish more clearly the sites of exogenous and/or endogenous opiate action.

One important anatomical consideration must be raised, namely, that what is called NRM in the rat does not correspond to the same structure in the cat. NRM was originally defined on a cytoarchitectural basis in the cat. It was presumed to correspond to the B3, serotonergic cell group of Dahlstrom and Fuxe (21) in the rat. Most rat atlases, however, illustrate NRM at the junction of the pyramids, with lateral wings arching over the pyramids. This is considerably different from the designation of NRM in the cat. Although recent 5-HT studies in the cat have revealed 5-HT containing neurons lateral to the cytoarchitecturally defined NRM, most studies restrict NRM to a medial zone in the medulla. It will be important to determine whether the lateral 5-HT neurons are part of the NRM, part of the Pgl, or more importantly, whether they differ in terms of their afferent and efferent connections and whether their functional roles are the same or different.

In addition to the hypothesized action of opiates at the midbrain and medullary levels, there is now considerable evidence, primarily from the laboratory of Yaksh (81), that opiates can exert their analgesic action via a direct effect on the spinal cord. There is considerable argument in the literature as to whether the spinal cord is the primary site of action after systemic injection or whether it only occurs at high doses. Whichever is true, this does not eliminate the fact that, at least from a clinical standpoint, the opiate action is powerful, reversed by naloxone, and thus provides a very important addition to clinical approaches to pain control.

The working hypothesis is that the analgesic action of opiates directly injected into the spinal cord reflects binding to opiate receptors located on primary afferent terminals, some of which probably contain substance P. In other words, the exogenous opiate would bypass the enkephalinergic interneuron in the spinal cord. In fact, recent in vivo studies have demonstrated that intrathecal injection of opiates blocks the release of substance P (45).

It has been suggested that the enkephalinergic interneuron in the spinal cord is at the end of the chain which begins at the periaqueductal gray and involves the 5-HT containing nucleus raphe magnus (7). Recent evidence, however, suggests that this may not be the case. For example, microinjection of opiates into PAG produces profound analgesia that is reversed by systemic, but not by intrathecal naloxone injection (80). In other words, the opiate receptors in the cord do not appear to be involved in the analgesia mediated from midbrain sites. In contrast, combined injection of the serotonin and norepinephrine antagonists, methysergide and phentolamine completely abolishes the analgesic affect of morphine injected into the PAG. Thus, it would appear that the enkephalin-containing interneuron in the spinal cord is an independent means of producing analgesia and is not activated by descending 5-HT or norepinephrine terminals.

As described above, some recent data from our laboratory have added a further twist to the role of the enkephalin-containing dorsal horn neurons. It is generally assumed that the enkephalin-interneuron is located in the substantia gelatinosa and that its axon terminates, to a great extent, on opiate receptors located on primary afferent terminals (51). Thus, the descending 5-HT terminal from NRM was assumed to terminate on the enkephalinergic neuron in the substantia gelatinosa. In our studies, however, we have localized numerous enkephalin-containing neurons in the marginal layer of the spinal dorsal horn (30). These neurons are much more intensely immunoreactive than those in the substantia gelatinosa. Since all marginal neurons are thought to be projection neurons, this finding also raises the possibility that there is a serotonergic, descending postsynaptic inhibition of enkephalin-containing neurons involved in pain transmission. In this case, the inhibition would not be reversed by naloxone.

Even more intriguing is the possibility that the marginal projection neuron, in addition to the substantia gelatinosa interneuron, is the source of an enkephalinergic input to the primary afferent opiate receptor. Although there is little evidence for a local axonal arborization of marginal neurons, a dendroaxonic relationship is conceivable. If the marginal neuron does feed back upon the primary afferent neuron, then a potentially important modulation of noxious input may be present at the first synapse. This inhibitory interaction could also be under descending monoaminergic control. Clearly a detailed analysis of aminergic-peptidergic interactions at the ultrastructural level is required before we can unravel the complex organization of the superficial dorsal horn, including its afferent input, and the descending systems which modulate its output.

Acknowledgement. I would like to express my appreciation to E.J. Glazer for helpful suggestions with the manuscript. I also thank A. Schilling for typing the manuscript. This work was supported by grant NS 14627, NSF BNS78-24762, Research Career Development Award NS 00364, and an Alfred P. Sloan Fellowship.

REFERENCES

(1) Abols, I.A., and Basbaum, A.I. 1979. Afferent input to the medullary reticular formation and nucleus raphe magnus (NRM) of the cat. An HRP study. Anat. Rec. 193: 467.

(2) Albe-Fessard, D.; Bovie, D.; Grant, G.; and Levante, A. 1975. Labelling of cells in the medulla oblongata and the spinal cord of the monkey after injections of horseradish peroxidase in the thalamus. Neurosci. Letters 1: 75-80.

(3) Atweh, S.F., and Kuhar, M.J. 1977. Autoradiographic localization of opiate-receptors in rat brain. I. Spinal cord and lower medulla. Brain Res. 124: 53-68.

(4) Barber, R.P.; Vaughn, J.E.; Saito, K.; McLaughlin, B.J.; and Roberts, E. GABAergic terminals in the substantia gelatinosa of the rat spinal cord. Brain Res. 141: 35-55.

(5) Barber, R.P.; Vaughn, J.E.; Slemmon, J.R.; Salvaterra, P.M.; Roberts, E.; and Leeman, S.E. 1979. The origin distribution and synaptic relationships of Substance P axons in rat spinal cord. J. Comp. Neurol. 184: 331-352.

(6) Basbaum, A.I.; Clanton, C.H.; and Fields, H.L. 1978. Three bulbospinal pathways from the rostral medulla of the cat. An autoradiographic study of pain modulating systems. J. Comp. Neurol. 178: 209-224.

(7) Basbaum, A.I., and Fields, H.L. 1978. Endogenous pain control mechanisms: Review and hypothesis. Annals Neurol. 4: 451-462.

(8) Basbaum, A.I., and Fields, H.L. 1979. The origin of descending pathways in the dorsolateral funiculus of the spinal cord of the cat and rat: Further studies on the anatomy of pain modulation. J. Comp. Neurol., in press.

(9) Basbaum, A.I.; Marley, N.J.E.; O'Keefe, J.; and Clanton, C.H 1977. Reversal of morphine and stimulus-produced analgesia by subtotal spinal cord lesions. Pain 3: 43-56.

(10) Beal, J. 1979. The ventral dendritic arbor of lamina I neurons in the adult primate spinal cord. Anat. Record 193: 479.

(11) Bennet, G.J.; Abdelmoumene, M.; Hayashi, H.; and Dubner, R. 1979. Morphology and physiology of Rexed's substantia gelatinosa (SG) and lamina I neurons intracellularly stained with HRP. Anat. Record 193: 480.

(12) Bennett, G.J.; Hayashi, H.; Abdelmoumene, M.; and Dubner, R. 1979. Physiological properties of stalked cells of the substantia gelatinosa intracellularly stained with horseradish peroxidase. Brain Res. 164: 285-289.

(13) Berkeley, K.J. 1976. Analysis of the border between N. ventralis lateralis and N. ventralis posterolateralis in the cat thalamus. Neurosci Abst. 1: 143.

(14) Boivie, J. 1971. The termination of the spinothalamic tract in the cat. An experimental study with silver impregnation methods. Exp. Br. Res. 12: 331-353.

(15) Boivie, J. 1979. An anatomical reinvestigation of the termination of the spinothalamic tract in the monkey. J. Comp. Neurol. 186: 343-370.

(16) Boivie, J., and Perl, E.R. 1975. Neural substrates of somatic sensation. In NTP International Review of Science, Physiology Series One, ed. C.C. Hunt, pp. 599-622. London: Butterworth.

(17) Burton, H., and Jones, E.G. 1976. The posterior thalamic region and its central projection in new world and old world monkeys. J. Comp. Neurol. 168: 249-302.

(18) Carstens, E., and Trevino, D.L. 1978. Laminar origins of spinothalamic projections in the cat as determined by the retrograde transport of HRP. J. Comp. Neurol. 182: 151-166.

(19) Casey, K.L. 1966. Nociceptive mechanisms in the thalamus of awake squirrel monkey. J. Neuro. physiol. 29: 727-750.

(20) Coggeshall, R.E.; Applebaum, M.L.; Fazen, M.; Stubbs III, T.B.; and Stykes, M.T. 1975. Unmyelinated axons in human ventral roots, a possible explanation for the failure of dorsal rhizotomy to relieve pain. Brain 98: 157-166.

(21) Dalström, A., and Fuxe, K. 1964. Evidence for the existence of monoamine containing neurons in the central nervous system. I. Demonstration of monoamines in the cell bodies of brain stem neurons. Acta Scand. 62: (Supp. 232) 1-55.

(22) Dennis, S.G., and Melzack, R. 1977. Pain signalling systems in the dorsal and ventral cord. Pain 4: 97-132.

(23) Dickenson, A.H.; Oliveras, J.L.; and Besson, J.M. 1979. Role of the nucleus raphe magnus in opiate analgesia as studied by the microinjection technique in the rat. Brain Res. 170: 95-112.

(24) Emson, P.C. 1979. Peptides as neurotransmitter candidates in the mammalian CNS. Prog. Neurobiol. 13: 61-116.

(25) Feldberg, W. 1976. The ventral surface of the brain: a scarcely explored region of pharmacological sensitivity. Neuroscience 1: 427-442.

(26) Fields, H.L., and Basbaum, A.I. 1978. Brainstem control of spinal pain transmission neurons. Ann. Rev. Physiol. 40: 193-221.

(27) Gallager, D.W., and Pert, A. 1978. Afferents to brainstem nuclei (brain stem raphe, nucleus reticularis pontis caudalis and nucleus gigantocellularis) in the rat as demonstrated by microiontophoretically applied HRP. Brain Res. 144: 257-276.

(28) Giesler, Jr., G.J.; Cannon, J.T.; Urca, G.; and Liebeskind, J.C. 1978. Long ascending projections from substantia gelatinosa Rolandi and the subjacent dorsal horn in the rat. Science 202: 984-986.

(29) Giesler, Jr., G.J.; Menerey, D.; and Basbaum, A.I. 1979. Differential origins of spinothalamic tract projections to medial and lateral thalamus in the rat. J. Comp. Neurol. 184: 107-126.

(30) Glazer, E.J., and Basbaum, A.I. 1979. Enkephalin perikarya in the marginal zone and sacral autonomic nucleus of the cat spinal cord. Neurosci. Abst. 5: 723.

(31) Glazer, E.J., and Basbaum, A.I. 1979. Immunocytochemical localization of leucine-enkephalin in cat CNS. Anat. Record. 193: 549.

(32) Gobel, S. 1976. Dendroaxonic synapses in the substantia gelatinosa glomeruli of the spinal trigeminal nucleus of the cat. J. Comp. Neurol. 167: 165-176.

(33) Gobel, S. 1978. Golgi studies of the neurons in layer I of the dorsal horn of the medulla (trigeminal nucleus caudalis). J. Comp. Neurol. 180: 375-394.

(34) Gobel, S. 1978. Golgi studies of the neurons in layer II of the dorsal horn of the medulla (trigeminal nucleus caudalis). J. Comp. Neurol. 180: 395-413.

(35) Gobel, S., and Binck, J.M. 1977. Degenerative changes in primary trigeminal axons and in neurons in nucleus caudalis following tooth pulp extirpations in the cat. Brain Res. 132: 347-354.

(36) Grant, G., and Arvidsson, J. 1975. Tranganglionic degeneration in trigeminal primary sensory neurons. Brain Res. 95: 265-279.

(37) Henry, J.L. 1976. Effects of substance P on functionally identified units in cat spinal cord. B.R. 114: 439-452.

(38) Hökfelt, T.; Elde, R.; Johansson, O.; Ljungdahl, A.; Schultzberg, M.; Fuxe, K.; Goldstein, M.; Nilsson, G.; Pernow, B.; Terenius, L.; Ganten, D.; Jeffcoate, S.L.; Rehfeld, J.; and Said, S. 1978. A distribution of peptide-containing neurons. In Psychopharmacology: A Generation of Progress, eds. M.A. Lipton, A. DiMascio and K.F. Killam, pp. 39-66. New York: Raven Press.

(39) Hökfelt, T.; Elde, R.; Johansson, O.; Luft, R.; Nilsson, G.; and Arimura, A. 1976. Immunohistochemical evidence for separate populations of somatostatin-containing and substance P-containing primary afferent neurons. Neurosci. 1: 131-136.

(40) Hökfelt, T.; Ljungdahl, A.; Steinbusch, H.; Verhofstad, A.; Nilsson, G.; Brodin, E.; Pernow, B.; and Goldstein, M. 1978. Immunohistochemical evidence of Substance P-like immunoreactivity in some 5-HT-containing neurons in the rat central nervous system. Neurosci. 3: 517-538.

(41) Hökfelt, T.; Ljungdahl, A.; Terenius, L.; Elde, R.; and Nilsson, G. 1977. Immunohistochemical analysis of peptide pathways possibly related to pain and analgesia: Enkephalin and Substance P. Proc. Natl. Acad. Sci. 74: 3081-3085.

(42) Hökfelt, T.; Terenius, T.; Kuypers, H.G.J.M.; and Dann, O. 1979. Evidence for enkephalin immunoreactive neurons in the medulla oblongata projecting to the spinal cord. Neurosci. Letters. 14: 55-60.

(43) Hunt, S.P.; Emson, P.C.; and Kelly, J.S. 1979. The immunohistochemical localization of met-enkephalin within the rat spinal cord: light and electron microscopic observation. Neurosci. Letter Suppl. 3: 20.

(44) Innis, R.B.; Correa, F.M.A.; Uhl, G.R.; Schneider, B.; and Snyder, S.H. 1979. Cholecystokinin octapeptide-like immunoreactivity: histochemical localization in rat brain. PNAS 76: 521-525.

(45) Jessel, T.M.; Mudge, A.W.; Leeman, S.E.; and Yaksh, T.L. 1979. Release of Substance P and somatostatin in vivo from primary afferent terminals in mammalian spinal cord. Neurosci. Abst. 5: 611.

(46) Kerr, F.W.L. 1975. Neuroanatomical substrates of nociception in the spinal cord. Pain 1: 325-356.

(47) Kerr, F.W.L. 1975. The ventral spinothalamic tract and other ascending systems of the ventral funiculus of the spinal cord. J. Comp. Neurol. 159: 335-356.

(48) Kerr, F.W.L., and Wilson, P.R. 1978. Pain. Ann. Rev. Neurosci. 1: 83-102.

(49) Kruger, L., and Albe-Fessard, D. 1960. Distribution of responses to somatic afferent stimuli in the diencephalon of the cat under chloralose anesthesia. Exp. Neurol. 2: 442-467.

(50) Kruger, L.E.; Perl, E.R.; and Sedivee, M.J. 1977. Electron microscopic study of mechanical nociceptor endings in cat skin. Anat. Record 193: 593.

(51) LaMotte, C. 1977. Distribution of the tract of Lissauer and the dorsal root fibers in the primate spinal cord. J. Comp. Neurol. 172: 529-561.

(52) LaMotte, C.; Pert, C.B.; and Snyder, S.H. 1976. Opiate receptor binding in primate spinal cord: distribution and changes after dorsal root section. Brain Res. 112: 407-412.

(53) Larsson, L.I., and Rehfeld, J.F. 1979. Localization and molecular heterogeneity of cholecystokinin in the central and peripheral nervous system. Brain Res. 165: 201-218.

(54) Light, A.R., and Metz, C.B. 1978. The morphology of the spinal cord efferent and afferent neurons contributing to the ventral roots of the cat. J. Comp. Neurol. 179: 501-516.

(55) Light, A.R., and Perl, E.R. 1979. Reexamination of the dorsal root projection to the spinal dorsal horn including observations on the differential termination of coarse and fine fibers. J. Comp. Neurol. 186: 117-132.

(56) Light, A.R., and Perl, E.R. 1979. Spinal termination of functionally identified primary afferent neurons with slowly conducting myelinated fibers. J. Comp. Neurol. 186: 133-150.

(57) Light, A.R.; Trevino, D.L.; and Perl, E.R. 1979. Morphological features of functionally defined neurons in the marginal zone and substantia gelatinosa of the spinal dorsal horn. J. Comp. Neurol. 186: 151-172.

(58) Lippman, H.H., and Kerr, F.W.L. 1972. Light and electron microscopic study of crossed ascending pathways in the anterolateral funiculus in the monkey. Brain Res. 40: 496-499.

(59) Ljungdahl, A.; Hokfelt, T.; and Nilsson, G. 1978. Distribution of Substance P-like immunoreactivity in the central nervous system of the rat. I. Cell bodies and nerve terminals. Neuroscience 3: 861-944.

(60) Mayer, D.J., and Liebeskind, J.C. 1974. Pain reduction by focal electrical stimulation of the brain: An anatomical and behavioral analysis. Brain Res. 68: 73-93.

(61) Mayer, D.J., and Price, D.D. 1976. Central nervous system mechanisms of analgesia. Pain 2: 379-404.

(62) Narotzky, R.A., and Kerr, F.W.L. 1978. Marginal neurons of the spinal cord: types, afferent synaptology and functional considerations. Brain Res. 139: 1-20.

(63) Olgart, L.; Hökfelt, T.; Nilsson, G.; and Pernow, B. 1977. Localization of Substance P-like immunoreactivity in nerves in the tooth-pulp. Pain 4: 153-160.

(64) Oliveras, J.L.; Guilbaud, G.; and Besson, J.M. 1979. A map of serotoninergic structures involved in stimulation producing analgesia in unrestrained freely moving cats. Brain Res. 164: 317-322.

(65) Oliveras, J.L.; Hosobuchi, Y.; Redjemi, F.; Guilbaud, G.; and Besson, J.M. 1977. Opiate antagonist, naloxone, strongly reduces analgesia induced by stimulation of a raphe nucleus (centralis inferior). Brain Res. 120: 221-230.

(66) Palkovits, M. 1978. Topography of chemically identified neurons in the central nervous system: A review. Acta Morphologica Acad. Sci. Hung. 26: 211-290.

(67) Pickel, V.M.; Reis, D.J.; and Leeman, S.E. 1977. Ultrastructural localization of substance P in neurons of rat spinal cord. Brain Res. 122: 534-540.

(68) Poggio, G.F., and Mountcastle, V.B. 1960. A study of the functional contributions of the lemniscal and spinothalamic systems to somatic sensibility. Bull. John's Hopkins Med. School. 106: 266-316.

(69) Ralston, H.J., and Ralston, D.D. 1979. The distribution of dorsal root axons in laminae I, II and III of the macaque spinal cord: A quantitative electron microscopy study. J. Comp. Neurol. 184: 643-684.

(70) Randic, M., and Miletic, V. 1978. Depressant actions of methionine-enkephalin and somatostatin in cat dorsal horn neurons activated by noxious stimuli. Brain Res. 152: 196-202.

(71) Ranson, S.W. 1913. The course within the spinal cord of the non-medullated fibers of the dorsal roots. A study of Lissauer's tract in the cat. J. Comp. Neurol. 23: 259-281.

(72) Reynolds, D.V. 1969. Surgery in the rat during electrical analgesia induced by focal brain stimulation. Science 164: 444-445.

(73) Satoh, M.; Akaike, A.; and Takagi, H. 1979. Excitation by morphine and enkephalin of single neurons of nucleus reticularis paragigantice1lularis in the rat: A probable mechanism of analgesic action of opiates. Brain Res. 169: 406.

(74) Snyder, R.L. 1977. The organization of the dorsal root entry zone in cats and monkeys. J. Comp. Neurol. 174: 47-69.

(75) Strick, P.L. 1975. Multiple sources of thalamic input to the primate motor cortex. Brain Res. 88: 372-377.

(76) Swanson, L.W., and McKellar, S. 1979. The distribution of oxytocin- and neurophysin-stained fibers in the spinal cord of the rat and monkey. J. Comp. Neurol. 188: 87-106.

(77) Uhl, G.R.; Kuhar, M.; and Snyder, S.H. 1977. Neurotensin: Immunohistochemical localization in rat central nervous system. PNAS 74: 4059-4063.

(78) Willis, W.D.; Haber, L.H.; and Martin, R.F. 1977. Inhibition of spinothalamic tract cells and interneurons by brain stem stimulation in the monkey. J. Neurophysiol. 40: 968-981.

(79) Willis, W.D.; Leonard, R.B.; and Kenshalo, Jr., D.R. 1978. Spinothalamic tract neurons in the substantia gelatinosa. Science 202: 980-988.

(80) Yaksh, T.L. 1979. Direct evidence that spinal serotonin and noradrenaline terminals mediate the spinal anti-nociceptive effects of morphine in the periaqueductal gray. Brain Res. 160: 180-185.

(81) Yaksh, T.L., and Rudy, T.A. 1978. Narcotic analgesics: CNS sites and mechanisms of action as revealed by intra-cerebral injection techniques. Pain 4: 299-360.

Pain and Society, eds. H.W. Kosterlitz and L.Y. Terenius, pp. 123-140.
Dahlem Konferenzen 1980. Weinheim: Verlag Chemie GmbH.

Segmental Neurophysiology of Pain Control

A. Iggo
Department of Veterinary Physiology, University of Edinburgh
Royal (Dick) School of Veterinary Studies
Summerhall, Edinburgh EH9 1QH, Scotland

Abstract. At the level of the spinal cord pain control is expressed by the interaction of an afferent input from stimulus-specified sensory receptors and from descending control emanating from the brain, with dorsal horn neurons. The nociceptors terminate in the superficial dorsal horn and activate neurons directly or indirectly at several levels of the gray matter. Some of the neurons are specifically excited by nociceptive afferents, whereas others are less specific and are also excited by sensitive mechanoreceptor afferents. Some of these neurons, in laminae I, IV, and V of the dorsal horn, send axons into ascending pathways. The excitability of these tract neurons is subject to inhibitory actions from both mechanoreceptor and nociceptor inputs at the segmental level and by descending axons. A scheme is described to account for the sensory interactions that occur. New information about the previously unrecorded substantia gelatinosa neurons is included in the scheme suggesting that they may have an important modulating function in the dorsal horn. Several problems are discussed, including the relation between the dorsal horn neuronal mechanism involved in putative pain mechanisms and those excited by the flexor reflex afferents.

INTRODUCTION

It is a truism that the spinal cord is involved with pain mechanisms, but considerable intellectual and experimental effort is required in establishing just what the involvement implies. The local or segmental mechanisms do not, by themselves, generate pain except in disorders. Instead the spinal cord, and more especially, its dorsal horn, provides the venue for interactions among entering and intrinsically generated neural activity that determines the output which is fed along ascending pathways to higher levels of brain. The entering activity has two major origins - a) incoming dorsal (and ventral) root afferent fibers bringing information from sensory receptors in the peripheral tissues of the body, and b) descending projections from more central regions of the nervous system, with as yet an ill-defined origin. These two sources of input interact in the spinal cord with intrinsic mechanisms and it is here that one of the major questions arises - by what means and to what extent do these interactions influence the sensory output in the ascending pathways?

Before embarking on that enquiry, it is worthwhile setting out some facts about the inputs. There has been considerable effort during the last two decades into the resolution of the conflicting views about the characteristics of the afferent inflow from peripheral sensory receptors, studied principally by recording unitary activity from the primary afferent fibers (7,22), and there is now a consensus that they can be categorized as mechanoreceptors, thermoreceptors, and nociceptors. This classification, together with the morpho-functional correlation that has emerged, is based on quantitative physical stimulation of the receptors but is also colored by psycho-physical correlates. As we shall see, the idea that 'touch is touch and pain is pain and ne'er the twain shall meet' is an idea that can be falsified, though to a certain extent it is implicit in the categorization of cutaneous receptors. The general thesis of a specification of function among the peripheral sensory receptors is borne out by contemporary work on the distribution of the afferent fibers in the spinal cord. The discovery that the small afferent fibers supplied diverse sensory receptors (21) began to undermine early ideas on the functional implication of Lissauer's tract and the superficial dorsal horn in pain. Ideas based, for example, on Ranson's (31) experiments revealed that the smaller axons in the dorsal roots entered and ended in the substantia gelatinosa and that cutting them abolished pseudo-affective responses in anesthetized animals. However, the development (14,24,33) and application (6,28), of intracellular staining techniques to functionally identified dorsal root afferent fibers has proved to be a potent analytical tool. This new approach has established that the various kinds of cutaneous (5,28) and muscle (4,8) mechanoreceptor with myelinated afferent fibers have distinctive morphological organization of their terminals in the gray matter of the spinal cord. The new knowledge thus provided further support for the codification of the receptors into functionally specific categories. Studies of the mechanical nociceptors with myelinated afferent fibers have added force to the general conclusions. Some of these axons are large enough to be penetrated by micropipette electrodes (28) filled with horseradish peroxidase (HRP), and they have a terminal distribution that is quite distinct from that of similar sized, but functionally different, axons from sensitive mechanoreceptors. By extrapolation it is reasonable to expect that the functionally diverse non-myelinated afferent fibers will also be found to have morphologically distinctive end-stations. Present evidence (26) indicates that the small myelinated and non-myelinated afferent fibers may have different end-stations in the superficial dorsal horn, although their functional attributes could not be established by the HRP staining methods used.

Two conclusions emerge from this work. First, the primary afferent fibers terminate in the dorsal horn, especially the finer ones that include the nociceptors. The larger cutaneous afferent fibers, innervating sensitive mechanoreceptors, also terminate in the dorsal horn, usually at deeper levels, and many also send collaterals that run in the dorsal columns to end in the dorsal column nuclei. Second, there is a reasonable firmness in the conclusion that the various kinds of sensory receptor defined by the morpho-functional characteristics of the receptors continue to have a well-defined physiological identity in the central nervous system. It would seem reasonable therefore to discard and not dis-inter theories, such as the temporo-spatial pattern theory (36), based as they are on non-specificity of the sensory receptors and afferent fibers, or those based on axonal diameter (29). Given the exact information about the afferent input and the existence of afferent fibers capable of signaling noxious or damaging stimulation of the periphery, the next logical step is to examine the characteristics of neural elements in the dorsal horn.

An immediate problem is the diversity of elements. The normal approach has been to use single-unit analytical techniques, originating in the classical micropipette electrode studies of Eccles and colleagues (3). Morphological studies have proved invaluable in providing a framework, but the basic problems remain that of identifying the neural elements from which single unit records are obtained and of obtaining unbiased samples. The need to make detailed studies of unit activity, combined with the small size of the nerve cells (axons ranging from 0.2 to about 12 μm and cell bodies ranging from 3 to about 60 μm in diameter) imposes rigorous constraints on the experiments. Much of the recent work has used paralyzed animal preparations in order to overcome movement artifact problems. This in turn leads to problems of anesthesia and in some laboratories to the use of spinal preparations, in which the interplay of ascending and descending controls is unavoidably absent. In terms of 'pain' or the 'pseudo-affective responses' commonly taken to be the counterpart of responses to pain, it is well-known that the spinal cord is subject to powerful descending control and, for example, that the flexion reflex is much exaggerated in spinal animals (16).

On the other hand, the use of freely-moving animals carrying devices for electrophysiological recording severely limits the precision of analysis and cell identification. This kind of approach may be most rewarding in testing hypotheses generated by the anesthetized paralyzed animal experiments.

NEURONS IN THE DORSAL HORN

There are many publications reporting neuronal activity in the dorsal horn and from these there emerges a conflicting array of results. Since the data obtained are strongly influenced by the results sought, or hypotheses tested, we should not be surprised. One encouraging feature of recent work is that laboratory technology has advanced to the stage where it is no longer necessary to limit the test stimuli to electrical stimulation of peripheral nerve trunks. Instead, there are good quantitative stimulators for mechanical (5) and thermal (2) excitation of sensory receptors so that the analysis is less hampered than previously by the mixed inhomogeneous barrages of afferent impulses that are initiated by nerve trunk stimulation. A recent example of the importance of the use of natural stimuli are the dorsal horn neurons reported by Light et al. (28), which could be excited by a particular kind of natural cutaneous stimuli, but which could not be excited by electrical stimulation of dorsal roots. This result probably arises from a concurrent or antecedent inhibitory action of afferent fibers excited by the nerve volley which was sufficient to prevent excitation by the slower excitatory afferent. (The study of pain lacks the good fortune of the monosynaptic motoneuron reflex studies in which a nearly pure population of the largest dorsal root axons were the afferent fibers).

Nevertheless, it continues to be necessary to use both natural and electrical stimuli in order to obtain adequate controls and for the proper identification of dorsal horn neurons.

NOCICEPTOR-DRIVEN DORSAL HORN NEURONS

From the purist viewpoint there are few studies that deal with this kind of neuron and we may properly ask whether such a search should be made. At once we are faced with the question - should we expect to find such neurons? It is possible to recognize two schools of thought (30), conveniently labeled the 'specifists' and the 'non-specifists.' This is significant since the standpoint of an investigator may influence not only the experiments he designs, but also his interpretation of the results.

An alternative approach, which I shall adopt, is to scan the literature and see what has been reported. It is at once apparent that noxious stimuli can excite dorsal horn neurons, as also can nerve volleys in small afferent fibers that include the nociceptors ((30) for review). But the responses are highly dependent on the experimental conditions. In spinal preparation there are large numbers of these nociceptor-driven neurons in laminae IV and V of the dorsal horn (34), but these neurons often become unresponsive if the spinal cord is intact (18). Since in the spinal animal, neurons in lamina IV and V may be unresponsive to noxious cutaneous or muscle stimuli, the neuronal population is not homogeneous. A classification of the neurons based exclusively on lamination (e.g., lamina V type neuron, etc.) is therefore untenable, since in any one lamina there is a diversity of neurons.

The nociceptor-driven neurons in lamina IV and V are non-specific in their input sensitivity since they can also be excited by the sensitive cutaneous mechanoreceptors with myelinated afferent fibers. This excitation is often monosynaptic, in keeping with the distribution of termination of the large myelinated cutaneous afferent fibers in this region of the dorsal horn (18). In addition, these myelinated afferent fibers often have a disynaptic inhibitory action on the same neurons (20). There is a complex interplay of excitatory and inhibitory actions. These interactions significantly influence the responses of the neurons. If electrical stimuli are used, the large afferent fibers can set up an inhibitory state that diminishes or abolishes the responses to later arriving impulses from the nociceptors (28). Indeed, even very powerful excitatory discharges evoked by an exclusive nociceptor afferent input can be completely suppressed by a concurrent input in the group II myelinated mechanoreceptor afferents (18).

The interconnections of the dorsal horn neurons remains an unsolved problem and, at present, the various attempts to suggest possible neuronal networks suffer the common weakness of a lack of solid evidence. On the one hand, there are laboratories which use natural stimuli, study dorsal horn electrophysiology and pharmacology and have a strong interest in ascending and descending pathways (e.g., (11,18,28,30,37)) and, on the other hand, there is the Scandinavian group led by Lundberg and Oscarsson who are also interested in ascending pathways but who take as their starting point the flexion reflex. These latter workers have developed the study of flexion reflexes and the afferents which drive them, for which they have coined the term flexion reflex afferents (19) or FRA. As yet the two main streams appear to be independent, although they must inevitably have common ground in the dorsal horn. The FRA group have made detailed intracellular studies: for example, Hongo, Janowska, and Lundberg (19) studied by this technique dorsal horn neurons that form part of the spinocervical tract and correspond to the lamina IV and V neurons just discussed. There is a clear need for a consensus in this area. The former group is attempting to define its input in terms of the sensory receptors whereas the latter group appears to be defining its afferent input by its effects, and so far no satisfactory amalgamation of the studies has been achieved.

SUPERFICIAL DORSAL HORN

Particular interest in the most superficial layers of the gray matter of the dorsal horn and its possible involvement in pain arises from the early work of Ranson (31), already referred to. Until about 10 years ago, the substantia gelatinosa and marginal layer of the dorsal horn were inaccessible to the unitary neurophysiological studies and as indicated above, most information about neuronal activity was restricted to lamina IV and deeper. Focal or evoked potential studies, and in particular the dorsal root potential, were used instead, combined with ablation and sectioning procedures.

It is now, however, possible to record unit neuron responses and there is a growing body of evidence to show that in the marginal layer (lamina I) there are neurons that are excited only by an input from the nociceptors. First reported by Christensen and Perl (13), there have been several confirmatory reports and they are now known to include at least two subclasses: 3a excited only by the myelinated mechanical nociceptors and 3b excited in addition by non-myelinated nociceptors (11). Once again the population of neurons is heterogeneous and includes thermosensory as well as probably nonspecific neurons (27).

SUBSTANTIA GELATINOSA (S.G.)

This region of the spinal cord is densely packed with small neurons. There may be as many as 100,000 in 1 mm^3 of S.G. Their small size has until quite recently defeated all attempts to record from them as units. There are now reports from several laboratories (12,28,35) of unit responses, with some uncertainty arising from the location of the recordings and, perhaps, an unwillingness to accept that what was previously undone may now be done. One difficulty is in labeling or marking the S.G. neurons. The techniques which succeed for the larger and deeper dorsal horn neurons depend on extrusion of the marker from the microelectrode and the very small tip diameters required for intracellular penetration of S.G. neurons have caused difficulties. There are recent reports that this has now been achieved in the S.G. (28), so that there is greater confidence in accepting claims of recording from neurons in the S.G. A variety of neuronal responses has been reported (12, 28,35), and although one may despair of introducing order at this stage of knowledge, there is sufficient information now available to make this a reasonable task. Some of the neurons have the characteristics of an exclusive specific nociceptor system, a finding which raises interesting questions of the role of the S.G. in pain mechanisms.

Interest in these S.G. neurons is sharpened by the interaction in dorsal horn neurons of innocuous and noxious cutaneous stimuli (see below). Accordingly, it is worth attempting to categorize the results reported so far. Several major groupings have been proposed:

Inverse neurons. These are the 100 or so S.G. neurons of Cervero et al. (10), a distinguishing feature being the presence of a background discharge that can be inhibited by appropriate cutaneous stimulation. The classes were made corresponding to the 3 classes of larger dorsal horn neurons, but responding in an opposite manner and called Inverse I - inhibited by light tactile stimulation; Inverse 2 - inhibited by both tactile and noxious stimuli; and Inverse 3 - inhibited by noxious stimuli. In each class the cells were excited by the alternative stimuli, i.e., Inverse I were excited by noxious stimuli, etc.

Habituating neurons. This is another major class reported (28,35). Some S.G. neurons are reported to have the remarkable property of responding to an initial tactile stimulus perhaps with a persistent discharge, but then develop a refractoriness to subsequent similar cutaneous stimuli, a phenomenon described as habituation.

The role of the S.G. remains enigmatic so long as we have only fragmentory reports on unit responses, although it clearly has a strong modulatory influence as Denny Brown et al. (15) established in their experiments on conscious primates. It may also have a decisive role in 'pain' transmission, since it also receives input from higher levels of the C.N.S. Present evidence, however, does not indicate for those S.G. neurons which have been tested (10) that there is a tonic descending control of the S.G.

INTRINSIC AND EXTRINSIC CONNECTIONS OF THE DORSAL HORN

The dorsal horn neurons are numerous, especially those of the S.G. and one important question that is germane to 'pain mechanisms' is: what are their synaptic relations? Electrophysiological evidence is meager, except in so far as some of the neurons clearly send axons to higher levels of the C.N.S. There are several well-defined routes: a) The spinothalamic tract, well-developed in primates (37) and much less so in the cat. Neurons in lamina I, IV, V, VII project into it and include examples of classes 1, 2, and 3. It is the class 3 (nociceptor-driven) neurons which appear to offer the most direct pathways (11), but strong arguments have also been made for the class 2 (or wide-dynamic range) neurons (30). One problem here is that these class 2 neurons are often under powerful selective tonic descending inhibition which may completely suppress their responses to noxious stimulation (18). This feature of their reactivity poses a problem in interpreting their role in pain. b) The spinocervical tract, well-developed in carnivores, carries information principally from tactile receptors but the cells can also often be excited by a nociceptor input, i.e., class 2 cells, and its sensory role is still undefined. c) The dorsal column pathway appears to be principally a tactile, rather than nociceptor path, but it contains postsynaptic elements, corresponding to class 2 cells. d) The FRA paths should also be taken into account although, as indicated earlier, we are uncertain of their homologies or concordance with the sensory nociceptor paths. e) Spinoreticular and other paths exist, still largely unexplored, but of renewed interest, in view of the existence in the brain stem of powerful mechanisms for modulating the sensory awareness of noxious stimuli (Besson; Casey, this volume).

There are then a variety of ascending pathways into which the dorsal horn neurons project, but it is becoming clear that many, perhaps the majority, of the dorsal horn neurons have only local targets. This conclusion is based partly on attempts to test for ascending projection by the method of antidromic electrical stimulation. Results of such tests indicate that many of all classes of neurons in the dorsal horn do not project. Are they concerned with modulating the activity of the projecting neurons? One puzzle here is that, on functional grounds, there may be little to distinguish a projecting from a non-projecting neuron, except that one sends an axon into an ascending path whereas another does not. What determines the fate of the axon?

New information about connectivity was obtained from intracellular staining of neurons and has shown a surprising abundance of axon collaterals as well as extensive dendritic spreading. This is so for SCT neurons and S.G. neurons and, if it is a general phenomenon, then the possibilities for local interactions in the dorsal horn would appear to be limitless!

MODULATION OF DORSAL HORN ACTIVITY

There is an abundance of excitatory and inhibitory interaction in the dorsal horn; reference has already been made to the excitatory effectiveness of natural tactile stimuli and ineffectiveness of electrical stimulation of dorsal roots containing the excitatory afferents (28). This result is explicable on the basis of an inhibitory action by fast fibers that blocks the subsequent excitatory action of later arriving impulses in the slow fibers, a conclusion long since reached by Zotterman (38) and others.

More recent work has directed attention to the effect of cutaneous afferent inflow on the response of dorsal horn neurons to noxious stimulation of the skin. An example of this kind of effect has been reported by Handwerker et al. (18). They used a purely noxious input due to radiant non-tactile heating of the skin which caused a powerful excitation of class 2 neurons in spinal cats and played against it an afferent input from cutaneous tactile receptors. Graded suppression of the response to noxious stimulation was found. Of particular interest was the kind of cutaneous receptor responsible; they were sensitive tactile receptors, with large (group II) myelinated axons, including the Type G hair follicle afferent units. The effect was observed whether the inhibitory stimulus came from the same or an adjacent receptive field and was evident whether or not the large myelinated fibers caused excitation on their own. The inhibitory action was at least in part postsynaptic. This result is of interest in view of its possible implication in the mechanisms of transcutaneous stimulation for the relief of pain, and possibly of acupuncture, although the action usually does not outlast the afferent inflow. The therapeutic procedures can be much more persistent, implying additional mechanisms.

A more widespread suppressive action involving activity reflected from the brain stem can be evoked by noxious stimuli (25) and this action can even be contralateral in contrast to the more localized ipsilateral segmental action described above.

INHIBITION OF SPECIFIC NOCICEPTOR-DRIVEN NEURONS

The class 3 neurons of lamina I offer the most straightforward example of 'pain' neurons in the spinal cord, since they can only be excited by an afferent input from nociceptors. But they too can be inhibited by segmental mechanisms, although they are more resistant than class 2 neurons. Cervero et al. (11) reported that class 3 neurons, strongly excited by mechano - or thermo - nociceptors or both, can have their discharges diminished or even, depending on the intensity of stimulation, abolished by an afferent input from cutaneous tactile receptors or even from other nociceptors. Once again the 'nociceptor' pathway turns out to be open to segmental influences from the tactile receptors.

Thus we see that the 'pain' mechanisms are complex, and furthermore, the tactile receptors are involved in the overall response, and so cannot be left out when considering the overall 'pain' mechanisms. At one level they almost certainly contribute to the spatial localization, at least of cutaneous pain, whereas, on another level, they must be seen as contributing to the control of pain.

DESCENDING ACTIONS

A consideration of the segmental mechanisms has to include at least a mention of the descending mechanisms, which are both excitatory and inhibitory. I will limit myself to the tonic descending action, which in anesthetized or decerebrate animal so strongly modifies the responses of the class 2 dorsal horn neurons (18). These neurons can be strongly excited in the spinal state by both tactile and noxious stimuli whereas, when the spinal cord is intact, their responses to noxious stimuli may be completely absent. In addition, the level of baçkground activity is much less with the cord intact. These results suggest that there is a tonic descending action which is active not only when the noxious stimulus is present, thus ruling out any spino - medullary - spinal reflex action. The origin of this striking inhibition is still an open question. What is of considerable interest is the apparent absence of this descending action on the class 3 nociceptor-driven dorsal horn neurons (11) or on the inverse S.G. neurons (10). The lack of tonic inhibition of the class 3 neurons is a further indication that they could provide a prompt and effective 'pain pathway.'

INTERNEURONAL MECHANISMS

What then of the segmental neuronal interplay? It is clear that we cannot take a simple view of the dorsal horn as only a switchboard or telephone relay, switching and combining the input. Instead it has to be seen as the stage for considerable interaction among neural events of both local and more remote origin. It is the portal through which the peripheral sensory inflow must inevitably be channeled since, apart from the numerically small number of ventral root afferent fibers, all the afferent fibers either end in the dorsal horn or send collateral branches into it. The output goes not only to the dorsal horn of adjacent and contralateral segments of the spinal cord but also ascends to the brain. In addition there are all the reflex responses, particularly the flexion reflexes, which are fed by the dorsal horn.

It may be unwise to rush into this complexity with generalizations, but without them there is no theoretical framework to guide future investigations. Inevitably they are incomplete, simply because knowledge is incomplete. A recent attempt in this field by Cervero and Iggo (9) is illustrated in Fig. 1. It is an attempt both at simplification and at synthesis. Some elements in the scheme are well-established, i.e., the dorsal horn neurons classes 1, 2, and 3, whereas others are more recently described and more controversial, i.e., S.G. neuron classes $\bar{1}$, $\bar{2}$, and $\bar{3}$. Nevertheless, there is evidence that they exist. The scheme suggests an interaction between the

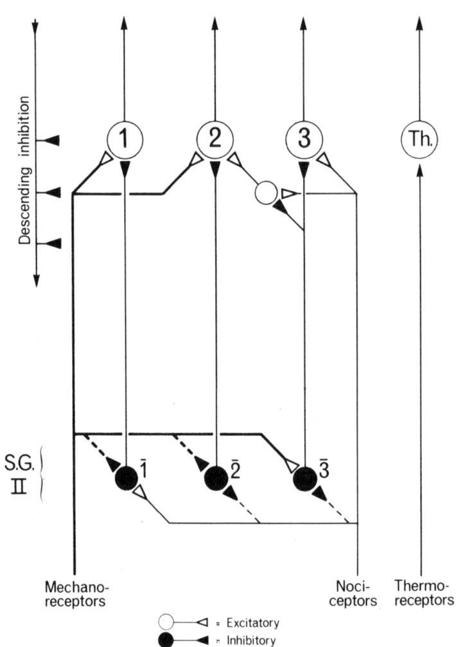

FIG. 1. - Reciprocal sensory interaction. Scheme to illustrate possible interactions among dorsal horn and substantia gelatinosa neurons, leading to a reciprocal interaction between afferent inputs from mechanoreceptors and nociceptors. S.G. = substantia gelatinosa neurons as classified by Cervero et al. (12); 1,2,3, and Th = classes of dorsal horn neurons according to Cervero et al. (11). (Cervero and Iggo (9)).

various elements that goes some way to accounting for the behavior of the neurons. One hypothetical feature of the scheme is the inhibitory action of the inverse S.G. neurons on the corresponding dorsal horn neurons; attempts to provide such evidence have so far failed.

The scheme then postulates a reciprocal sensory interaction among the major groups of cutaneous receptors. It does not deal with the finer detail of more restricted interactions within these major groups, such as the primary afferent depolarization of tactile receptors reported by Jänig et al. (23), nor does it attempt to assess the extent to which the inhibitory actions are pre- or postsynaptic. These are open questions. This model and others like it do no more than provide a theoretical or conceptual framework, as an aid to further analysis. It at least has the merit of a fairly solid foundation in established experimental work and can be seen as a successor to previous attempts at accounting for changes in the excitability of putative 'pain pathway neurons,' such as Barron and Matthews dorsal root potential (1), remote inhibition of Frank, (17), primary afferent depolarization (PAD) (32) and Melzack and Wall's gate hypothesis (29).

Into these various interneuronal actions we must now insert the chemical agents that operate at the synapses, or even more generally on the neurons. I hope that what has been laid out in this paper will prove useful as a framework for the pharmacological account to follow.

REFERENCES

(1) Barron, D.H., and Matthews, B.H.C. 1938. The interpretation of potential changes in the spinal cord. J. Physiol. (Lond.) 92: 276-321.

(2) Beck, P.W.; Handwerker, H.O.; and Zimmermann, M. 1974. Nervous outflow from the cat's foot during noxious radiant heat stimulation. Brain Res. 67: 373-386.

(3) Brock, L.G.; Coombs, J.S.; and Eccles, J.C. 1952. The recording of potentials from motoneurons with an intracellular electrode. J. Physiol. 117: 431-460.

(4) Brown, A.G., and Fyffe, R.E.W. 1978. The morphology of group la afferent fibre collaterals in the spinal cord of the cat. J. Physiol. 274: 111-127.

(5) Brown, A.G., and Iggo, A. 1967. A quantitative study of cutaneous receptors and afferent fibres in the cat and rabbit. J. Physiol. 193: 707-733.

(6) Brown, A.G.; Rose, P.K.; and Snow, P.J. 1977. The morphology of hair follicle afferent collaterals in the spinal cord of the cat. J. Physiol. 272: 779-797.

(7) Burgess, P.F., and Perl, E. 1973. Cutaneous mechanoreceptors and nociceptors. In Handbook of Sensory Physiology, ed. A. Iggo, vol. II, pp. 29-78. Heidelberg: Springer.

(8) Burke, R.E.; Walmsley, B.; and Hodgson, J.A. 1979. HRP anatomy of group la afferent controls on alpha motoneurons. Brain Res. 160: 347-352.

(9) Cervero, F., and Iggo, A. 1978. Reciprocal sensory interaction in the spinal cord. J. Physiol. 284: 84-85P.

(10) Cervero, F.; Iggo, A.; and Molony, V. 1979. An electrophysiological study of neurons in the substantia gelatinosa Rolandi of the cat's spinal cord. Q. J. exp. Physiol. 64: 297-314.

(11) Cervero, F.; Iggo, A.; and Ogawa, H. 1976. Nociceptor-driven dorsal horn neurons in the lumbar spinal cord of the cat. Pain 2: 5-24.

(12) Cervero, F.; Molony, V.; and Iggo, A. 1977. Extracellular and intracellular recordings from neurons in the substantia gelatinosa Rolandi. Brain Res. 136: 565-569.

(13) Christensen, B.N., and Perl, E.R. 1970. Spinal neurons specifically excited by noxious or thermal stimuli: marginal zone of the dorsal horn. J. Neurophysiol. 33: 293-307.

(14) Cullheim, S., and Kellerth, J.O. 1976. Combined light and electron microscopical tracing of neurons, including axons and axon terminals, after intracellular injection of horseradish peroxidase. Neurosci. Lett. 2: 307-313.

(15) Denny-Brown, D.; Kirk, E.J.; and Yanagisawa, N. 1973. The tract of Lissauer in relation to sensory transmission in the dorsal horn of spinal cord in the Macaque monkey. J. comp. Neurol. 151: 175-200.

(16) Eccles, R.M., and Lundberg, A. 1959. Supraspinal control of interneurones mediating spinal reflexes. J. Physiol. 147: 565-584.

(17) Frank, K., and Fuortes, M.G.F. 1957. Presynaptic and postsynaptic inhibition of monosynaptic reflexes. Fed. Proc. 16: 39-40.

(18) Handwerker, H.O.; Iggo, A.; and Zimmermann, M. 1975. Segmental and supraspinal actions on dorsal horn neurons responding to noxious and non-noxious skin stimuli. Pain 1: 147-165.

(19) Holmqvist, B.; Lundberg, A.; and Oscarsson, O. 1960. Supraspinal inhibitory control of transmission to three ascending spinal pathways influenced by the flexion reflex afferents. Arch. ital. Biol. 98: 60-80.

(20) Hongo, T.; Jankowska, E.; and Lundberg, A. 1966. Convergence of excitatory and inhibitory action on interneurones in the lumbosacral cord. Exp. Brain Res. 1: 338-358.

(21) Iggo, A. 1960. Cutaneous mechanoreceptors with afferent C fibres. J. Physiol. 152: 337-353.

(22) Iggo, A. 1974, Cutaneous receptors. In The Peripheral Nervous System, ed. J.I. Hubbard, pp. 347-404. New York, London: Plenum Press.

(23) Jänig, W.; Schmidt, R.F.; and Zimmermann, M. 1968. Two specific feedback pathways to the central afferent terminals of phasic and tonic mechanoreceptors. Exp. Brain Res. 6: 116-129.

(24) Jankowska, E.; Rastad, J.; and Westman, J. 1976. Intracellular application of horseradish peroxidase and its light and electron microscopical appearance in spinocervical tract cells. Brain Res. 105: 557-562.

(25) LeBars, D.; Dickenson, A.H.; and Besson, J.-M. 1979. Diffuse noxious inhibitory controls (DNIC). I. Effects on dorsal horn convergent neurons in the rat. Pain 6: 283-304.

(26) Light, A.R., and Perl, E.R. 1979a. Reexamination of the dorsal root projection to the spinal dorsal horn including observations on the differential termination of coarse and fine fibers. J. comp. Neurol. 186: 117-132.

(27) Light, A.R., and Perl, E.R. 1979b. Spinal termination of functionally identified primary afferent neurons with slowly conducting myelinated fibers. J. comp. Neurol. 186: 133-150.

(28) Light, A.R.; Trevino, D.L.; and Perl, E.R. 1979. Morphological features of functionally defined neurones in the marginal zone and substantia gelatinosa of the spinal dorsal horn. J. comp. Neurol. 186: 151-172.

(29) Melzack, R., and Wall, P.D. 1965. Pain mechanisms: A new theory. Science 150: 971-979.

(30) Price, D.D., and Dubner, R. 1977. Neurons that subserve the sensory-discriminative aspects of pain. Pain 3: 307-338.

(31) Ranson, S.W. 1915. Unmyelinated nerve-fibres as conductors of protopathic sensation. Brain 38: 381-389.

(32) Schmidt, R.F. 1973. Control of the access of afferent activity to somatosensory pathways. In Handbook of Sensory Physiology, ed. A. Iggo, vol. 1, pp. 151-206. Berlin, Heidelberg, New York: Springer Verlag.

(33) Snow, P.K.; Rose, P.J.; and Brown, A.G. 1976. Tracing axons and axon collaterals in spinal neurones using intracellular injection of horseradish peroxidase. Science N.Y. 191: 312-313.

(34) Wall, P.D. 1960. Cord cells responding to touch, damage and temperature of the skin. J. Neurophysiol. 23: 197-210.

(35) Wall, P.D.; Merrill, E.G.; and Yaksh, T.L. 1979. Responses of single units in laminae 2 and 3 of cat spinal cord. Brain Res. 160: 245-260.

(36) Weddell, G. 1960. Studies related to the mechanism of common sensibility. In Cutaneous Innervation, ed. W. Montagna, pp. 112-160. Oxford, London, New York, Paris: Pergamon Press.

(37) Willis, W.D. 1976. Spinothalamic system: physiological aspects. In Advances in Pain Research and Therapy, eds. J.J. Bonica and D. Albe-Fessard, vol. 1, pp. 215-223. New York: Raven Press.

(38) Zotterman, Y. 1939. Touch, pain and tickling: an electrophysiological investigation on cutaneous sensory nerves. J. Physiol. 95: 1-28.

Pain and Society, eds. H.W. Kosterlitz and L.Y. Terenius, pp. 141-160.
Dahlem Konferenzen 1980. Weinheim: Verlag Chemie GmbH.

Pharmacological Aspects of Segmental Pain Control

W. Zieglgänsberger
Max-Planck-Institut für Psychiatrie
8000 München 40, F. R. Germany

Abstract. Neurons in the dorsal horn of the mammalian spinal cord are known to relay afferent nociceptive information to rostral structures. Descending pathways originating from various supraspinal sites control this transmission at the segmental level. The action of narcotic analgesics is determined by a direct inhibitory action on spinal and supraspinal neurons concerned with pain transmission. Furthermore, there is evidence that pathways which reduce the activity of these relay neurons may be activated by opioids. Serotonergic, noradrenergic and dopaminergic transmitter mechanisms might be involved in these actions, which can be triggered by electrical stimulation and by microinjections of opioids into certain mesencephalic and diencephalic sites.

The recent introduction of sensitive histochemical and biochemical analytical methods has shown that sites in the spinal cord and in other areas of the central nervous system concerned with nociception are very rich in neuropeptides. Peptidergic neurons, e.g., in the substantia gelatinosa of the spinal cord or the trigeminal nuclear complex are ideally located to gain control over incoming nociceptive messages. Current research suggests that among these probably predominantly inhibitory acting interneurons there are enkephalinergic ones. Systemically and microintophoretically applied opioids reduce the firing rate of most neurons in the dorsal horn activated either synaptically or chemically by application of putative excitatory transmitters such as L-glutamate and substance P. This peptide has been demonstrated in primary afferent fibers and in axons and cell bodies in dorsal horn layers. The histochemical demonstration of the inhibitory acting peptide somatostatin in afferent fibers led to the speculation that this peptide might mediate primary afferent inhibition. Recently, neurotensin-containing axons and cell bodies were demonstrated in the dorsal horn. The role of this excitatory acting neuropeptide is unknown.

Several lines of evidence strongly suggest that various other peptides extracted from central and peripheral neuronal structures may function as chemical messengers in the spinal cord. However, no single peptide can yet be considered a proven neurotransmitter or neuromodulator in the mammalian CNS.

INTRODUCTION

Although not conclusive in every aspect, neurons in the marginal layer and the nucleus proprius (lamina IV,V,VI) of the dorsal horn of the spinal cord may be considered integral parts of the nociceptive system in the mammalian central nervous system. It is well established that nociceptive messages are not only relayed by these neurons but are modulated by segmental and descending influences (for review see (11,22,47, 48,58,93,106)). The heterogeneous population of small interneurons commonly addressed as substantia gelatinosa is most likely a site for inhibitory control ((60); for review see (47,82,93)). Most of these interneurons possess axons that branch abundantly and project to the dendritic tree of neurons located deeper in the dorsal horn. Their terminals form characteristic glomerulus-shaped contacts with dendritic spines, structures which may be involved in integrative and modulatory processes.

The dorsal horn of the spinal cord of all species investigated so far is among the richest in neuroactive peptides. Some of them were previously found only in the peripheral nerves of the intestinal tract or in hormone-producing cells. In the following, evidence will be provided that neuroactive peptides are likely parts of the somatosensory system. The extensive discussion here of a spinal site for a modulation of nociceptive information from the periphery should not overshadow the role of supraspinal mechanisms, which includes the predominantly depressant effect of serotonergic, noradrenergic, and dopaminergic pathways upon dorsal horn neuronal activity ((9,27,36, 97,); see also Basbaum, this volume).

THE ENDOGENOUS OPIOID SYSTEM IN THE SPINAL CORD

Enkephalin, Site of Action. Pre- Versus Postsynaptic Sites

Since the first reports of depressant effects of opioid alkaloids on nociceptive flexor reflexes (see (95)), a spinal site of action was established. The effects of systemically, topically, and iontophoretically applied opioids (for review see (9,64,97,101)) are mainly inhibitory on dorsal horn cells including those involved in nociception. Since the isolation, characterization, and synthesis of methionine- and leucine-enkephalin ((41); for review see (5,51,88,89)) there has been a great number of studies on the endogenous opioid systems, including studies of the electrophysiological effects of these compounds (for review see (64,101)). With few exceptions, the major action on neurons sensitive to opioid peptides is a decrease in excitability. These depressant actions are at least partially reversed by the opiate antagonist naloxone. It has been proposed that the depressant effects are produced via presynaptic action where the release of excitatory transmitter is decreased by opiates, and/or via postsynaptic effects by which the efficacy of an excitatory neurotransmitter, e.g., L-glutamate released from primary afferents, is decreased. Depending on the location, both mechanisms may be important in the overall effect of opioids.

Most studies suggest a clear postsynaptic effect of opioids. This is indicated in, e.g., neurons in laminae IV and V and motoneurons in the spinal cord where depolarization produced by L-glutamate (102) was markedly reduced by opioids (98,100, 105). No change in membrane potential or input resistance of these cells was produced during the application of opiates. The mechanism of this action is thought to be mainly due to a modulation of the chemically excitable Na-channel by the opioids. Recently, these findings were corroborated by studies performed in tissue cultures of spinal neurons (3). Furthermore, iontophoretically applied opioids decrease the rate of rise of EPSPs evoked by afferent fiber stimulation (98) and the facilitation produced by trains of pulses is abolished after systemic application (45). The typical postsynaptic response to afferent stimulation involved 3 separate responses: (a) a short latency high amplitude EPSP usually eliciting a few spikes, (b) an IPSP following the fast EPSP, (c) slowly rising EPSPs which most likely originate from small fiber input. These slowly rising EPSPs resembled synaptic activity induced by high intensity electrical stimulation of brain sites and of peripheral nerves ((31,73) and citations therein) and by noxious heat stimulation (Zieglgänsberger et al., unpublished observations). A decrease in rise time of EPSPs might be expected to be much more effective in blocking spike initiation triggered by slow synaptic potentials rather than those produced with powerful fast excitatory potentials. Similar observations have been made in cortical (81) and striatal neurons (28). The extracellular discharge pattern of cortical and striatal neurons following electrical stimulation of the ipsilateral of contralateral cortex was similar to that found in spinal neurons. With a latency of 3-25 ms, a series of action potentials were recorded; this was followed by a silent period of 10-80 ms and finally a late response was recorded which went on for 1-2 s. Similar to the effect in spinal cord neurons, opiate alkaloids and methionine-enkephalin (intravenously and/or iontophoretically applied) selectively blocked the late response in these cells.

Also these effects are most likely mediated via postsynaptic receptors as indicated by the finding that enkephalin also blocked the increase in firing rate produced by L-glutamate. It therefore seems possible to explain the differential effect of opiates on small fiber activation by a postsynaptic change in the rise time of the synaptic potentials. A differential effect on synaptic potentials originating from small caliber fiber stimulation rather than those from larger fibers would then explain the well-known selectivity of opioids on pain messages.

Current research suggests that in addition to postsynaptic opiate receptors, opiate-sensitive sites might also be located on terminals of primary afferent fibers. It has been observed that dorsal root rhizotomy decreases the number of binding sites for opioids by about 50% (53). Electrophysiological studies which favor such an additional presynaptic site of action (12,45) were performed in cat spinal cord or in cultured dorsal root ganglia (see below). A preferential decrease in the excitability of small unmyelinated (C- and A-delta) afferents has been recorded employing Wall's technique following systemic or iontophoretic applications of opioids (13,77,78) to cats.

In cultured dorsal root ganglia, the action of opiates has been studied by several groups. Stimulation of these cells with an extracellular electrode resulted in a complex multi-unit potential recorded in the dorsal horn areas of fetal mouse spinal cord explants (15). This multi-unit potential was markedly attenuated by low concentrations (100 nM) of opioids in a naloxone-sensitive and stereospecific manner. In another study, synaptic potentials were recorded intracellularly in cultured spinal neurons by stimulation of single dorsal root ganglion cells with intracellular current injection (56). Iontophoretic application of opiates onto these spinal neurons induced a significant decrease in synaptically evoked potentials. This effect was interpreted as being mediated via presynaptically located receptors. Another action of opiates and opioid peptides on cultured dorsal root ganglion cells was to decrease the duration of the action potential (63). This effect is thought to be due to interference with calcium conductance, however, other ion species have not yet been ruled out. Biochemical and pharmacological data suggest an important role of calcium in the actions of opioids in the nervous system. Experimental evidence that morphine and opioid peptides interfere with the presynaptic release of transmitter via a Ca^{++}-dependent mechanism was obtained most recently from studies performed in the mouse vas deferens, a tissue where presynaptic effects of opiates are well established ((43); for review see (64)). This supports the hypothesis that opiates reduce the availability of calcium ions necessary for the stimulus-release coupling in presynaptic terminals.

The Substantia Gelatinosa ROLANDI: An Enkephalinergic Gating System?

Enkephalinergic control mechanisms of substantia gelatinosa neurons have been inferred from findings in different laboratories (see also (105)).

The dorsal horn of all species investigated to date contains a large number of opiate binding sites (2,53,71). Histochemical studies have demonstrated cell bodies and axons containing enkephalin in this region ((23,40,94); see also Basbaum, this volume). Ultrastructural studies have shown that these neurons do not form axo-axonic contacts (24), which will be necessary for the presynaptic inhibitory mechanism suggested from pharmacological studies (44). Assuming then that enkephalins are neuromodulators reducing the efficacy of excitatory transmission, it might be postulated that the peptide should be released more like a local hormone influencing larger areas of the target neurons. No clear topographic relationship between the releasing cell and the target structure, in this case the dendrites of neurons located deeper in the dorsal horn, is to be expected (see also (105)). Interestingly, the inhibitory action on the discharge rate of these neurons was more pronounced when the opioids were applied to supposedly dendritic sites in laminae II-III (21).

It has been hypothesized that enkephalin-releasing neurons were in the sample of spontaneously active units recorded extra- and intracellularly from the substantia gelatinosa (14); see also Iggo, this volume). These neurons were inhibited by C-fiber activation and activated by A-fiber stimulation. If these neurons tonically released enkephalin, a nociceptive stimulus would reduce the inhibitory tone on cells originating in the spinothalamic system and facilitate the perception of noxious stimuli. The alerting function of such a stimulus may suggest it to be physiologically relevant. A-fiber stimulation would have the opposite effect: a reduction of nociception. Since microiontophoretically appled naloxone mainly excites dorsal horn cells, it may be assumed that the enkephalinergic system is tonically active. However, the hyperalgesic effects of systemically applied naloxone are generally not very marked and only demonstrable under certain experimental conditions (for refs. see (105)). This indicates that the tonic activity of the enkephalinergic system is quite low, although it cannot be excluded that naloxone is relatively inactive against endogenous enkephalin. Furthermore, since naloxone has actions other than those which involve interaction with the opioid receptors, such experiments ought to be controlled by studies with the (+)-naloxone which does not interact with these receptors but shares most of the unspecific actions of its pharmacologically active isomer (29). In the proposed enkephalinergic control system, descending pathways could either act directly on ascending neurons or via activation or inhibition of enkephalinergic neurons in the substantia gelatinosa. Only parts of the descending inhibition induced by electrical stimulation would then be naloxone-reversible (see below).

β-Endorphin

Recently, it became apparent that despite the fact that β-endorphin contains the sequence of methionine-enkephalin, the two systems are generically independent of each other. No β-endorphin-reactive material has been demonstrated in the spinal cord. That does not exclude a role of β-endorphin in this structure, e.g., following stress-induced release from the pituitary (76), but it should then be hormone-like. Several lines of evidence suggest that besides the enkephalins and endorphins other endogenous substances might play a role in the control of nociception (see (36,70)).

Other Peptide Candidates Involved in Somatosensory Perception

Substance P

There are several sites where there is growing evidence that substance P acts as a neurotransmitter substance as postulated already by Lembeck (54) (for refs. see (105)). Substance P immunoreactivity is found generally in small unmyelinated fibers associated with afferent nerve pathways but also in cell bodies in the dorsal horn (39,40). At all sites tested, substance P is mainly excitatory on neuronal discharge activity. Using intracellular recordings from spinal neurons of cat, the increase in excitability is associated with depolarization (50,52,104). The action of substance P is longlasting and obviously does not involve a conductance change of the postsynaptic (somatic) membrane. Short pulses of L-glutamate applied from the same pipette became more effective in evoking cell firing (104). The ionic mechanism of the depolarization has not been established. It has been suggested that substance P may excite exclusively nociceptive neurons (35). Although still an attractive hypothesis, more recent experimental findings shed some doubt on such a selective action ((105), and citations therein). Furthermore, evidence was provided that enkephalin and substance P most likely do not interact via axo-axonic synapses (20) in the dorsal horn (see above). The observed inhibitory action of enkephalin upon substance P induced neuronal activity may be attributed to a functional antagonism between these two peptides. The physiological significance of such an interaction is still obscure.

Somatostatin

The localization of somatostatin-like immunoreactivity at sites in the central and peripheral nervous system is probably not related to hormonal regulation and gives somatostatin a place among other neuroactive peptides (37,38,49). This peptide is found in nerve terminals of the spinal cord as has been demonstrated by immunohistochemistry (72) and in subcellular fraction studies (26). The action of somatostatin has been studied at several sites in the peripheral and central nervous systems, including the dorsal and ventral roots of frog spinal cord (69), cells in the laminae I-III of rat spinal cord (61), cortex, hypothalamus, cerebellum (75), hippocampus (19), and myenteric plexus of the guinea-pig ileum (96). With the exception of the hippocampus where somatostatin was reported to excite pyramidal cells (19), other studies indicate that it decreases neuronal excitability by a mechanism involving a conductance increase of the postsynaptic membrane. The inhibitory action of somatostatin on neurons in the dorsal horn and the close proximity of these neurons may be taken as evidence in favor of a role in primary afferent inhibition.

Neurotensin

The distribution of neurotensin in the CNS has been determined using radioimmunoassay and immunohistochemical techniques (49,91,92). Neuronal cell bodies and axons containing neurotensin-immunoreactive material were found in structures including the substantia gelatinosa, trigeminal nucleus, amygdala, anterior pituitary and hypothalamic nuclei.

Some preliminary electrophysiological studies on the action of neurotensin on neurons in the CNS have been made. Neurons in several areas which have a relatively high density of binding sites for, and high levels of, neurotensin were studied. These areas include frontal cortex, hippocampus, striatum and lateral thalamus (103) and laminae I-IV of the spinal cord (62). The predominant effect produced by iontophoretically applied neurotensin was an increase in firing rate with a time course similar to that of substance P. The physiological role of neurotensin is still obscure.

Descending Systems Involved in the Modulation of Nociceptive Input

The link between the descending serotonergic and monoaminergic systems and opioid- or stimulus-induced antinociception is well established (for review see, e.g., (1,9,36,58,70,97); and Basbaum; Besson, this volume). However, various other pathways using still unknown transmitters could be involved in both opioid- and stimulus-induced modulation of nociceptive input. Current research suggests that they exert their modulatory influence on the spinal neurons as well as on rostral structures (27).

An indirect effect of opioids via activation of descending inhibitory pathways was first postulated by Takagi (85). Single unit recordings in the dorsal horn have established the inhibitory function of such pathways ((4,7,32,55,67,84); for review see (58)).

How the activation of descending pathways is brought about is still unknown. Since opioids are generally inhibitory, such an activating action might be due to disinhibition comparable to mechanisms observed in the hippocampus (99). Excitatory effects on several groups of neurons in the brain stem following systemic (18,66) or iontophoretic application (79,86) have been observed.

Serotonin-containing neurons descending from the ventral raphe complex have been demonstrated to impinge on dorsal horn neurons ((17,68), and citations therein). Microiontophoretic application of serotonin onto spinal neurons reduces their discharge activity, a finding consistent with an inhibitory role of these pathways (6,33,74).

The main contributions of the descending noradrenergic system derive from the nucleus reticularis lateralis (16) and the locus coeruleus (65). Electrical stimulation of the bulbar reticular formation of the rabbit (nucleus reticularis paragigantocellularis) inhibits the firing of neurons located in lamina V of the dorsal horn (8,84). These neurons are also inhibited by iontophoretically applied noradrenaline (6,25,33). Although direct locus coeruleus projections to the spinal cord exist (30), mechanisms involving noradrenergic, serotonergic, and enkephalinergic links operative in concert might be postulated for the antinociceptive action observed after electrical stimulation of this structure (57,83).

Acute and chronic opioid actions are closely related to dopaminergic mechanisms (see (10,87)). The studies performed by Jurna and co-workers established the involvment of the nigrostriatal feedback system in the antinociception ((34,46), and citations therein). A synopsis of the most complex data obtained by various groups of investigators gives credence to the belief that stimulation of the dopamine-system inhibits opioid-induced antinociception also at the spinal level, whereas depression of this system by dopamine antagonists potentiates the effects of the narcotic analgesics (for refs. see (59,90)).

CONCLUSION

From the present data it can be concluded that opioids have direct inhibitory actions on structures throughout the part of the neuroaxis which receives input from nociceptive pathways. These sites may include structures which make important contributions to opioid actions by modifying the affective and motivational tone. The opiate-induced antinociception may furthermore be related to the activation of descending inhibitory control systems operative in the spinal cord. The analysis of the functional relevance of peptidergic mechanisms involved in somatosensory perception will remain a most exciting area of research.

REFERENCES

(1) Akil, H.; Watson, S.J.; Holman, R.B.; and Barchas, J.D. 1978. Parallels between the neuromodulator mechanisms of stimulation analgesia and morphine analgesia. In Factors Affecting the Action of Narcotics, eds. M.I. Adler, L. Manara and R. Samanin, pp. 565-578. New York: Raven Press.

(2) Atweh, S.F., and Kuhar, M.J. 1977. Autoradiographic localization of opiate receptors in rat brain. I. Spinal cord and lower medulla. Brain Res. 124: 53-67.

(3) Barker, J.L.; Neal, J.H.; Smith, T.G., Jr.; and Macdonald, R.C. 1978. Opiate peptide modulation of amino acid responses suggest novel form of neural communication. Science 199: 1451-1453.

(4) Barnes, C.D.; Fung, S.J.; and Adams, W.L. 1979. Inhibitory effect of substantia nigra on impulse transmission from nociceptors. Pain 6: 207-215.

(5) Beaumont, A., and Hughes, J. 1979. Biology of opioid peptides. Ann. Rev. Pharm. Tox. 19: 245-267.

(6) Belcher, G.; Ryall, R.W.; and Schaffner, R. 1978. The differential effect of 5-hydroxytryptamine, noradrenaline and raphe stimulation on nociceptive and non-nociceptive dorsal horn interneurones in the cat. Brain Res. 151: 307-321.

(7) Bennett, H.G.J., and Mayer, D.J. 1976. Effects of microinjected narcotic analgesics into the periaqueductal gray (PAG) on the response of rat spinal cord dorsal horn interneurones. Proc. Soc. Neurosci. 2: 928.

(8) Besson, J.M.; Guilbaud, G.; and Le Bars, D. 1975. Descending inhibitory influences exerted by the brain stem upon the activities of dorsal horn lamina I cells induced by intra-arterial injection of bradykinin into the limbs. J. Physiol. (Lond.) 248: 725-732.

(9) Besson, J.M., and Le Bars, D. 1978. Effect of morphine on the transmission of painful messages at the spinal level. In Factors Affecting the Action of Narcotics, eds. M.I. Adler, L. Manara and R. Samanin, pp. 103-124. New York: Raven Press.

(10) Bläsig, J. 1978. On the role of brain catecholamines in acute and chronic opiate action. In Developments in Opiate Research, ed. A. Herz, pp. 279-356. New York: Dekker.

(11) Brown, A.G. 1973. Ascending and long spinal pathways dorsal columns spinocervical tract and spinothalamic tract. In Handbook of Sensory Physiology II, ed. A. Iggo pp. 321-331. Berlin-Heidelberg-New York: Springer

(12) Calvillo, O. 1976. Presynaptic effects of opiates and their antagonists in the spinal cord of the cat. Proc. Can. Fed. Biol. Soc. 19: 171.

(13) Carstens, E.; Tulloch, I.F.; Zieglgänsberger, W.; and Zimmermann, M. 1979. Presynaptic excitability changes induced by morphine in single cutaneous afferent C- and A-fibers. Pflügers Arch. 379: 143-147.

(14) Cervero, F.; Molony, V.; and Iggo, A. 1977. Extra- and intracellular recordings from neurones in the substantia gelatinosa Rolandi. Brain Res. 136: 565-569.

(15) Crain, S.M.; Peterson, E.R., Crain, B.; and Simon, E.J. 1977. Selective opiate depression of sensory evoked synaptic networks in dorsal horn regions of spinal cord cultures. Brain Res. 133: 162-166.

(16) Dahlström, A., and Fuxe, K. 1964. Evidence for the existence of monoamine neurons in the central nervous system. I. Demonstration of monoamines in the cell bodies of brain stem neurons. Acta Phys. Scand. 64, Suppl. 231: 1-55.

(17) Dahlström, A., and Fuxe, K. 1965. Evidence for the existence of monoamine neurons in the central nervous system. II. Experimentally induced changes in the intraneuronal levels of bulbospinal neuron systems. Acta. Phys. Scand. 64, Suppl. 247: 1-85.

(18) Deakin, J.F.W.; Dickenson, A.H.; and Dostrovsky, J.O. 1977. Morphine effects on raphe magnus neurones. J. Physiol. (Lond.) 267: 43-45P.

(19) Dodd, J., and Kelly, J.F. 1978. Is somatostatin an excitatory transmitter in the hippocampus? Nature 273: 674-675.

(20) Duggan, A.W.; Griesmith, B.T.; Headley, P.M.; and Hall, J.G. 1979. Lack of effect by substance P at sites in the substantia gelatinosa where met-enkephalin reduces the transmission of nociceptive impulses. Neurosci. Lett. 12: 313-317.

(21) Duggan, A.W.; Hall, J.G.; and Headley, P.M. 1976. Morphine, enkephalin and the substantia gelatinosa. Nature (Lond.) 264: 456-458.

(22) Dykes, R.W. 1975. Nociception. Brain Res. 99: 229-245.

(23) Elde, R.; Hökfelt, T.; Johansson, O.; and Terenius, L. 1976. Immunohistochemical studies using antibodies to leucine-enkephalin: initial observations on the nervous system of the rat. Neuroscience 1: 349-351.

(24) Emson, P.C.; Hunt, S.P.; Rehfeld, J.F.; and Fahrenkrug, J. 1979. Neurochemical studies on several brain peptides. In Regulation and Function of Neural Peptides, ed. M. Trabucchi. New York: Raven Press, in press.

(25) Engberg, I., and Ryall, R.W. 1966. The inhibitory action of noradrenaline and other monoamines on spinal neurones. J. Physiol. (Lond.) 185: 298-308.

(26) Epelbaum, J.; Brazeau, P.; Tsang, D.; Brawery, J.; and Martin, J.B. 1977. Subcellular distribution of radioimmunoassayable somatostatin in rat brain. Brain Res. 126: 309-323.

(27) Fields, H.L., and Basbaum, A. 1978. Brain stem control of spinal pain transmission neurones. Ann. Rev. Physiol. 40: 193-221.

(28) Fry, J.P., and Zieglgänsberger, W. 1979. Comparison of the effects of GABA and enkephalin on synaptically evoked activity in the rat striatum. Applied Neurophys. 42: 54-56.

(29) Fry, J.P.; Zieglgänsberger, W.; and Herz, A. 1979. A demonstration of naloxone-precipitated opiate withdrawal on single neurones in the morphine-tolerant/dependent rat brain. Brit. J. Pharm. in press.

(30) Hancock, M.B., and Fougerousse, C.L. 1976. Spinal projections from the nucleus locus coeruleus and nucleus subcoeruleus in the cat and monkey as demonstrated by retrograde transport of horse radish peroxidase. Brain Res. Bull. 1: 229-234.

(31) Handwerker, H.O.; Iggo, A.; and Zimmermann, M. 1975. Segmental and supraspinal actions on dorsal horn neurons responding to noxious and non-noxious skin stimulation. Pain 1: 147-165.

(32) Hayes, R.L.; Price, D.D.; Ruda, M.; and Dubner, R. 1979. Suppression of nociceptive responses in the primate by electrical stimulation of the brain or morphine administration; behavioral and electrophysiological comparisons. Brain Res. 167: 417-421.

(33) Headley, P.M.; Duggan, A.W.; and Griesmith, B.T. 1978. Selective reduction of noradrenaline and 5-hydroxytryptamine of nociceptive responses of cat dorsal horn neurones. Brain Res. 145: 185-200.

(34) Heinz, G., and Jurna, I. 1979. The anti-nociceptive effect of reserpine and haloperidol mediated by the nigrostriatal system: Antagonism by naloxone. Naunyn-Schmiedeberg's Arch. Pharmacol. 306: 97-100.

(35) Henry, J.L. 1976. Effects of substance P on functionally identified units in cat spinal cord. Brain Res. 114: 431-451.

(36) Herz, A. 1978. Sites of opiate action in the central nervous system. In Developments in Opiate Research, ed. A. Herz, pp. 153-191. New York: Dekker.

(37) Hökfelt, T.; Efendic, S.; Hellerström, C.; Johannsson, O.; Luft, R.; and Arimura, A. 1975. Cellular localization of somatostatin in endocrine-like cells and neurons of the rat with special references to the A. cells of the pancreatic islets and the hypothalamus. Acta Endocrinologica Suppl. 200: 5-41.

(38) Hökfelt, T.; Elfuin, L.G.; Elde, R.; Schultzberg, M.; Goldstein, M.; and Luft, R. 1977. Occurrence of somatostatin-like immunoreactivity in some peripheral sympathetic noradrenergic neurons. Proc. Natl. Acad. Sci. 74: 3587-3591.

(39) Hökfelt, T.; Kellerth, J.O.; Nilsson, G.; and Pemow, B. 1975. Experimental immunohistochemical studies on the localization and distribution of substance P in cat primary sensory neurones. Brain Res. 100: 235-252.

(40) Hökfelt, T.; Ljungdahl, A.; Terenius, L.; Elde, R.; and Nilsson, G. 1977. Immunohistochemical analysis of peptide pathways possibly related to pain and analgesia: Enkephalin and substance P. Proc. Acad. Sci. 74: 3081-3085.

(41) Hughes, J.; Smith, T.W.; Kosterlitz, H.W.; Forthergill, L.A.; Morgan, B.A.; and Morris, H.R. 1975. Identification of two related pentapeptides from the brain with potent opiate agonist activity. Nature 258: 577-579.

(42) Hunt, S.P.; Emson, P.C.; and Kelly, J.S. 1979. The immunohistochemical localization of met-enkephalin within the rat spinal cord: Light and electronmicroscopic observations. Neurosci. Lett. Suppl. 3: 200.

(43) Illes, P.; Zieglgänsberger, W.; and Herz, A. 1979. Normorphine inhibits neurotransmission in the mouse vas deferens by a calcium-dependent mechanism. Neurosci. Lett. Suppl. 3: 238.

(44) Jessel, T.M., and Iversen, L.L. 1977. Opiate analgesics inhibit substance P release from rat trigeminal nucleus. Nature (Lond.) 268: 549-551.

(45) Jurna, I.; Grossmann, W.; and Theres, C. 1973. Inhibition by morphine of repetitive activations of cat spinal motoneurones. Neuropharmacology 12: 983-993.

(46) Jurna, I.; Heinz, G.; Blinn, G.; and Nell, T. 1978. The effect of substantia nigra stimulation and morphine on α-motoneurones and the tail-flick response. Europ. J. Pharmacol. 51: 239-250.

(47) Kerr, F.W.L. 1975. Neuroanatomical substrates of nociception in the spinal cord. Pain 1: 325-356.

(48) Kerr, F.W.L., and Casey, K.L. 1978. Pain. Neurosci. Res. Prog. 16: 1, MIT Press.

(49) Kobayashi, R.M.; Brown, M.; and Vale, W. 1977. Regional distribution of neurotensin and somatostatin in rat brain. Brain Res. 126: 584-588.

(50) Konishi, S., and Otsuka, M. 1974. The effects of substance P and other peptides on spinal neurones of the frog. Brain Res. 65: 397-410.

(51) Kosterlitz, H.W. 1979. Endogenous opioid peptides and the control of pain. Psychol. Med. 9: 1-4.

(52) Krnjević, K. 1977. Effects of substance P on central neurones in cats. In Substance P, eds. U.S. von Euler and B. Pernow, pp. 217-230. New York: Raven Press.

(53) La Motte, C.; Pert, C.B.; and Snyder, S.H. 1976. Opiate receptor binding in primate spinal cord distribution and changes after dorsal root section. Brain Res. 112: 407-412.

(54) Lembeck, F. 1953. Zur Frage der zentralen Übertragung afferenter Impulse. III. Das Vorkommen und die Bedeutung der Substanz P in den dorsalen Wurzeln des Rückenmarks. Naunyn-Schmiedeberg's Arch. Pharmacol. 219: 107-213.

(55) Liebeskind, J.C.; Giesler, G.J.; and Urca, G. 1976. Evidence pertaining to an endogenous mechanism of pain inhibition in the central nervous system. In Sensory Functions of the Skin of Primates, with Special Reference to Man, ed. J. Zottermann. Wenner-Gren Internat. Symp. Series. Oxford: Pergamon Press.

(56) Macdonald, R.L., and Nelson, P.G. 1978. Specific-opiate induced depression of transmitter release from dorsal root ganglion cells in culture. Science 199: 1449-1451.

(57) Margalit, D., and Segal, M. 1979. A pharmacologic study of analgesia produced by stimulation of the locus coeruleus. Psychopharmacology 62: 169-173.

(58) Mayer, D.J., and Price, D.D. 1976. Central nervous system mechanisms of analgesia. Pain 2: 379-404.

(59) McGilliard, K.L., and Takemori, A.E. 1979. The effect of dopaminergic modifiers on morphine-induced analgesia and respiratory depression. Europ. J. Pharmacol. 54: 61-68.

(60) Melzack, R., and Wall, P.D. 1965. Pain mechanisms: A new theory. Science 150: 971-979.

(61) Miletić, V.; Kavacs, M.S.; and Randić, M. 1977. Actions of somatostatin and methionine-enkephalin on cat dorsal horn neurons activated by noxious stimuli. Neuroscience Abs. 3: 488.

(62) Miletić, V., and Randić, M. 1978. Excitatory action of neurotensin on cat dorsal horn neurons in Lamina I-III. Abst. 7th Intern. Cong. Pharmacol., 472.

(63) Mudge, A.W.; Leemann, S.E.; and Fischbach, G.D. 1979. Enkephalin inhibits release of substance P from sensory neurones in cultures and decreases action potential duration. Proc. Natl. Acad. Sci. 76: 526-530.

(64) North, R.A. 1979. Opiates, opioid peptides and single neurones. Life Sci. 24: 1527-1546.

(65) Nygren, L.G., and Olson, L. 1977. A new major projection from locus coeruleus: the main source of noradrenergic nerve terminals in the ventral and dorsal columns of the spinal cord. Brain Res. 132: 85-93.

(66) Oleson, T.D., and Liebeskind, J.C. 1975. Relationship of neuronal activity in the raphe nuclei of the rat to brain stimulation-produced analgesia. Physiologist 18: 338-342.

(67) Oliveras, J.L.; Besson, J.M.; Guilbaud, G.; and Liebeskind, J.C. 1974. Behavioral and electrophysiological evidence of pain inhibition from midbrain stimulation in the cat. Exp. Brain Res. 20: 32-44.

(68) Oliveras, J.L.; Bourgoin, S.; Hery, F.; Besson, J.M.; and Hamon, M. 1977. The topographical distribution of serotonergic terminals in the spinal cord of the cat: biochemical mapping by the combined use of microdissection and microassay techniques. Brain Res. 138: 393-406.

(69) Padjen, A.L. 1977. Effects of somatostatin on frog spinal cord. Neuroscience Abs. 3: 411.

(70) Pert, A. 1978. Central sites involved in opiate actions. In The Bases of Addiction, ed. J. Fishman, pp. 299-332. Berlin: Dahlem Konferenzen. Life Sci. Rep. 8.

(71) Pert, C.B.; Kuhar, M.J.; and Snyder, S.H. 1975. Autoradiographic localization of the opiate receptor in rat brain. Life Sci. 16: 1849-1854.

(72) Petrusz, P.; Sar, M.; Grossman, G.H.; and Kizer, J.S. 1977. Synaptic terminals with somatostatin-like immunoreactivity in the rat brain. Brain Res. 137: 181-187.

(73) Price, D.D.; Hull, C.D.; and Buchwald, N.A. 1971. Intracellular responses of dorsal horn cells to cutaneous and sural nerve A and C fiber stimuli. Exp. Neurol. 33: 291-309.

(74) Randić, M., and Yu, H.H. 1976. Effects of 5-hydroxytryptamine and bradykinin in cat dorsal horn neurons activated by noxious stimuli. Brain Res. 111: 197-203.

(75) Renaud, L.P.; Martin, J.B.; and Brazeau, P. 1975. Depressant action of TRH, LH-RH, and somatostatin on activity of central neurones. Nature 255: 233-235.

(76) Rossier, J.; French, E.D.; Rivier, C.; Ling, N.; Guillemin, R.; and Bloom, F.E. 1977. Foot shock induced stress increases ß-endorphin levels in blood but not brain. Nature 270: 618-620.

(77) Sastry, B.R. 1978. Morphine and met-enkephalin effects on sural A δ afferent terminal excitability. Europ. J. Pharmacol. 50: 269-273.

(78) Sastry, B.R. 1979. Presynaptic effects of morphine and methionine-enkephalin in feline spinal cord. Neuropharmacology 18: 367-375.

(79) Satoh, M.; Akaike, A.; and Takagi, H. 1979. Excitation by morphine and enkephalin of single neurons of nucleus reticularis paragigantocellularis in the rat: a probable mechanism of analgesic action of opioids. Brain Res. 169: 406-410.

(80) Satoh, M.; Nakamura, N.; and Takagi, H. 1971. Effects of morphine on bradykinin-induced unitary discharges in the spinal cord of the rabbit. Europ. J. Pharmacol. 16: 245-250.

(81) Satoh, M.; Zieglgänsberger, W.; Fries, W.; and Herz, A. 1974. Opiate agonist-antagonist interaction at cortical neurones of naive and tolerant/dependent rats. Brain Res. 82: 378-382.

(82) Schmidt, R.F. 1971. Presynaptic inhibition in the vertebrate central nervous system. Erg. Physiol. 63: 20-101.

(83) Segal, M., and Sandberg, D. 1977. Analgesia produced by electrical stimulation of catecholamine nuclei in the rat brain. Brain Res. 123: 369-372.

(84) Takagi, H.; Doi, T.; and Kawasaki, K. 1975. Effects of morphine, l-dopa, tetrabenazine on the lamina V cells of the spinal cord. Life Sci. 17: 67-72.

(85) Takagi, H.; Matsumara, M.; Yanai, A.; and Ogiu, K. 1955. The effect of analgesics on the reflex activity of the cat. Jap. J. Pharmacol. 4: 176-187.

(86) Takagi, H.; Satoh, M.; Akaike, A.; Shibata, T.; Yajima, H.; and Ogawa, H. 1978. Analgesia by enkephalins injected into the nucleus reticularis gigantocellularis of rat medulla oblongata. Europ. J. Pharmacol. 49: 113-116.

(87) Takemori, A.E. 1976. Pharmacologic factors which alter the action of narcotic analgesics and antagonists. Ann. N.Y. Acad. Sci. 281: 262-280.

(88) Terenius, L. 1978. Endogenous peptides and analgesia. Ann Rev. Pharm. Tox. 18: 189-204.

(89) Teschemacher, H.J. 1978. Endogenous ligands of opiate receptors (endorphins). In Developments in Opiate Research, ed. A. Herz, pp. 67-151. New York: Dekker.

(90) Tulunay, F.C.; Yano, T.; and Takemori, A.E. 1976. The effect of biogenic amine modifiers on morphine analgesia and its antagonism by naloxone. Europ. J. Pharmacol. 35: 285-291.

(91) Uhl, G.; Kuhar, M.J.; and Snyder, S.H. 1977. Neurotensin, a central nervous system peptide: Apparent receptor binding in brain membranes. Brain Res. 130: 299-313.

(92) Uhl, G., and Snyder, S.H. 1976. Regional and subcellular distribution of brain neurotensin. Life Sci. 19: 1827-1832.

(93) Wall, P.D. 1973. Dorsal horn electrophysiology. In Handbook of Sensory Physiology II, ed. A. Iggo, pp. 253-270. Berlin-Heidelberg-New York: Springer.

(94) Watson, S.J.; Akil, H.; and Barchas, J.D. 1977. Immunocytochemical localization of opiate peptides and beta-lipotropin in rat brain. Proc. Neurosci. 976.

(95) Wikler, A. 1950. Sites and mechanisms of action of morphine and related drugs in the central nervous system. Pharm. Rev. 2: 435-503.

(96) Williams, J.T., and North, R.A. 1979. Inhibition of firing of myenteric neurons by somatostatin. Brain Res. 155: 165-168.

(97) Yaksh, T.L., and Rudy, T.A. 1978. Narcotic analgesics: CNS sites of action as revealed by intracerebral injection techniques. Pain 4: 299-359.

(98) Zieglgänsberger, W., and Bayerl, J. 1976. The mechanism of inhibition of neuronal activity by opiates in the spinal cord of the cat. Brain Res. 115: 111-128.

(99) Zieglgänsberger, W.; French, E.D.; Siggins, G.B.; and Bloom, F.E. 1979. Opioid peptides may excite hippocampal pyramidal neurons by inhibiting adjacent inhibitory interneurons. Science 205: 415-417.

(100) Zieglgänsberger, W., and Fry, J.P. 1976. Actions of enkephalin on cortical and striatal neurones of naive and morphine tolerant/dependent rats. In Opiates and Endogenous Opioid Peptides, ed. H.W. Kosterlitz, pp. 231-238. Amsterdam: Elsevier/North-Holland Biomedical Press.

(101) Zieglgänsberger, W., and Fry J.P. 1978. Actions of opioids on single neurons. In Developments in Opiate Research, ed. A. Herz, pp. 193-239. New York: Dekker.

(102) Zieglgänsberger, W., and Puil, E.A. 1973. Actions of glutamic acid on spinal neurones. Exp. Brain Res. 17: 35-49.

(103) Zieglgänsberger, W.; Siggins, G.; Brown, M.; Vale, W.; and Bloom, F.E. 1978. Actions of neurotensin upon single neurone activity in different regions of the rat brain. Abst. 7th Intern. Cong. Pharmacol. 126.

(104) Zieglgänsberger, W., and Tulloch, I.F. 1979. Effects of substance P on neurones in the dorsal horn of the spinal cord. Brain Res. 166: 273-282.

(105) Zieglgänsberger, W., and Tulloch, I.F. 1979. The effects of methionine- and leucine-enkephalin on spinal neurones of the cat. Brain Res. 167: 53-64.

(106) Zimmermann, M. 1976. Neurophysiology of nociception. In Neurophysiology II. Int. Rev. of Physiol, ed. R. Porter, vol. 10, pp. 179-221. Baltimore-London-Tokyo: University Park Press.

Pain and Society, eds. H.W. Kosterlitz and L.Y. Terenius, pp. 161-182.
Dahlem Konferenzen 1980. Weinheim: Verlag Chemie GmbH.

Supraspinal Modulation of the Segmental Transmission of Pain

J.-M. R. Besson
Unité de Recherches de Neurophysiologie Pharmacologique
INSERM (U. 161), 75014 Paris, France

Abstract. The transmission of nociceptive messages at the spinal level is strongly modulated by descending influences originating in the brain stem. Studies, centered on dorsal horn convergent neurons activated by both innocuous and noxious stimuli, underlined the major role played by the periaqueductal gray matter and the nucleus raphe magnus. The preferential inhibitory effects on noxious activities of dorsal horn neurons caused by the stimulation of both of these areas could serve as a neurophysiological basis for an explanation of the powerful antinociception induced by such stimulations in freely moving animals and in man. These effects are mediated via the dorsolateral funiculus of the spinal cord which contains numerous fibers originating in the nucleus raphe magnus. However, several investigations indicate that these descending actions are not exclusively mediated by serotonergic mechanisms. The high density of raphe magnus projections at the level of the spinal cord, especially in the substantia gelatinosa of Rolando, suggests a possible participation of enkephalinergic interneurons in these controls. However, the implication of endogenous opiates in these phenomena and the modality of activation of these systems under normal or pathological conditions are still under discussion.

INTRODUCTION

Numerous investigations have demonstrated that descending pathways from the upper centers of the CNS can modify sensory or motor functions at the spinal level. The study of their influences on the activity of dorsal horn neurons driven by noxious inputs started at the end of the 1960s and has clearly established the effectiveness of the inhibitory descending systems in the modulation of nociceptive messages. The mechanisms involved in these phenomena, mainly originating in the cortex and the brain stem, are still extensively studied in an attempt to find a neurophysiological basis for the behavioral and clinical findings that stimulation produces antinociception and for the explanation of some mechanisms underlying the analgesic effects of morphine. In this presentation we will successively consider the influences of the cortex and more importantly those of brain stem areas - periaqueductal gray matter (PAG) and the raphe nuclei - the stimulation of which has powerful antinociceptive effects in freely moving animals and humans. Studies on the effects of descending controls on dorsal horn neurons receiving noxious inputs have centered on those neurons known variously as lamina V type, class 2, wide dynamic range, polymodal or convergent units. These cells receive both A and C fiber inputs and correspondingly respond to peripheral and deep stimuli in both the innocuous and noxious ranges. The neurons responding only to superficial noxious stimuli (class 3 units, according to Iggo (44)) which are located in laminae I and II, have been rarely studied in this respect.

DESCENDING CORTICAL PATHWAYS

In the cat, primary afferent depolarization, an index of presynaptic inhibition, can be evoked by electrical stimulation of the primary sensorimotor cortex, the SII area (5,20), and the orbital cortex (1); various anatomical studies suggest that the descending effects are mediated via the pyramidal tract, but may also be relayed in the brain stem. Direct evidence of these descending inhibitory effects has been obtained by recording from single units in the dorsal horn. Stimulation of the pyramidal tract and the orbital cortex (80) were found to inhibit strongly the activity of lamina IV type cells (class 1 cells activated only by non-noxious cutaneous stimulation) and, to a lesser extent, of convergent units;

some of these latter ones were clearly excited or responded by a mixed excitatory-inhibitory effect. Some neurons inhibited by pyramidal tract stimulation were found to ascend in the dorsolateral column (31); similarly, primary and secondary somato-sensory areas (16,19) were found to induce profound inhibition on neurons at the origin of the spinocervical tract (SCT).

Although the orbital cortex has been shown to depress the responses of convergent neurons to sustained pinch, no systematic attempts have been made in these studies to consider the corticofugal effects on responses induced by noxious stimuli on dorsal horn neurons. More relevant is the study of Coulter et al. (26) who found in the monkey that electrical stimulation of either the pre- or post-central gyrus in the hindlimb area produced a depression of the activity of convergent spinothalamic tract neurons (STT) recorded at the lumbar level. These cortical descending influences acted on the responses to low threshold natural stimulation (hair movements, skin displacement), while they showed little or no effect on the slowly adapting responses to intense mechanical or thermal stimulation. Interestingly, none of the 4 STT cells examined in the marginal layer of the spinal cord were influenced by cortical stimulation. The time course of these inhibitory effects was roughly parallel to those of various activities generally considered to reflect presynaptic inhibitory mechanisms; however, a postsynaptic site of action could not be ruled out even if IPSPs were only infrequently obtained in dorsal horn neurons after pyramidal stimulation (54).

From a functional point of view, these cortical areas may be involved in a negative feed-back loop by controlling their own afferents; on the basis of the preferential effect of stimulation of the sensorimotor cortex on responses of convergent STT neurons to non-noxious stimuli, corticofugal effects have been interpreted "as a switching of these neurons from detectors of weak stimuli to detectors of intense stimuli" (26). However further investigations, including the exploration of other areas, are needed in order to investigate the role of the cerebral cortex in the spinal modulation of cutaneous inputs.

DESCENDING PATHWAYS ORIGINATING IN THE BRAIN STEM

Initial studies have shown that stimulation of wide areas of the brain stem induces presynaptic inhibition of cutaneous afferent fibers and that electrical stimulation of the mesencephalic tegmentum and central pontobulbar core produce an inhibition of various activities of units located in the dorsolateral fasciculus supposedly in the SCT (76). Another approach to these systems was the use, mainly in decerebrate preparations of a reversible cold block of the spinal cord rostral to the recording site in order to gauge the degree of tonic descending influences on these cells by comparing their response characteristics before and during the temporary spinalization. In decerebrate animals, thoracic cold block was found to increase the excitability, spontaneous activity, and receptive field size of lumbar convergent neurons (77). These effects were due to descending effects from supraspinal levels and not intraspinal influences, because spinal sections at C_1 produce very similar effects. Other workers confirmed these general findings and furthermore found preferential effects on reponses to noxious stimuli: a clear enhancement during cold block was observed for responses of convergent neurons to radiant heat and to C fibers while responses to weak mechanical stimuli were unaffected (38). Descending tonic inhibitory effects on responses to noxious radiant heat were also described in the rat; correspondingly, when the spinal cord was blocked, the threshold of these neurons to thermal stimuli was reduced (61). More precisely, preferential effects on responses of SCT neurons to heavy pressure, pinch, and noxious radiant heat have been described (14,15,24). Similarly the excitatory effects on SCT neurons of nociceptive chemical stimulation of the gastrocnemius-soleus muscle were of minor importance in the decerebrate state but clearly revealed or enhanced during the temporary spinalization by cold block (41). These findings are in good agreement with our previous observations related to the bradykinin-induced activity of convergent units in the spinal and decerebrate cat (12). Although in the cat (25), weaker descending influences have also been described on neurons exclusively driven by noxious stimuli, further information is required on the effects of descending controls on these neurons. In any case, all the studies related to convergent neurons clearly demonstrate the existence, the strength, and the tonicity of the descending inhibitory controls of supraspinal origin. More recent studies have considered the neuronal effects induced by brain stem areas, the stimulation of which produces profound antinociceptive effects in man and animals. The fact that stimulation of these brain stem areas exert powerful effects on spinal (57) or trigeminal (67) reflexes evoked by noxious stimulation suggests that antinociception may be partly mediated by the activation of descending inhibitory actions on those spinal dorsal horn and trigeminal neurons which appear to participate in the central transmission of noxious messages. The findings related to stimulation that produces antinociception have recently been reviewed extensively (11,33,50,56), and this presentation will be limited mainly to the pertinent electrophysiological investigations. From the extensive mapping studies (63) we performed on the chronic cat, which included 300 stimulation sites spread over the whole brain stem between the mesencephalon and the medulla, it appears that two areas play a major role in stimulation-induced antinociception: namely, the PAG as initially reported by Reynolds (1971) and extensively studied by Mayer et al. (57), and the raphe nuclei, consisting of the nucleus raphe dorsalis (DRN) at the level of the PAG, the nucleus centralis superior and the more ventral raphe centralis inferior comprising nucleus raphe pontis and nucleus raphe magnus. The most powerful effects are obtained from the nucleus raphe magnus (NRM) (66).

Stimulation of the PAG

The powerful behavioral antinociceptive effects induced by stimulation of the PAG in the cat prompted our group to study in this species in acute experiments the effects of PAG stimulation on dorsal horn neuronal activity (51,62). Inhibitory effects were rarely found on neurons only activated by non-noxious cutaneous stimuli whereas 88% of convergent neurons had their activity depressed by the central stimulation. The activities inhibited were those induced by noxious radiant heat, the long latency response to intense electrical simulation of the receptive field and, as a preferred experimental procedure, the responses of the neurons to strong cutaneous mechanical stimulation. The inhibitions were in most cases profound, generally causing depression of the evoked neuronal activity by at least 50%; the inhibitory effects outlasted the period of stimulation by only several seconds. In several experiments the response to noxious stimuli was almost abolished while the response of the same cell to innocuous stimuli was unaffected. Confirmation of these effects has been obtained recently (23,29), when it was found that ventral PAG stimulation decreases the slope of the curve of discharge to noxious radiant heat against temperature without changing the extrapolated threshold (23); in another study, however, such preferential effects on noxious responses were rarely observed after PAG stimulation (29). In addition, recent electrophysiological studies (52,75,84) showing a depression of trigeminal neuronal responses to tooth pulp stimulation by PAG correlate well with our earlier study (67) in which we reported that PAG stimulation in chronic cats produces a preferential inhibition of a nociceptive trigeminal reflex.

The inhibition of neuronal responses by PAG stimulation is obviously not a prerequisite for antinociception as the effective sites in the electrophysiological studies include the whole PAG and adjacent reticular areas. In contrast, behavioral studies have shown that the effective sites in producing antinociception are confined to the ventral PAG within and around the DRN. However pharmacological observation (36) revealed that only the neuronal inhibitions caused by stimulation of sites producing antinociception are antagonized by intravenous D-lysergic acid diethylamide (LSD) which has been shown to inhibit the firing of serotonergic raphe neurons; methysergide, a putative serotonin (5-HT) antagonist, has similar properties (21). Furthermore, depletion of 5-HT by p-chlorophenylalanine (pCPA) reduces the inhibitory effects of PAG stimulation on dorsal horn neurons (21). These electrophysiological approaches agree well with behavioral studies which demonstrate a considerable reduction in stimulation-induced antinociception by pCPA pretreatment (3) and a partial antagonism by LSD (39). They suggest that 5-HT neurons are a main link in these inhibitory phenomena although the pathways involved are not clearly understood. There is no clear evidence for direct spinal projections from the PAG and it is well-known that the DRN has dense rostral projections, suggesting a possible action on supraspinal transmission and perception of pain. In this connection the observation is of importance that stimulation of the PAG produces a modality-specific inhibition of neurons located in the nucleus gigantocellularis of the lower brain stem which respond to noxious stimulation (60). This effect could be attributed to a direct projection from the PAG, but strong support for the idea of the involvement of descending pathways arises from experiments in animals where chronic unilateral sectioning of the dorsolateral funiculus (DLF) reduces the antinociceptive effect of stimulation of the PAG when noxious stimuli are applied to the cutaneous areas ipsilateral and caudal to the lesion (7,8). Since there is a paucity of direct spinal projections from the PAG, it may be concluded from these experiments that the antinociceptive effect caused by stimulation of the PAG are relayed by other stuctures. The major candidate for this role is the nucleus raphe magnus (NRM). Stimulation of this structure has a powerful antinociceptive effect in chronic animals (66) and, as will be discussed later, produces inhibitions of dorsal horn neurons. The NRM has dense projections to the spinal cord via the dorsolateral funiculus (DLF), and there is both anatomical and electrophysiological evidence for projections from the PAG or DRN to the NRM (see Basbaum, this volume). However, the lesioning of the DLF does not provide definitive evidence for an action of the PAG via the NRM as the DLF does not exclusively contain fibers from the NRM and the studies have only been made in chronic animals. An investigation of the effect of sectioning of the DLF on the inhibitions by the PAG of the dorsal horn neurons is required as is the effect of PAG stimulation after destruction of the NRM from both behavioral and electrophysiological approaches.

Stimulation of the NRM

Since our initial work (49) reporting strong inhibitory effects on convergent neurons following NRM stimulation, many studies have confirmed these findings in the cat (7,10,29,34,37,43,52,58), monkey (9,79), and rat (73) using responses of the neurons to intense mechanical stimuli or noxious heat. In general, the effects observed last longer than those obtained with PAG stimulation. As regards the selectivity of the inhibitions, we found several neurons had their responses to weak mechanical stimuli unaffected (37), a finding recently confirmed in the cat (29) but not in the monkey (79). However, when peripheral nerves were stimulated, NRM stimulation was found to influence more effectively the responses due to activation of thin myelinated afferent fibers than those due to activation of large fibers (79). We have found similar effects in the rat and, in addition, observed powerful reductions of the activity due to activation of unmyelinated fibers (74). This preferential effect of NRM stimulation on dorsal horn neuronal responses to noxious inputs may result from differences in the synaptic efficiency of large ($A\alpha\beta$) and thin ($A\delta$ and C) afferent fiber inputs. When the responses of neurons only driven by non-noxious stimuli are considered, NRM stimulation had no effect in two studies (34, 37) but, in a third report, sometimes influenced responses to light touch but rarely those due to hair movement (10).

The inhibition of the convergent neurons is especially relevant to the reduction of pain transmission to higher centers as some of these neurons convey nociceptive messages in the spinothalamic (9,79) and spinoreticular (59) tracts. All these data agree well with numerous studies demonstrating dense descending projections via the DLF from the NRM; these are discussed by A. Basbaum (this volume). Importantly, stimulation of the DLF produces powerful inhibitions of spinocervical tract neurons in decerebrate cats; the inhibitions were more effective against the activity produced by stimulation of thin myelinated and unmyelinated fibers (17,18). Correspondingly, lesions of the DLF abolish the neuronal inhibitions induced by NRM stimulation (7,34,79) but surprisingly the effect of DLF lesions on antinociception produced by NRM stimulation has not been investigated.

Involvement of 5-HT in the Descending Control Systems of the Brain Stem

The involvement of serotonergic mechanisms in the modulation of spinal transmission by the brain stem has been widely studied; however many problems remain to be resolved. Inital evidence originated from Lundberg's group who showed a role for 5-HT in tonic descending inhibitions on flexor reflex afferents in the decerebrate cat. This inhibition is reduced but not blocked by raphe lesions and is partially reversed by 5-HT antagonists (see refs. in (30)). The remaining, presumably nonserotonergic, inhibitory effects after raphe destruction probably act via the dorsal reticulospinal tract which is rapidly conducting, unlike the serotonergic fibers which are thought to be unmyelinated (27). In recent studies, the characterization of raphe spinal neurons by antidromic activation from the spinal cord (6,32,53,78) leads to the conclusion that the conduction velocities of these axons are generally incompatible with unmyelinated axons. Similarly, with the exception of a few neurons (10), the latency of the inhibitory effects induced by NRM stimulation are also inconsistent with the conduction velocities of unmyelinated axons. If we consider, as has been suggested by Dahlström and Fuxe (27), 5-HT fibers to be unmyelinated, the results obtained with NRM stimulation are not in favor of the involvement of 5-HT. However, caution is necessary. First, it is well-known that the electrical threshold of myelinated fibers is lower than that of unmyelinated fibers; consequently studies using antidromic activation from the spinal cord would overestimate the number of large fibers. Second, NRM stimulation may simultaneously activate myelinated and unmyelinated pathways which would result in an overlapping in their inhibitory effects; thus, in these conditions it is possible to determine only the latency of the earlier inhibition due to activation of large fibers. Third, some 5-HT fibers may be myelinated. Although uncertain, this would be a peculiarity of the NRM since projections from rostral raphe nuclei have been shown to be generally unmyelinated. To resolve these discrepancies more precise studies are required, including pharmacological identification of raphe spinal neurons. An additional problem has been raised by the use of 5-HT antagonists in experiments on inhibition of dorsal horn neurons by NRM stimulation: negative effects of cinanserin in the rat (74), methysergide in the cat (10), and cinanserin, methysergide and cyproheptadin in the monkey (Willis, personal communication) on this inhibition have been reported. Whilst such negative results question the ability of these agents to antagonize the inhibitory effects of 5-HT, a possible explanation might also be that the pharmacological block is overridden by the unphysiological effects of electrical stimulations. Interestingly, the inhibitions of dorsal horn neurons by PAG stimulation, believed to be relayed via the NRM, can be blocked by LSD or methysergide (21,36). In addition, clearer results have been obtained in rats completely depleted of 5-HT by pCPA pretreatment: in these animals NRM stimulation produced markedly weakened inhibitory effects on dorsal horn neurons (74). PAG stimulation is also less effective in pCPA-treated animals. However, it must be pointed out that even in animals with no spinal 5-HT, NRM stimulation still produces inhibitory effects on some neurons, indicating that these descending influences are not exclusively mediated by 5-HT pathways. The effect of pCPA in these electrophysiological studies agrees well with behavioral evidence for a role of 5-HT in antinociception. Thus, depletion of 5-HT by pCPA markedly reduces the antinociceptive effects of PAG stimulation (3). Furthermore, in cats (64), the tolerance to antinociceptive effects induced by NRM stimulation is reversed by

5-HTP, the precursor of 5-HT. In the same way, it is well-known that 5-HT has a role in the antinociception caused by opiates (recently reviewed in (11,33,50,56)). Interestingly, the antinociceptive effects of microinjection of morphine into the PAG is reduced by methysergide and cinanserin (81) and that obtained from the NRM by cinanserin (28). Somewhat indirect evidence for a role of 5-HT in descending inhibitions due to NRM stimulation is the finding that application of 5-HT on dorsal horn neurons by iontophoresis (10,40,70) causes a preferential depression of neuronal responses to noxious stimuli. These cells included some at the origin of the spinothalamic tract (45,46). Correspondingly, direct application of 5-HT into the subarachnoid space of the spinal cord has behavioral antinociceptive effects and a similar application of a variety of 5-HT agonists and antagonists has the expected, appropriate actions (82). Since it is generally admitted that there are no spinal 5-HT containing interneurons, these findings fit well with the idea of a 5-HT descending inhibitory system originating in the brain stem and acting at the spinal level. Finally NRM stimulation accelerates the turnover of spinal 5-HT, a finding which suggests that the neuronal inhibitions and antinociception are related to the 5-HT release from spinal terminals (13).

Site of Action of the Descending Raphe System

There is a high density of both raphe magnus projections and 5-HT terminals in the dorsal horn, particularly in the substantia gelatinosa of Rolando (SGR) which also contains substance P terminals, high levels of opiate receptors, enkephalinergic neurons and terminals (see this volume). These morphological observations point to a variety of possible interactions at this level, especially as 5-HT or opiates are more potent in modulating the dorsal horn activities when applied iontophoretically to the SGR rather than to deeper laminae (40). The involvement of enkephalinergic neurons in descending inhibitory controls is supported by the fact that the inhibitory effects induced by NRM stimulation on C fiber-evoked activity in convergent neurons are partially reversed (by 30%) by naloxone administration (73); but no effect was found in another study (29). However, the reversing effect of naloxone we found at the cellular level correlates well with the reduction by this drug of the behavioral antinociceptive effects of NRM stimulation (65). As far as electrophysiological investigations on inhibitions due to PAG stimulation are concerned, naloxone has been reported to have no effect (22), a finding which may relate to the weakness (4,68) or absence (35,83) of effects of this drug reported in the behavioral studies on PAG stimulation. To summarize, it seems that there is clearer evidence for an involvement of opiates in the antinociceptive effects of NRM than of PAG stimulation when tested against acute pain in animals. However, in the case of human chronic pain, electrical stimulation of the PAG or the periventricular gray produces analgesia which is reduced by naloxone (2,42,72) and so presumably mediated by opiate mechanisms. The need for an animal model for chronic pain is highlighted by these discrepancies.

The precise mechanism of these inhibitory effects is not well understood. Primary afferent depolarization, an index of presynaptic inhibition, on various fibers has been reported to be induced by NRM stimulation (52,55,69). In contrast, a postsynaptic action may be suggested by the occurrence of IPSPs, which can occasionally be evoked by stimulation of the medial brain stem (54), the depression by NRM stimulation of the excitations produced by DL-homocysteic acid (10), and the inhibition by iontophoretically applied 5-HT of the responses of dorsal horn neurons to excitatory amino acids (10,45).

CONCLUSION

The general conclusion from these studies is that controls emanating from brain stem areas play a major role in the modulation of nociceptive messages at the spinal level. The key areas in these effects seem to be those rich in serotonergic cell bodies, notably n. raphe dorsalis and the n. raphe magnus which is at the origin of the raphe-spinal system. An outstanding problem is how these "analgesic systems" are naturally activated, but it is generally believed that they act as a negative feedback loop on neurons activated by noxious stimuli. However, an alternative hypothesis based on the existence of diffuse noxious inhibitory controls has been proposed recently (47,48): although the experimental results obtained from manipulations of the "analgesic systems" were not questioned, it was suggested that their real physiological role might be to bring out the transmission of pain messages, thus providing an alerting signal for nocifensive reactions.

REFERENCES

(1) Abdelmoumène, M.; Besson, J.M.; and Aléonard, P. 1970. Cortical areas exerting presynaptic inhibitory action on the spinal cord in cat and monkey. Brain Res. 20: 327-329.

(2) Adams, J.E. 1976. Naloxone reversal of analgesia produced by brain stimulation in the human. Pain 2: 161-166.

(3) Akil, H., and Mayer, D.J. 1972. Antagonism of stimulation-produced analgesia by p-CPA, a serotonin synthesis inhibitor. Brain Res. 44: 692-697.

(4) Akil, H.; Mayer, D.J.; and Liebeskind, J.C. 1976. Antagonism of stimulation-produced analgesia by naloxone, a narcotic antagonist. Science 191: 961-962.

(5) Andersen, P.; Eccles, J.C.; and Sears, T.A. 1962. Presynaptic inhibitory action of cerebral cortex on spinal cord. Nature (Lond.) 194: 740-743.

(6) Anderson, S.D.; Basbaum, A.I.; and Fields, H.L. 1977. sponse of medullary raphé magnus neurons to peripheral stimulation and the systemic opiates. Brain Res. 123: 363-368.

(7) Basbaum, A.I.; Clanton, C.H.; and Fields, H.L. 1976. Opiate and stimulus produced analgesia: functional anatomy of a medullospinal pathway. Proc. Natl. Acad. Sci. (Wash.) 73: 4685-4688.

(8) Basbaum, A.I.; Marley, N.J.E.; O'Keefe, J.; and Clanton, C.H. 1977. Reversal of morphine and stimulus-produced analgesia by subtotal spinal cord lesions. Pain 3: 43-56.

(9) Beal, J.E.; Martin, R.F.; Applebaum, A.E.; and Willis, W.D. 1976. Inhibition of primate spinothalamic tract neurons by stimulation in the region of nucleus raphé magnus. Brain Res. 114: 328-333.

(10) Belcher, G.; Ryall, R.W.; and Schaffner, R. 1978. The differential effects of 5-hydroxytryptamine, noradrenaline and raphé stimulation on nociceptive and non-nociceptive horn interneurons in the cat. Brain Res. 151: 307-321.

(11) Besson, J.M.; Dickenson, A.H.; Le Bars, D.; and Oliveras, J.L. 1979. Opiate analgesia: the physiology and pharmacology of spinal pain systems. In Advances in Pharmacolgy and Therapeutics, ed. C. Dumont, vol. 5, Neuropsychopharmacology, pp. 61-81. Oxford: Pergamon Press.

(12) Besson, J.M.; Guilbaud, G.; and Le Bars, D. 1975. Descending inhibitory influences exerted by the brain stem upon the activities of dorsal horn lamina V cells induced by intra-arterial injection of bradykinin into the limbs. J. Physiol. (Lond.) 248: 725-739.

(13) Bourgoin, S.; Bruxelle, J.; Oliveras, J.L.; Besson, J.M.; and Hamon, M. 1979. Accelerated turn-over of spinal 5-HT by electrical stimulation of the posterior raphé nuclei in the rat. Abstract of the Satellite Symposium of the International Society for Neurochemistry: Serotonin. Athens.

(14) Brown, A.G. 1970. Descending control of the spinocervical tract in decerebrate cats. Brain Res. 17: 152-155.

(15) Brown, A.G. 1971. Effects of descending impulses on transmission through the spinocervical tract. J. Physiol. (Lond.) 219: 103-125.

(16) Brown, A.G.; Coulter, J.D.; Rose, P.K.; Short, A.D.; and Snow, P.J. 1977. Inhibition of spinocervical tract discharges from localized areas of the sensorimotor cortex in the cat. J. Physiol. (Lond.) 264: 1-16.

(17) Brown, A.G.; Haman, W.C.; and Martin,III, H.F. 1973. Descending influences on spinocervical tract cell discharges evoked by non-myelinated cutaneous afferent nerve fibres. Brain Res. 53: 218-221.

(18) Brown, A.G.; Kirk, E.J.; and Martin,III, H.F. 1973. Descending inhibition of transmission through the spinocervical tract. J. Physiol. (Lond.) 230: 689-765.

(19) Brown, A.G., and Short, A.D. 1974. Effects from the somatic sensory cortex on transmission through the spinocervical tract. Brain Res. 74: 338-341.

(20) Carpenter, D.; Lundberg, A.; and Norrsell, U. 1963. Primary afferent depolarization evoked from the sensorimotor cortex. Acta Physiol. Scand. 59: 126-142.

(21) Carstens, E.; Fraunhoffer, M.; and Zimmermann, M. 1979. Evidence that serotonin (5-HT) mediates inhibition from midbrain periqueductal gray, but not reticular formation, of spinal nociceptive transmission in cat. Neurosci. Letters, Suppl. 3: S 258.

(22) Carstens, E.; Klumpp; and Zimmermann, M. 1979. The opiate antagonist, Naloxone, does not effect descending inhibition from midbrain of nociceptive spinal neuronal discharges in the cat. Neurosci. Letters 11: 323-327.

(23) Carstens, E.; Yokota, T.; and Zimmermann, M. 1979. Inhibition of spinal neuronal responses to noxious skin testing by stimulation of mesencephalic periacqueductal gray in the cat. J. Neurophysiol. 42: 558-568.

(24) Cervero, F.; Iggo, A.; and Molony, V. 1977. Responses of spinocervical tract neurons to noxious stimulation of the skin. J. Physiol. (Lond.) 267: 537-558.

(25) Cervero, F.; Iggo, A.; and Ogawa, H. 1976. Nociceptor-driven dorsal horn neurons in the lumbar spinal cord of the cat. Pain 2: 5-24.

(26) Coulter, J.D.; Maunz, R.A.; and Willis, W.D. 1974. Effects of stimulation of sensorimotor cortex on primate spinothalamic neurons. Brain Res. 65: 351-356.

(27) Dahlström, A., and Fuxe, K. 1965. Evidence for the existence of monoamine neurons in the central nervous system. II - Experimentally induced changes in the intraneuronal amine levels of bulbospinal neuron systems. Acta Physiol. Scand. Suppl. 64, 247: 5-36.

(28) Dickenson, A.H.; Oliveras, J.L.; and Besson, J.M. 1979. Role of the nucleus raphé magnus in opiate analgesia as studied by the microinjection technique in the rat. Brain Res. 170: 95-111.

(29) Duggan, A.W., and Griersmith, B.T. 1979. Inhibition of the spinal transmission of nociceptive information of supraspinal stimulation in the cat. Pain 6: 149-161.

(30) Engberg, I.; Lundberg, A.; and Ryall, R.W. 1968. Is the tonic decerebrate inhibition of reflex paths mediated by monoaminergic pathways? Acta Physiol. Scand. 72: 123-133.

(31) Fetz, E.E. 1968. Pyramidal tract effects in the cat lumbar dorsal horn. J. Neurophysiol. 81: 69-80.

(32) Fields, H.L., and Anderson, S.D. 1978. Evidence that raphe spinal neurons mediate opiate and midbrain stimulation-produced analgesia. Pain 5: 333-349.

(33) Fields, H.L., and Basbaum, A.I. 1978. Brain stem control of spinal pain transmission neurons. Ann. Rev. Physiol. 40: 193-221.

(34) Fields, H.L.; Basbaum, A.I.; Clanton, C.H.; and Anderson, S.D. 1977. Nucleus raphé magnus inhibition of spinal cord dorsal horn neurons. Brain Res. 126: 441-453.

(35) Gebhart, G.F., and Toleikis, J.R. 1978. An evaluation of stimulation produced analgesia in the cat. Exp. Neurol. 62: 570-579.

(36) Guilbaud, G.; Besson, J.M.; Oliveras, J.L.; and Liebeskind, J.C. 1973. Suppression by LSD of the inhibitory effect exerted by dorsal raphé stimulation on certain spinal cord interneurons in the cat. Brain Res. 61: 417-422.

(37) Guilbaud, G.; Oliveras, J.L.; Giesler, Jr., G.; and Besson, J.M. 1977. Effects induced by stimulation of the centralis inferior nucleus of the raphé on dorsal horn interneurons in cat's spinal cord. Brain Res. 126: 355-360.

(38) Handwerker, H.O.; Iggo, A.; and Zimmermann, M. 1975. Segmental and supraspinal actions on dorsal neurons responding to noxious and non-noxious skin stimuli. Pain 1: 147-165.

(39) Hayes, R.L.; Newlon, P.G.; Rosecrans, J.A.; and Mayer, D.J. 1977. Reduction of stimulation-produced analgesia by lysergic acid diethylamide a depressor of serotonergic neural activity. Brain Res. 122: 367-372.

(40) Headley, P.M.; Duggan, A.W.; and Griersmith, B.T. 1978. Selective reduction by noradrenaline and 5-hydroxytryptamine of cat dorsal horn neurons. Brain Res. 145: 185-189.

(41) Hong, S.K.; Kniffki, K.D.; Mense, S.; Schmidt, R.F.; and Wendisch, M. 1979. Descending influences on the responses of spinocervical tract neurons to chemical stimulation of fine muscle afferents. J. Physiol. (Lond.) 290: 129-140.

(42) Hosobuchi, Y.; Adams, J.E.; and Linchitz, R. 1977. Pain relief by electrical stimulation of central gray matter in humans, and its reversal by naloxone. Science 197: 183-186.

(43) Hu, J.W., and Sessle, B.J. 1979. Trigeminal nociceptive and non nociceptive neurons: brain stem intranuclear projections and modulation by orofacial, periacqueductal and nucleus raphé magnus stimuli. Brain Res. 170: 547-552.

(44) Iggo, A. 1974. Activation of cutaneous nociceptors and their actions on dorsal horn neurons. In Advances in Neurology, ed. J.J. Bonica, vol. 4, Pain, pp. 1-9. New York: Raven Press.

(45) Jordan, L.M.; Kenshalo, D.R.; Martin, R.F.; Haber, L.H.; and Willis, W.D. 1978. Depression of primate spinothalamic tract neurons by iontophoretic application of 5-hydroxytryptamine. Pain 5: 135-142.

(46) Jordan, L.M.; Kenshalo, D.R.; Martin, R.F.; Haber, L.H.; and Willis, W.D. 1979. Two populations of spinothalamic tract neurons with opposite responses to 5-hydroxytryptamine. Brain Res. 164: 342-346.

(47) Le Bars, D.; Dickenson, A.H.; and Besson, J.M. 1979. Diffuse noxious inhibitory controls (DNIC). I - Effects on dorsal horn convergent neurons in the rat. Pain 6: 283-304.

(48) Le Bars, D.; Dickenson, A.H.; and Besson, J.M. 1979. Diffuse noxious inhibitory contols (DNIC). II - Lack of effect on non-convergent neurons, supraspinal involvement and theoretical implications. Pain 6: 305-327.

(49) Le Bars, D.; Menétrey, D.; Conseiller, C.; and Besson, J.M. 1974. Comparaison chez le chat spinal et le chat décérébré, des effets de la morphine sur les activités des interneurones de type V de la corne dorsale de la moelle. C.R. Acad. Sci. (Paris) 279: 1369-1371.

(50) Liebeskind, J.C.; Giesler, Jr., G.; and Urca, G. 1976. Evidence pertaining to an endogenous mechanism of pain inhibition in the central nervous system. In Sensory Functions of the Skin in Primates, ed. I. Zotterman, pp. 561-573. Oxford: Pergamon Press.

(51) Liebeskind, J.C.; Guilbaud, G.; Besson, J.M.; and Oliveras, J.L. 1973. Analgesia from electrical stimulation of the periacqueductal gray matter in the cat: behavioral observations and inhibitory effects on spinal cord interneurons. Brain Res. 50: 441-446.

(52) Lovick, T.A.; West, D.C.; and Wolstencroft, J.H. 1977. Interactions between brain stem raphe nuclei and the trigeminal nuclei. In Pain in the Trigeminal Region, eds. D.J. Anderson and B. Matthews, pp. 307-317. Amsterdam: Elsevier/North-Holland.

(53) Lovick, T.A.; West, D.C.; and Wolstencroft, J.H. 1978. Responses of raphé spinal and other bulbar raphé neurons stimulation of the periacqueductal gray in the cat. Neurosci. Letters 8: 45-49.

(54) Lundberg, A. 1964. Supraspinal control of transmission in reflex paths to motoneurons and primary afferents. In Progress in Brain Research, eds. J.C. Eccles and P. Schadé, vol. 12, pp. 197-221. Amsterdam: Elsevier/North-Holland.

(55) Martin, R.F.; Haber, L.H.; and Willis, W.D. 1979. Primary afferent depolarization of identified cutaneous fibers following stimulation in medial brain stem. J. Neurophysiol. 42: 779-790.

(56) Mayer, D.J., and Price, D.D. 1976. Central nervous system mechanisms of analgesia. Pain 2: 379-404.

(57) Mayer, D.J.; Wolfe, T.L.; Akil, H.; Carder, B.; and Liebeskind, J.C. 1971. Analgesia from electrical stimulation in the brain stem of the rat. Science 174: 1351-1354.

(58) Mc Creery, D.B.; Bloedel, J.R.; and Hames, E.G. 1979. Effects of stimulating in raphé nuclei and in reticular formation on response of spinothalamic neurons to mechanical stimuli. J. Neurophysiol. 42: 166-182.

(59) Menétrey, S.; Chaouch, A.; and Besson, J.M. 1979. Location and properties of lumbar spinoreticular tract neurons in the rat. Neurosci. Letters, Suppl. 3: S 262.

(60) Morrow, T.J., and Casey, K.L. 1976. Analgesia produced by mesencephalic stimulation: effect on bulboreticular neurons. In Advances in Pain Research and Therapy, eds. J.J. Bonica and D. Albe-Fessard, pp. 503-510. New York: Raven Press.

(61) Necker, R., and Hellon, R.F. 1978. Noxious thermal input from the rat tail: modulation by descending inhibitory influences. Pain 4: 231-242.

(62) Oliveras, J.L.; Besson, J.M.; Guilbaud, G.; and Liebeskind, J.C. 1974. Behavioral and electrophysiological evidence of pain inhibition from midbrain stimulation in the cat. Exp. Brain Res. 20: 32-44.

(63) Oliveras, J.L.; Guilbaud, G.; and Besson, J.M. 1979. A map of serotoninergic structures involved in stimulation producing analgesia in unrestrained freely moving cats. Brain Res. 164: 317-322.

(64) Oliveras, J.L.; Hosobuchi, Y.; Guilbaud, G.; and Besson, J.M. 1978. Analgesia by electrical stimulation of the feline nucleus raphé magnus: development of tolerance and its reversal by 5-HTP. Brain Res. 146: 404-469.

(65) Oliveras, J.L.; Hosobuchi, Y.; Redjemi, F.; Guilbaud, G.; and Besson, J.M. 1977. Opiate antagonist, naloxone, strongly reduces analgesia induced by stimulation of a raphé nucleus (centralis inferior). Brain Res. 120: 221-229.

(66) Oliveras, J.L.; Redjemi, F.; Guilbaud, G.; and Besson, J.M. 1975. Analgesia induced by electrical stimulation of the inferior centralis nucleus of the raphé in the cat. Pain 1: 139-145.

(67) Oliveras, J.L.; Woda, A.; Guilbaud, G.; and Besson, J.M. 1974. Inhibition of jaw opening reflex by electrical stimulation of the periacqueductal gray matter in the awake, unrestrained cat. Brain Res. 72: 328-331.

(68) Pert, A., and Walter, M. 1976. Comparison between naloxone reversal of morphine and electrical stimulation induced analgesia in the rat mesencephalon. Life Sciences 19: 1023-1032.

(69) Proudfit, H.K., and Anderson, E.G. 1974. New long latency bulbospinal evoked potentials blocked by serotonin antagonists. Brain Res. 65: 542-546.

(70) Randic, M., and Yu, H.H. 1976. Effects of 5-hydroxytryptamine and bradykinin in cat dorsal horn neurons activated by noxious stimuli. Brain Res. 111: 197-203.

(71) Reynolds, D.V. 1969. Surgery in the rat during electrical analgesia induced by focal brain stimulation. Science 164: 444-445.

(72) Richardson, D.E., and Akil, H. 1977. Pain reduction by electrical brain stimulation in man: chronic self stimulation in the periacqueductal gray matter. J. Neurosurg. 47: 184-194.

(73) Rivot, J.P.; Chaouch, A.; and Besson, J.M. 1979. The influence of naloxone on the C fiber response of dorsal horn neurons and their inhibitory control by raphé magnus stimulation. Brain Res., in press.

(74) Rivot, J.P.; Chaouch, A.; and Besson, J.M. 1979. Caractéristiques électrophysiologiques et pharmacologiques du controle exercé par le noyau raphé magnus sur la transmission spinale des messages nociceptifs. J. Physiol. (Paris), in press.

(75) Sessle, B.J.; Dubner, R.; Greenwood, L.F.; and Lucier, G.E. 1976. Descending influences of periaqueductal gray matter and somatosensory cerebral cortex on neurones in trigeminal brain stem nuclei. Canad. J. Physiol. Pharmacol. 54: 66-69.

(76) Taub, A. 1964. Local, segmental and supraspinal interaction with a dorsolateral spinal cutaneous afferent system. Exp. Neurol. 10: 357-374.

(77) Wall, P.D. 1967. The laminar organization of dorsal horn and effects of descending impulses. J. Physiol. 188: 403-423.

(78) West, D.C., and Wolstencroft, J.H. 1977. Electrophysiological identification of raphé spinal neurones in the cat. J. Physiol. 29: 265.

(79) Willis, W.D.; Haber, L.H.; and Martin, R.F. 1977. Inhibition of spinothalamic tract cells and interneurons by brainstem stimulation in the monkey. J. Neurophysiol. 40: 968-981.

(80) Wyon-Maillard, M.C.; Conseiller, C.; and Besson, J.M. 1972. Effects of orbital cortex stimulation on dorsal horn interneurons in the cat spinal cord. Brain Res. 46: 71-83.

(81) Yaksh, T.L.; Du Chateau, J.; and Rudy, T.A. 1976. Antagonism by methysergide and cinanserin of the antinociceptive action of morphine administered into the periaqueductal gray. Brain Res. 104: 367-372.

(82) Yaksh, T.L., and Wilson, P.R. 1975. Spinal serotonin terminal system mediates antinociception. J. Pharmacol. Exp. Ther. 208: 446-453.

(83) Yaksh, T.L.; Young, J.C.; and Rudy, T.A. 1976. An inability to antagonize with naloxone the elevated nociceptive thresholds resulting from electrical stimulation of the mesencephalic central gray. Life Sciences 18: 1193-1198.

(84) Yokota, T., and Hashimoto, S. 1976. Periaqueductal gray and tooth pulp afferent interaction on units in caudal medulla oblongata. Brain Res. 117: 508-512.

Pain and Society, eds. H.W. Kosterlitz and L.Y. Terenius, pp. 183-200.
Dahlem Konferenzen 1980. Weinheim: Verlag Chemie GmbH.

Supraspinal Mechanisms in Pain: The Reticular Formation

K. L. Casey
Department of Physiology, University of Michigan
Medical School, Ann Arbor, MI 48109, USA

Abstract. Pain is an experience with sensory-discriminative and motivational-affective components. Neurons forming the spinothalamic projection to ventrolateral thalamus have physiological properties suited for the mediation of the sensory-discriminative component of pain. The action of this system provides a basis for localizing noxious stimuli in time, space, and along a continuum of intensities and submodalities. Neurons projecting to the reticular formation lack these physiological properties. It is suggested here, on the basis of the available anatomical and physiological evidence, that the reticular formation responds to nociceptor input by establishing, as a behavioral mode, a constellation of protective autonomic and somatomotor reactions which characterize pain behavior and which mediate the motivational and affective component of pain.

INTRODUCTION

Acute pain is an adaptive warning of impending or actual tissue damage. It interrupts ongoing behavior, directs attention to the site of injury, and motivates behavior to escape from the offending stimulus. Chronic, intractable pain is an equally compelling but typically maladaptive state often associated with profound affective disturbances in patients. These descriptions emphasize two major features of pain which must be considered in attempting to understand the underlying neural mechanisms. First, pain is a somatic or visceral sensation which can be localized in time, space, and along a continuum of intensities; like other sensations pain has discriminative features. Second, pain is unpleasant; unlike most other sensations, it has an affective dimension which is a necessary component of the experience. A neurophysiology of pain must ultimately account for both the discriminative and affective features of pain.

ASCENDING CENTRAL PATHWAYS

Since pain is an experience which has discriminative and affective dimensions and includes autonomic and somatomotor responses, it is not surprising that this diversity is reflected by the underlying anatomy (39) and physiology (15). The diagram in Figure 1 shows the major features of the ascending systems now thought to be important in mediating pain and pain-related behavior.

Two anatomically and physiologically distinct types of neurons receive input from nociceptive afferents and send axons toward the brain via the contralateral spinothalamic tract (27). Many of the cells capping the dorsal margin of the substantia gelatinosa (marginal cells of Waldeyer) respond exclusively to noxious stimuli and transmit impulses to substantia gelatinosa and to contralateral thalamus. Most neurons deeper in the dorsal horn have a wide dynamic range of response; they are excited by large-diameter myelinated touch-pressure afferents and respond with increasing frequency as stimulus intensity is brought into the noxious range. Axons of the deeper cells project to the reticular formation of the brain stem as well as to the contralateral thalamus. The major features of this description apply also to the caudal portion of the trigeminal sensory nucleus which receives nociceptive input from the face.

THE SPINOTHALAMIC SYSTEM

The spinothalamic tract (STT) neurons comprise the classical pain pathway projecting directly to the posterior lateral thalamus. The trigeminal counterpart is the trigeminothalamic tract. The responses of these dorsal horn or caudal trigeminal nucleus neurons to noxious stimuli suggest that there should be a substantial population of posterior lateral thalamic neurons which are exclusively or differentially responsive to nociceptor input. It is rather surprising, then, that recordings of neural activity in animals have revealed a relatively small proportion of nociceptive neurons, possibly because of the anesthetics often used

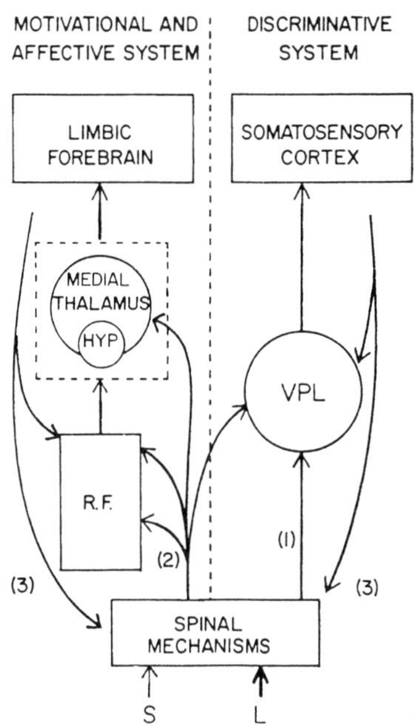

FIG. 1 - Diagram of neural systems important in pain and pain modulation. Small diameter nociceptive afferents (S) and larger diameter non-nociceptive fibers (L) activate spinal mechanisms leading to the generation of impulses ascending to higher centers. Neurons in the ventrobasal thalamus (ventralis posterolateralis shown here: VPL) receive input from fibers of the dorsal column-medial lemniscal system (1) and from that portion of ventrolateral spinal cord (2) forming the spinothalamic tract. Projection of these neurons to the somatosensory cortex provides the basis for the discriminative aspects of somesthesis, possibly including pain. Other fibers ascending from the ventrolateral spinal cord (2) send projections into the brain stem reticular formation (RF) and to the medial thalamus. Ascending reticular formation fibers also project to the medial thalamus and hypothalamus where they may influence limbic forebrain mechanisms subserving the motivational and affective components of pain. Both discriminative and motivational-affective systems are modulated by descending pathways (3) acting at thalamic, brain stem, and spinal levels.
(From: Postgrad. Med. 1973. 53: 58-63)

in such experiments or because certain neurons have been missed by sampling errors (11, 31, 47). The posterolateral thalamus has been electrically stimulated or destroyed in human and in animal experiments, and the results suggest that other pathways and structures must play an equally important and necessary role in pain mechanisms. In the human, for example, reports of pain accompanying posterolateral thalamic stimulation are surprisingly rare - and lesions in this area may result in a "thalamic syndrome" in which normally innocuous stimuli have an unpleasant or even severely painful quality (58). Furthermore, there is little clinical and experimental evidence to indicate that the cortical projections of posterolateral thalamic neurons are critical for pain perception; surgical extirpation of this cortical tissue has been notably unsuccessful in relieving clinical pain (58). Neurophysiological observations have, however, established that nociceptive information is transmitted to the posterolateral thalamus and associated cortex (17, 31), and there is general agreement that the neurons of this system mediate the discriminative aspects of pain.

On the evidence at hand, it is reasonable to suggest that the direct STT system subserves the discriminative aspects of pain, permitting the organism to recognize that potential or actual tissue damage has occurred, to localize it in space and time, and perhaps to recognize the physical nature of the stimulus (thermal, mechanical, chemical).

THE SPINORETICULAR SYSTEM

Dorsal horn neurons projecting to the medullary or mesencephalic reticular formation form the spinoreticular tract (SRT). A comparable system originates from the caudal portion of the trigeminal nucleus. Neurophysiological experiments performed in several different laboratories have shown that a substantial proportion of brain stem reticular formation neurons respond either differentially or exclusively to noxious stimuli (15). Most often, the response of these neurons resembles that of the deeper dorsal horn cells with a wide dynamic range; there is a relatively weak response to innocuous stimuli but a longer and more intense discharge when noxious stimuli are applied. Similar responses have been recorded from neurons of the medial thalamus which receive input via reticulothalamic projections; some of these medial thalamic neurons may also receive input from STT neurons. Many of these reticular and medial thalamic neurons respond to innocuous somatic stimuli and some are activated by visual and auditory inputs. Furthermore, reticular formation neurons typically respond to stimulation anywhere within an extensive area of the body surface. it is unlikely that such cells could encode the spatial information necessary to localize pain. The output of reticular neurons is similarly extensive. Many, if not most, of these cells have multifocal axonal projections to the thalamus, spinal cord, and within the brain stem. Many experiments have shown that the reticular formation is not simply a sensory pathway; reticular neurons undoubtedly mediate motor and autonomic responses to the various inputs they receive. What functions, then, might this system subserve?

THE RETICULAR FORMATION AND PAIN

Limitations of time and space in most research reports or reviews preclude serious speculation about the significance of nociceptor afferent input to reticular formation neurons. Consequently, many authors focus on some aspect of reticular formation structure or function, relate that to some aspect of pain, and suggest, for example, that reticular formation neurons responding to noxious stimuli may mediate diffuse pain, or burning pain, or chronic pain - or that these neurons instead regulate motor or autonomic responses to pain, or attenuate pain by functioning as part of an endogenous control system. I will not attempt to review these arguments or the evidence in their support; Bowsher (6) has recently reviewed in detail the relevant anatomy and physiology of the reticular formation. Instead, I will state my own conceptual bias, and some of the evidence on which it is based, hoping that this will stimulate the formulation of more precise working hypotheses to guide future experiments.

Pain As a Behavioral Mode

Over a decade ago, Kilmer and his associates developed computer models of the reticular formation based primarily on the Scheibel's anatomical studies (52, 53) and some assumptions about the biological function of these neurons (33). The thesis underlying the Kilmer models is that the reticular formation commits a vertebrate to one or another mode of behavior. According to the authors: "An animal is said to be in a mode if the main focus of its attention throughout its central nervous system (CNS) is on doing the things of that mode" ((33), p. 280).

Although there is general agreement that sleep and waking are distinct modes or states of CNS function under reticular formation control, it is unlikely that a division of all waking behavior into similarly distinct modes would be widely accepted today. However, there are circumstances in which external or internal events completely command the organism's attention and lead to a limited number of stereotyped responses or behaviors involving sensory, motor and automonic function. The rapid recruitment of all these components of behavior into a specific pattern would seem to qualify such a response as a behavioral mode, distinct from behavioral adjustments requiring only a change in motor control or a shift of sensory focus, for example.

Tissue damage, or threat of tissue damage, could be considered a trigger for one type of modal behavior. Noxious stimuli may, of course, be ignored if the input from nociceptive afferents is small or if other events command the organism's behavior and produce, in effect, an analgesic state. Usually, however, strong noxious stimuli elicit global behavioral changes. Tissue damage interrupts ongoing behavior, shifts the focus of sensory attention to the origin of nociceptive afferent discharge, facilitates protective motor reflexes, and elicits autonomic responses. This behavior is accompanied by the unpleasant somatic or visceral sensation we call pain. The behavior normally elicited by strong noxious stimuli, then, would probably be among those waking behaviors which could reasonably be called modal.

If some waking behaviors are modal and if pain behavior is among them, what evidence suggests that the reticular formation provides the neural machinery for switching the organism into that mode? Two major lines of evidence seem essential; a) reticular formation neurons should be organized for coadunate action to effect coherent and specific changes in sensory, motor, and autonomic function, and b) reticular formation neurons should be strongly influenced by noxious stimuli and their activation or inactivation should produce corresponding changes in pain behavior.

Interactive Organization of Reticular Formation

The intrinsic organization of the reticular formation is consistent with the view that reticular activation can affect synchronously many components of behavior. Cytoarchitectural studies (45, 55) show that the reticular formation is composed of several nuclear groups with cell bodies of distinctive shape and size. Silver stain studies, however, reveal some common and unifying structural features superimposed on this morphological heterogeneity. Following the cytoarchitectural classification of dendritic patterns proposed by Ramon-Moliner (48), Ramon-Moliner and Nauta (49) identified a core of isodendritic neurons extending through the medulla and mesencephalon. With a few exceptions, this isodendritic core comprises the reticular formation of the brain stem. The axonal projections of these cells are typically quite long, extending substantial distances along the rostro-caudal axis of the brain stem; reticular formation neurons with only short axons are apparently rarely, if ever, found. Along their course, the axons send collaterals to the spinal cord, the diencephalon, other reticular neurons, and to various sensory and motor nuclei of the brain stem. The reticular formation, then, is not a diffuse network of short-axoned neurons forming a multisynaptic chain. Rather, neurons comprising the isodendritic core appear organized to distribute information quickly to muliple foci throughout a substantial portion of the neuraxis, from the diencephalon through the spinal cord.

Physiological studies show that reticular formation neurons can mediate motor, autonomic, and sensory functions. Although there are circumscribed regions which have specialized functions, there is also evidence for substantial interaction, providing a basis for unified operations of the reticular core. Berntson and Micco (4) have extensively reviewed the evidence that many complex behaviors are organized by mechanisms intrinsic to the brain stem. The reticular formation is known to be essential for the coordination of the motor components of the behaviors of animals experimentally deprived of forebrain function (23). Medullary and pontine reticular neurons also regulate various aspects of spinal motor (50) and respiratory activity (51). Reticular formation neurons in these same regions, however, also mediate autonomic functions. Clusters of cells within several medullary and pontine reticular nuclei have been shown to project directly to the intermediolateral nucleus of the spinal cord where they excite or inhibit cardioacceleratory neurons (27). Direct electrical stimulation within some of these bulboreticular sites evokes activity in the splanchnic nerve (22) and the superior cervical ganglion (56).

Sensory functions may also be strongly affected by bulboreticular neurons in sites eliciting somatomotor and autonomic effects. For example, certain midline raphe nuclei of the medulla have been shown to receive input from the carotid sinus and aortic depressor nerves (18) and to mediate substantial changes in blood pressure and heart rate (1). Other physiological and behavioral studies, however, have emphasized the finding that electrical stimulation within these same cell groups markedly depresses the nociceptive responses of certain dorsal horn cells and produces analgesia (37). Numerous other studies have demonstrated reticular control over somatic, auditory, and visual sensory systems (35) from sites within the cytoarchitectural boundaries of those implicated in motor or autonomic control. Finally, reticular formation neurons in these same sites also have axons projecting rostrally to the upper brain stem or diencephalon (5, 7, 9, 19, 36, 42, 49).

The evidence, then, indicates that neurons within a given cytoarchitectural territory can affect somatomotor, autonomic, and sensory function. The intrinsic interneuronal connections and the distribution of physiological properties of reticular formation neurons also suggest that different groups of cells can act coadunatively to produce the constellation of changes which would characterize a shift into a behavioral mode.

Neurophysiological and Behavioral Evidence for Pain-Related Functions of Reticular Formation

There is abundant evidence that nociceptor afferents are among the most effective inputs influencing the discharge of a substantial population of reticular formation neurons (6). Investigators from several laboratories have demonstrated, in cat and rat, an exclusive or differential effect of mechanical, thermal, or chemical noxious stimuli on neurons of the medullary and mesencephalic reticular formation (3, 10, 12, 20, 21, 24, 34, 59, 60). By recording from single cells in awake animals, it has also been possible to correlate the somatic activation of medullary reticular neurons with escape behavior in the cat (14) and to show, in rat, that some of these cells develop responses to innocuous stimuli which have been paired with noxious shock (57).

Electrical stimulation within various groups of reticular formation neurons has been shown repeatedly to either elicit or markedly attenuate pain behavior in cat, rat, or monkey depending on the site of stimulation. Aversive reactions have been produced by stimulation in the medullary nucleus gigantocellularis (13, 28, 29) and mesencephalic tegmentum (43). Analgesia has been elicited by stimulation in the dorsal raphe nuclei of the midbrain and the raphe magnus of the medulla (37), and neurophysiological studies (38) have shown that stimulation within either the nucleus raphe magnus or the adjacent gigantocellular reticular formation results in a complex modulation of the excitability of spinothalamic tract neurons.

The reticular formation has been shown to be an important site for the action of analgesic drugs. Local injection of morphine into various reticular sites produces anti-nociception; whether this is due to the activation of pain inhibitory mechanisms acting elsewhere or the attenuation of local neuronal responses to noxious input has not been determined (37). Systemic injections of morphine have also been shown to inhibit some reticular formation neurons, excite others, and reduce neuronal responses to noxious input (25, 44).

Destructive lesions within the reticular formation are known to affect pain behavior. Melzack et al. (41) found that medial mesencephalic lesions attenuated pain reactions of cats in the immediate post-lesion period, but later resulted in increased reactivity to noxious stimuli. Kelley and Glusman (30) found that laterally placed midbrain lesions reduced the operant responses of cats to electrical shocks. Halpern and Halverson (26) found that lesions in the gigantocellular nucleus of the medulla significantly increased the latency and electrical shock threshold of escape (barrier crossing) in cats; similar observations have been reported by Anderson and Pearl (2). In a series of experiments now in progress (16), we have observed that unilateral, moderately sized lesions in the paramedian medullary reticular formation of cats can markedly reduce unlearned escape responses to noxious thermal pulses. Control observations show that the effect is not due to motor impairment.

The evidence cited above leaves little doubt that a significant population of neurons in the reticular formation is strongly influenced by nociceptor input and is an important determinant of pain behavior and, presumably, some aspects of pain experience. There is reason to suggest that reticular neurons with ascending projections may mediate the affective and motivational dimension of the pain experience (40). The medial thalamus and hypothalamus, which receive reticular input, both project to limbic system forebrain structures, such as the cingulate gyrus and hippocampal formation, which are known to play an important role in motivational and affective mechanisms. Selective lesions within limbic forebrain structures of humans and animals, for example, have been shown to markedly attenuate the aversive quality of noxious stimuli without interfering with the discriminative aspects of somesthesis. The effect of narcotic analgesics on reticular formation neurons (46) may also account, in part, for the reduction of suffering in clinical pain while preserving much of the discriminative ability to recognize noxious stimuli.

The neural system mediating motivational and affective mechanisms is not a specialized pain pathway. Many other inputs are important determinants of affective state and can motivate behavior. Pain, however, is an especially compelling experience, so it is reasonable to expect that nociceptive afferents would be among the major inputs to a system which may determine affective and motivational states.

Input As a Determinant of the Mode of Reticular Formation Function

The function of reticular formation cells cannot be related exclusively to pain or to one dimension of pain mechanisms. In the absence of noxious input, some of these neurons must contribute to various aspects of other ongoing behavior and their activity must be determined by regional input variables peculiar to that population. For example, the activity of some of these neurons is highly correlated with specific movements or with REM sleep when noxious input is absent (54); the function of others is likely to be related to autonomic control (27) or to modulation of other sensory inputs (35) during a variety of behaviors. Rather, the evidence suggests that tissue damage recruits this functionally heterogeneous but strongly interactive population into a characteristic pattern of coherent activity.

From what is currently known of the anatomy and physiology of the reticular formation, the statement of Brodal (8) seems as appropriate now as it was over 20 years ago:

"The reticular formation is not diffusely organized but is subdivided into several regions which differ with regard to their cytoarchitecture, fibre connexions and intrinsic organization. These regions, however, cannot be considered as being independent of each other, since their fibre connexions provide ample possibilities for interaction and collaboration between the various regions" (p.74).

The evidence indicates that input from nociceptive afferents would be among the events promoting the collaborative interaction mentioned in this statement.

SUMMARY COMMENT

It is unlikely that the role of the reticular formation in pain mechanisms will be adequately understood in terms of independent motor, sensory, or autonomic functions or only in relation to some aspect of pain as an experience. Current evidence supports Brodal's (8) contention that the reticular formation should not be considered a collection of independent centers. So far as pain mechanisms are concerned, the more heuristic view may be that this isodendritic core is a federation of pluripotential and functionally heterogeneous neurons brought into coherent activity by noxious stimuli to establish, as a behavioral mode, the constellation of protective responses and the aversive experience which are essential components of pain.

Acknowledgement. Supported by grants NS12015 and NS12581 from the National Institutes of Health (USPHS).

REFERENCES

(1) Adair, J.R.; Hamilton, B.L.; Scappaticci, K.A.; Helke, C.J.; and Gillis, R.A. 1977. Cardiovascular responses to electrical stimulation of the medullary raphe area of the cat. Brain Res. 128: 141-145.

(2) Anderson, K.V., and Pearl, G.S. 1975. Long-term increases in nociceptive thresholds following lesions in feline nucleus reticularis gigantocellularis. Abstracts, First World Congress on Pain (IASP), Florence.

(3) Becker, D.P.; Gluck, H.; Nulsen, F.E.; and Jane, J.A. 1969. An inquiry into the neurophysiological basis for pain. J. Neurophysiol. 30: 1-13.

(4) Berntson, G.G., and Micco, D.J. 1976. Theoretical review. Organization of brainstem behavioral systems. Brain Res. Bull. 1: 471-483.

(5) Bobillier, P.; Petitjean, F.; Salvert, D.; Ligier, M.; and Seguin, S. 1975. Differential projections of the nucleus raphe dorsalis and nucleus raphe centralis as revealed by autoradiography. Brain Res. 85: 205-210.

(6) Bowsher, D. 1976. Role of the reticular formation in responses to noxious stimulation. Pain 2: 361-378.

(7) Bowsher, D.; Mallart, A.; Petit, D.; and Albe-Fessard, D. 1968. A bulbar relay to the centre median. J. Neurophysiol. 31: 288-300.

(8) Brodal, A. 1957. The Reticular Formation of the Brain Stem. Anatomical Aspects and Functional Correlations. Springfield, IL: C.C. Thomas.

(9) Brodal, A., and Rossi, G.F. 1955. Ascending fibers in brain stem reticular formation of cat. Arch. Neurol. Psychiat. 74: 68-87.

(10) Burton, H. 1968. Somatic sensory properties of caudal bulbar reticular neurons in the cat (Felis domestica). Brain Res. 11: 372-375.

(11) Casey, K.L. 1966. Unit analysis of nociceptive mechanisms in the thalamus of the awake squirrel monkey. J. Neurophysiol. 29: 727-750.

(12) Casey, K.L. 1969. Somatic stimuli, spinal pathways, and size of cutaneous fibers influencing unit activity in the medial medullary reticular formation. Exp. Neurol. 25: 35-56.

(13) Casey, K.L. 1971. Escape elicited by bulboreticular stimulation in the cat. Int. J. Neurosci. 2: 15-28.

(14) Casey, K.L. 1971. Somatosensory responses of bulboreticular units in awake cat: Relation to escape-producing stimuli. Science 173: 77-80.

(15) Casey, K.L. 1978. Neural mechanisms of pain. In Handbook of Perception, eds. E.C. Carterette and M.P. Friedman, vol. VIB, pp. 183-230. New York: Academic Press.

(16) Casey, K.L., and Morrow, T.J. 1978. Responses of cats to thermal pulses: Effect of thalamic and reticular formation lesions. Abstracts, vol. 1, Second World Congress on Pain (IASP), Montreal.

(17) Craig, A.D., and Burton, H. 1979. Spinothalamic terminations in the ventroposterolateral nucleus of the cat. Soc. for Neurosci. Abstracts. 5: 705.

(18) Crill, W.E., and Reis, D.J. 1968. Distribution of carotid sinus and depressor nerves in cat brain stem. Am. J. Physiol. 214: 269-276.

(19) Eccles, J.C.; Nicoll, R.A.; Taborikova, H.; and Willey, T.J. 1975. Medial reticular neurons projecting rostrally. J. Neurophysiol. 38: 531-538.

(20) Eickhoff, R.; Handwerker, H.O.; McQueen, D.S.; and Schick, E. 1978. Noxious and tactile input to medial structures of midbrain and pons in the rat. Pain 5: 99-113.

(21) Goldman, P.L.; Collins, W.F.; Taub, A.; and Fitzmartin, J. 1972. Evoked bulbar reticular unit activity following delta fiber stimulation of peripheral somatosensory nerve in cat. Exp. Neurol. 37: 597-606.

(22) Gootman, P.M., and Cohen, M.I. 1971. Evoked splanchnic potentials produced by electrical stimulation of medullary vasomotor regions. Exp. Brain Res. 13: 1-14.

(23) Grillner, S. 1975. Locomotion in vertebrates: Central mechanisms and reflex interaction. Physiol. Rev. 55: 247-304.

(24) Guilbaud, G.; Besson, J.M.; Oliveras, J.L.; and Wyon-Maillard, M.C. 1973. Modifications of the firing rate of bulbar reticular units (nucleus gigantocellularis) after intra-arterial injection of bradykinin into limbs. Brain Res. 63: 131-140.

(25) Haigler, H.J. 1976. Morphine: Ability to block neuronal activity evoked by a nociceptive stimulus. Life Sci. 19: 841-858.

(26) Halpern, B.P., and Halverson, J.D. 1974. Modification of escape from noxious stimuli after bulbar reticular formation lesions. Behav. Biol. 11: 215-229.

(27) Henry, J.L., and Calaresu, F.R. 1974. Excitatory and inhibitory inputs from medullary nuclei projecting to spinal cardioacceleratory neurons in the cat. Exp. Brain Res. 20: 485-504.

(28) Keene, J.J., and Casey, K.L. 1970. Excitatory connection from lateral hypothalamic self-stimulation sites to escape sites in medullary reticular formation. Exp. Neurol. 28: 155-166.

(29) Keene, J.J., and Casey, K.L. 1973. Rewarding and aversive brain stimulation: opposite effects on medial thalamic units. Physiol. Behav., pp. 283-287.

(30) Kelly, D.D., and Glusman, M. 1968. Aversive thresholds following midbrain lesions. J. Comp. Physiol. Psychol. 66: 25-34.

(31) Kenshalo, D.R.; et al. 1979. Responses of VPL_c neurons in the primate thalamus to noxious thermal stimuli. Soc. for Neurosci. Abstracts 5: 612.

(32) Kerr, F.W.L. 1975. Neuroanatomical substrates of nociception in the spinal cord. Pain 1: 325-356.

(33) Kilmer, W.L.; McCulloch, W.S.; and Blum, J. 1969. A model of the vertebrate central command system. Int. J. Man-Mach. Stud. 1: 279-309.

(34) LeBlanc, H.J., and Gatipon, G.B. 1974. Medial bulboreticular response to peripherally applied noxious stimuli. Exp. Neurol. 42: 264-273.

(35) Livingston, R.B. 1959. Central control of receptors and sensory transmission systems. In Handbook of Physiology, ed. W.S. Fields, vol. 1, pp. 741-760. Washington, D.C.: American Physiological Society.

(36) Magni, F., and Willis, W.D. 1963. Identification of reticular formation neurons by intracellular recording. Arch. ital. Biol. 101: 681-702.

(37) Mayer, D.J., and Price, D.D. 1976. Central nervous system mechanisms of analgesia. Pain 2: 379-404.

(38) McCreery, D.B.; Bloedel, J.R.; and Hames, E.G. 1979. Effects of stimulating in raphe nuclei and in reticular formation on response of spinothalamaic neurons to mechanical stimuli. J. Neurophysiol. 42: 166-183.

(39) Mehler, W.R.; Feferman, M.E.; and Nauta, W.J.H. 1960. Ascending axon degeneration following anterolateral cordotomy. An experimental study in the monkey. Brain 83: 718-750.

(40) Melzack, R., and Casey, K.L. 1968. Sensory, motivational, and central control determinants of pain. In The Skin Senses ed. E.R. Kenshalo, pp. 423-443. Springfield, IL: C.C. Thomas

(41) Melzack, R.; Stotler, W.A.; and Livingston, W.K. 1958. Effects of discrete brain stem lesions in cats on perception of noxious stimulation. J. Neurophysiol. 21: 353-367.

(42) Nauta, W.J.H., and Kuypers, H.G.J.M. 1958. Some ascending pathways in the brain stem reticular formation. In Reticular Formation of the Brain, eds. H.H. Jasper and L.D. Proctor, pp. 3-30. Boston: Little, Brown & Co.

(43) Olds, M.E., and Olds, J. 1963. Approach-avoidance analysis of rat diencephalon. J. Comp. Neurol. 120: 259-295.

(44) Oleson, T.D.; Twonbly, D.A.; and Liebeskind, J.C. 1978. Effects of pain-attenuating brain stimulation and morphine on electrical activity in the raphe nuclei of the awake rat. Pain 4: 211-230.

(45) Olszewski, J. 1954. The cytoarchitecture of the human reticular formation. In The Brain Mechanisms of Consciousness, eds. E.D. Adrian, F. Bremer, and H.H. Jasper. Springfield, IL: C.C. Thomas.

(46) Pert, A., and Yaksh, T. 1974. Sites of morphine-induced analgesia in the primate brain: relation to pain pathways. Brain Res. 80: 135-140.

(47) Poggio, G.F., and Mountcastle, V.B. 1963. The functional properties of ventrobasal thalamic neurons studied in unanesthetized monkeys. J. Neurophysiol. 26: 775-806.

(48) Ramon-Moliner, E. 1962. An attempt at classifying nerve cells on the basis of their dendritic patterns. J. Comp. Neurol. 119: 211-227.

(49) Ramon-Moliner, E., and Nauta, W.J.H. 1966. The isodendritic core of the brain stem. J. Comp. Neurol. 126: 311-336.

(50) Rossi, G.F., and Zanchetti, A. 1957. The brain stem reticular formation. Anatomy and physiology. Arch. ital. Biol. 95: 199-435.

(51) Salmoiraghi, G.C. 1963. Functional organization of brain stem respiratory neurons. Ann NY Acad. Sci. 109: 571-585.

(52) Scheibel, M.E., and Scheibel, A.B. 1968. Structural substrates for integrative patterns in the brain stem reticular core. In Reticular Formation of the Brain, eds. H.H. Jasper, L.D. Proctor, R.S. Knighton, W.C. Noshay and R.T. Costello, pp. 31-68. Boston: Little, Brown & Co.

(53) Scheibel, M.E., and Scheibel, A.B. 1968. The brain stem reticular core - an integrative matrix. In Systems Theory and Biology, ed. M.D. Mesarovic, pp. 261-285. New York: Springer Verlag.

(54) Siegel, J.M., and McGinty, D.J. 1977. Pontine reticular formation neurons: relationship or discharge to motor activity. Science 196: 678-680.

(55) Taber, E. 1961. The cytoarchitecture of the brain stem of the cat. I. Brain stem nuclei of cat. J. Comp. Neurol. 116: 27-69.

(56) Taylor, D.G., and Gebber, G.L. 1972. Functional organization of brain stem vasomotor area. Fed. Proc. 31: 377.

(57) Vertes, R.P., and Miller, N.E. 1976. Brain stem neurons that fire selectively to a conditioned stimulus for shock. Brain Res. 103: 229-242.

(58) White, J.C., and Sweet, W.H. 1969. Pain and the Neurosurgeon: A Forty-Year Experience. Springfield, IL: C.C. Thomas.

(59) Wolstencroft, J.H. 1964. Reticulospinal neurons. J. Physiol. (London) 174: 91-108.

(60) Young, D.W., and Gottschaldt, K.M. 1976. Neurons in the rostral mesencephalic reticular formation of the cat responding specifically to noxious mechanical stimulation. Exp. Neurol. 51: 628-636.

Pain and Society, eds. H.W. Kosterlitz and L.Y. Terenius, pp. 201-222.
Dahlem Konferenzen 1980. Weinheim: Verlag Chemie GmbH.

The Role of Endogenous Opiates in Pain Control

H. Akil and S. J. Watson
Mental Health Research Institute, University of Michigan
Ann Arbor, MI 48109, USA

Abstract. This paper broadly reviews the current evidence implicating the endogenous opioids in pain modulation, bearing in mind the complexity of brain endorphins. It points to the existence of both opioid and non-opioid mechanisms of analgesia. It puts forth a working model for pain control suggesting complex interactions between pain transmission and pain inhibition via opioid and non-opioid mechanisms. Discussion of the model points to the pitfalls of using naloxone reversibility as the only criterion of involvement of endogenous opioids in an analgetic phenomenon. It is used as a springboard for evolving criteria for determining whether or not activation of endogenous opioids is the mechanism underlying a given type of analgesia.

INTRODUCTION

In this paper, we will present a brief overview of the current findings implicating endogenous opioids in pain regulation, as well as those pointing to their lack of involvement. While this will not be an exhaustive literature review, we hope to use it to highlight the difficulties we face, both conceptually and empirically. This will constitute a springboard for presenting a working model of pain transmission in which we can begin to delineate endogenous opioid and non-opioid components of inhibition of pain. The model will also serve as a starting point for establishing the criteria necessary to classify an analgesic phenomenon as "opioid-mediated."

Before embarking on this overview, however, it is necessary to summarize briefly our current understanding of the physiology of opioid peptides in the Central Nervous System. This will constitute the broad framework against which we will evaluate the evidence to date, and within which we can project our future goals.

MULTIPLICITY OF ENDOGENOUS OPIOID SYSTEMS

The discovery and sequencing of the enkephalins (30) was rapidly followed by the realization that endogenous opioid systems in brain were quite complex. β-Endorphin (βEP) was identified in pituitary soon thereafter (34). Several hypotheses about the relationship between enkephalins and βEP were entertained. For example, it was possible that βEP was a pituitary hormone, whereas the enkephalins would be brain neurotransmitters. Alternatively, βEP may also exist in brain but function as an enkephalin precursor. However, immunohistochemical and biochemical studies showed that neither hypothesis was completely accurate. βEP did exist in brain as well as in the pituitary, but not as an enkephalin precursor. Rather, it appeared to have a separate distribution, quite distinct from that of the enkephalins (9,12,52). While the enkephalins were distributed in multiple cell groups throughout the brain and down to the spinal cord (21,53), βEP could be localized in a single cell group in the arcuate nucleus of the hypothalamus. This βEP system projected via long axons to several limbic structures including areas such as the medial thalamus, and periaqueductal central gray (all critical integration areas for pain modulation). The two enkephalins (methionine- and leucine-enkephalin) could not be distinguished from each other in terms of overall distribution and were also in areas such as the central gray, as well as in Laminae I and V of the spinal cord. However, the distribution of both enkephalins and βEP was not restricted to those brain regions classically implicated in pain physiology. These peptides can also be found in other subcortical regions involved in endocrine regulation or motor integration.

A further dimension was added when it was discovered that βEP and its precursor, β-Lipotropin (βLPH), were stored in the same pituitary cells as ACTH and were in fact derived from a common precursor molecule, pro-opiocortin or 31K (36). We and others have since demonstrated that the 31K system also exists in brain (43,50,51,52,54). The βEP-containing neuron also contains ACTH and αMSH. Within them the biosynthesis appears to resemble what is seen in the intermediate lobe of the pituitary: the 31K precursor is cleaved into a 16K N-Terminus fragment (function unknown), then $ACTH_{1-39}$, and βLPH. The latter two peptides are further processed to αMSH (N-acetyl $ACTH_{1-13}$ amide) and βEP (βLPH 61-91) (20). We can, indeed, visualize both the precursor, intermediates (16K, ACTH, βLPH), and the final products (βEP and αMSH).

Thus, the brain contains at least three endogenous opioid peptides, the two enkephalins localized in what resembles interneurons or short local circuits, and βEP in a single wide-ranging system. The latter peptide co-exists with αMSH and derives from a common precursor. Whether βEP and αMSH are co-released in brain and what their potential interaction is remain to be determined. However, uncovering these modulations is likely to be extremely important in our understanding of the role of this system in pain regulation. Finally, the complexity of the endogenous pathways would lead one to expect some differences in their associated receptors. The hypothesis of multiple opiate receptors has been advanced by Martin et al. (37). While we shall not elaborate on it here, it is yet another variable which may complicate our understanding of modulation of pain by endogenous opioids.

STUDIES OF ENDOGENOUS OPIOIDS AND PAIN INHIBITION

Administration of Opioid Peptides

The most obvious reason to expect a role of endogenous opioids in pain derives from the analgesic effect of opiates and opioid peptides when pharmacologically administered. While enkephalin has a transient analgesic effect (10), βEP produces much longer lasting analgesia (15). The effect of both peptides is prevented by the administration of the opiate antagonist naloxone, an important criterion for implicating the opiate receptor.

It should be noted, however, that the pharmacological administration of either family of opioids may lead to the activation of opiate receptors in sites which are not typically recruited by these peptides under physiological conditions. For example, βEP administration may activate opiate receptors in nucleus gigantocellularis, whereas endogenous βEP may not. Since the opiate receptor "cross reacts" with several endogenous opioids, we cannot conclude that any given opiate typically produces pain inhibition just because its pharmacological administration does. Nor can we state that βEP is more important because it is a more potent analgesic. While this may be due to a difference in rate of breakdown of the two peptides, or in the rate of dissociation from the receptor (1), it is difficult to determine at this point which are the more critical substances in pain control. Indeed, analgesia is an extreme state of pain regulation, often undesirable. It is possible to conceive of enkephalins as controlling acute pain and producing rapid but short-lived changes, while βEP modulates the "set point" and longer lasting effects.

The foregoing discussion does point to some of the difficulties of attributing a physiological role based on direct pharmacological administration of opioid peptides. An alternative approach is to attempt to alter the functions of endogenous opioids by blocking the receptor and examining the subsequent effects on pain responsiveness. Thus, a number of studies using the opiate antagonist, naloxone, have been recently published.

Naloxone's Effect on Pain Responsivness

In 1974, Jacob and his co-workers (31) demonstrated that naloxone administration produces hyperalgesia on the hot plate test. One interpretation of this finding is that pain responsiveness is under inhibitory control of endogenous opioids, and that their blockade results in hypersensitivity to pain. If this were the case, then other types of pain tests should be similarly affected. Yet, there are several negative reports using other tests in rat and man (25,26). While there are some reports of naloxone causing hyperalgesia in the tail flick test (11), the effect tends to be small. In man, naloxone has had little effect on experimental pain (26), although there are reports of naloxone effects in some experimental situations and in clinical pain, as well as reversal of placebo effects (16,32,33). There is also a recent report of patients who are congenitally insensitive to pain showing some pain responsiveness after naloxone injection (19). The above findings are all new, require replication, and typically involve situations where pain responsiveness has swung away from homeostasis. Nonetheless, naloxone remains, generally speaking, relatively impotent in producing significant hyperalgesia in animals or in man.

The small effects of naloxone fly in the face of a hypothesis which would place endogenous opioids at a critical junction in circuits modulating pain responsiveness. One possible explanation is that the endogenous opioid modulation of pain is not tonic - rather opioids have to be activated by some environmental or physiological stimulus before they exhibit their modulation of pain. Under this hypothesis, certain types of pain tests, such as the hot plate test employed by Jacob et al. (31), would succeed in activating endogenous opioids resulting in naloxone-reversible increases in pain threshold. Other potential hypotheses which might account for the discrepant effects of naloxone on pain responsiveness could incorporate multiple pain inhibitory mechanisms with complex interactions. Such a model will be proposed and discussed shortly.

Opioids and Stimulation-Produced Analgesia

Before turning to a model, however, it may be useful to address the first hypothesis and explore some of the possible ways that endogenous opioids could be activated, and whether they appear to produce naloxone-reversible analgesia. The most direct activation would result from direct stimulation of opioid pathways within the brain. This, of course, is far from physiological. However, our work on stimulation-produced analgesia (SPA) in animals and man (5,41,46,47) does point to the importance of endogenous opioids in the control of pain. SPA in rats is known to produce naloxone reversible analgesia (3,4) and to be cross-tolerant with morphine (38). SPA has been employed to alleviate intractable pain in over thirty human patients. The stimulation site is medial, immediately adjacent to the ventricular system. The analogous sites in lower animals are extremely rich in endogenous opioids, particularly βEP. We (5) and Hosobuchi et al. (28) have reported that this analgesia can be reversed by naloxone: this was congruent with our previous animal findings (3,4) which had led us to suggest that SPA is accompanied by a release of endogenous opioids.

We therefore undertook the study of the C.S.F. from stimulated human patients to determine whether stimulation which leads to pain relief is correlated with the release of endogenous opioids. In two separate studies, we examined levels of enkephalin-like material and of βEP-like immunoreactivity before and after analgetic electrical stimulation in our patients (6,7). In the first study, enkephalin-like material was characterized on two chromatographic methods which separated it from βEP and was measured with two bioassays which recognized opiate-like material, the opiate binding assay, and the vas-deferens bioassay. In the second study, we employed a specific radioimmunoassay which recognized βEP but not methionine enkephalin (8). Both studies demonstrated a significant rise in opioid peptides during twenty minutes of stimulation. Enkephalin-like material was elevated by approximately 50%, whereas βEP-like material was dramatically increased (up to 20-30-fold). In a very similar study, Hosobuchi et al. (29) have also demonstrated a substantial rise in βEP immunoreactivity upon electrical stimulation in humans.

While the studies with SPA have been critical in suggesting a role of endogenous opioids in pain regulation, they also began to point to the complexities of pain modulation. Even the first studies of naloxone's effect on SPA in rat (3,4) showed that only a fraction of the animals exhibited naloxone-reversible analgesia. Other animals, which were not easily distinguishable by any other means, had a high degree of analgesia which remained totally resistant to the effects of naloxone.

Furthermore, other investigators could not produce reversal of of SPA with naloxone (55). However, recently, we have begun to uncover some of the complicating factors involved in this paradigm. A report at the 1978 Neuroscience meeting by Stein suggested that naloxone-reversibility of SPA and self-stimulation was highly dependent on current parameters. More recent work in the laboratory of Liebeskind (45) demonstrates that naloxone reversibility is site-specific. Stimulation of ventral central gray leads to naloxone-reversible analgesia, whereas more dorsal sites appear resistant to naloxone's effect. It is possible that stimulation of sites presynaptic to an enkephalinergic or endorphinergic synapse cause naloxone-reversible analgesia, whereas stimulation of a post-synaptic site would produce naloxone-resistant analgesia. However, it is also likely that there are mechanisms of pain inhibition which do not involve opioids at all. That such probably exists is further indicated by studies described below.

Stress-Induced Analgesia

If we entertain the hypothesis that endogenous opioid control over pain is tonically "silent," then it must be engaged by physiological or environmental events. We and others (2,27, 35) have shown that stress can bring about changes in pain responsiveness, including a high degree of analgesia. We (2,35) demonstrated that footshock stress resulted in a rise in endogenous opioid levels in brain, and that the analgesia was partially prevented by naloxone. Recently, Frederickson and co-workers (23) have shown a rise in enkephalin immunoreactivity upon heat stress, and this effect exhibited a circadian rhythm congruent with that of naloxone's effect on pain responsiveness in the hot plate test (22).

While the view of stress-induced activation of the endogenous opioid system is attractive, it is too simplistic. Whereas naloxone is capable of reversing the analgesic effects of stress in our hands ((2) and unpublished data) and those of others (13), the effect is at best partial, and other researchers using shorter stress do not see any naloxone effects (27). Furthermore, stress-induced analgesia exhibits cross-tolerance with morphine in the hands of one group studying mice (18), but does not exhibit cross-tolerance in our hands (9) or those of Bodnar and co-workers (14). In fact, we have observed a dramatic enhancement in stress-induced analgesia in opiate-tolerant rats (9), a paradoxical finding which has been recently replicated by others. Thus, the partial effects of naloxone and the paradoxical effects of tolerance of morphine on stress-induced analgesia point to the need for a more complex model of pain regulation.

Other Modes of Inducing Analgesia and the Relation to Endogenous Opioids

Placebo effects on pain have been reported to be naloxone reversible (32), whereas hypnotic analgesia does not appear to be (24). Mayer and co-workers (40) were the first to report that acupuncture analgesia is naloxone-reversible in man and Pomeranz and co-workers (44) have demonstrated a similar phenomenon in mice.

Bodnar and his co-workers have studied several other methods of inducing analgesia including the use of insulin hypoglycemia and shown that many of them can be partially or totally resistant to naloxone.

Among the above paradigms, however, few, if any, have directly correlated changes in levels of endogenous opioids with changes in pain responsiveness. In fact, the work studying pain responsiveness and endogenous opioids directly consists merely of the above-reported studies on SPA and release of endogenous opioids and the pioneering work performed by Terenius and co-workers (43, 49). These authors have demonstrated that opioids in the C.S.F., some of them still unidentified, appeared to be lower in some patients suffering from chronic pain. They have evolved a classification of pain syndromes and a correlation between them and certain opioid-containing fractions in human C.S.F.

In summary, the evidence for a role of endogenous opioids in pain inhibition can be stated as follows:

1) Pharmacological administration of endogenous opioids causes analgesia.

2) Some chronic pain patients exhibit decreased levels of opioids in C.S.F.
3) Analgesic electrical stimulation is correlated with release of opioids in C.S.F.
4) Naloxone produces complex effects partially or totally preventing SPA, stress-induced analgesia, acupuncture and placebo analgesia, and altering threshold to clinical pain and to some animal tests. On the other hand, naloxone fails to reverse analgesia in animals undergoing electrical stimulation at certain sites or responding to stress, fails to reverse hypnosis analgesia and does not appear to alter experimental pain in man.
5) Cross-tolerance of some analgesias with morphine has only been studied in a few paradigms. Such cross-tolerance occurs with SPA but shows paradoxical interaction with stress-induced analgesia and acupuncture analgesia.

Thus, most studies suggest that even if endogenous opioids are involved in pain regulation, one must invoke non-opioid mechanisms of analgesia as well (c.f. (39)). Furthermore, many of the conclusions appear to depend primarily on the use of naloxone, with little other evidence. While naloxone-reversibility could be construed as necessary, we will discuss below why it may not be sufficient to implicate endogenous opioids in any given analgesic phenomenon.

A WORKING MODEL FOR PAIN MODULATION

From the foregoing discussion, it appears clear that we are in need of defining criteria for calling an analgesic phenomenon opioid in nature. Is naloxone reversibility a necessary and sufficient condition? Can it, alone, be the basis for classifying analgesic phenomena as "opioid" and "non-opioid"? In order to address these issues, we are suggesting a model of pain modulation which takes into consideration the information we already possess and hopes to integrate the apparent complexities many researchers have encountered.

It should be stated here that this is merely a working model. We know much too little about many facets of this problem to have any certainty in assigning circuitry, directionality, or determining the critical components in such a model. One of our main goals is to show the reader how a reasonable working hypothesis can be evolved which points to the pitfalls of using naloxone as a sole criterion for determining the opioid nature of an analgesic phenomenon. We hope to use the model to evolve reasonable criteria for dissecting apart opioid and non-opioid mechanisms and for putting in perspective the role of endorphinergic mechanisms in pain control. Specifically, we are using it to address the following questions:

1) How do opioid and non-opioid mechanisms of analgesia relate to each other and how do their interactions affect pain transmission and perception?
2) Why does naloxone, which reverses opiate alkaloids, readily exhibit minimal effects on many baseline pain behaviors and partial effects on many analgesic phenomena?
3) How is it possible to have an analgesic phenomenon which is susceptible to naloxone blockade but not to opiate tolerance?
4) Can we evolve criteria for teasing apart opioid from non-opioid mechanisms?

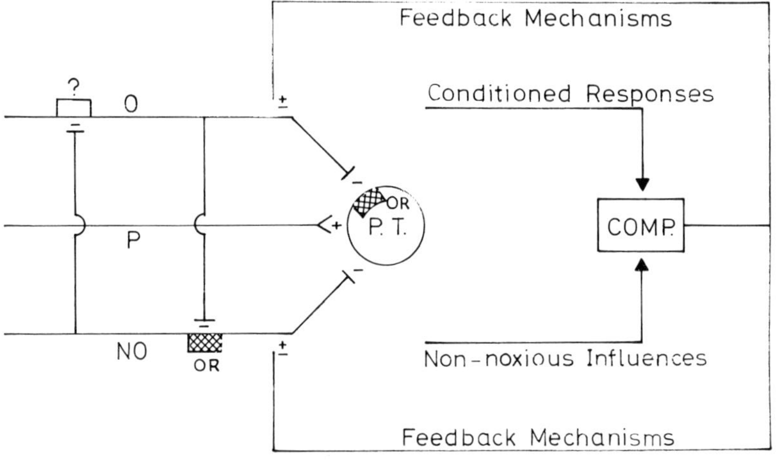

FIG. 1 - A schematic diagram of the working model.

The circle in the middle labelled PT represents pain transmission. The model depicts PT as being determined by three major factors: P = pain input, O = opioid pain inhibitory system, and NO = a non-opioid pain inhibitory system. Pain input would facilitate pain transmission, whereas O and NO are antinociceptive mechanisms and would therefore inhibit pain transmission. Pain inhibition by the opioid system would be mediated via an opiate receptor (OR) at a critical junction, depicted here on PT. Moreover, O and NO are not likely to function in isolation. They are seen as interacting with each other, possibily by mutual inhibition, in order to prevent extreme and long lasting analgesia and to maintain the organism's critical ability to respond to pain. Here again, the modulation of NO by O would be mediated via an opiate receptor (OR on NO). Pain transmission, in turn, would be integrated with other inputs and via comparator mechanisms modulate both opioid and non-opioid systems, allowing them to become more or less active. The large arrows in the scheme point to some of the influences on the comparator circuit which affect its feedback onto O and NO - perceptual events, the subject's mood or drive state, non-noxious but possibly stressful influences, and conditioned or anticipatory responses resulting from the organism's history with pain in general, and the noxious event in particular.

A number of points should be made before discussing the implications of the model. First, the modulation of pain in this manner is not necessarily localized in one site within the C.N.S. Rather, these interactions are likely to take place at several levels of the neuraxis, from the first synapse in the spinal cord to the midbrain, limbic structures, thalamus, and even cortex. Second, each of the components, P, O, NO, are not thought to involve a single connection or neurotransmitter. Rather, they represent multisynaptic systems, some involving opioids at a critical junction (O), while others do not (NO). Finally, while this model does not address the controversy of "pain as a modality" versus "pain as a pattern of inputs," it accepts the notion that pain transmission is a highly modifiable event. As such, it is consistent with the broader principles of the Gate Control Theory (42). Its main goal, however, is to define the role of opioid vs. non-opioid mechanisms of pain control.

According to this working model, what can we expect if we administer naloxone to an otherwise "normal" animal and test for pain responsiveness? While naloxone may block the opiate receptor on PT, thus decreasing the inhibitory effect of the O system, the opiate receptor on NO would be blocked as well. This would release NO from inhibition, allowing it to become more active and restoring an ideal balance at the level of PT. We may, therefore, effect little or no change in pain responsiveness. This does not mean that we would never expect naloxone to affect pain threshold. There are states or behaviors where the relative importance of O in modulating PT is much greater, where non-opioid mechanisms may not compensate adequately, and where naloxone would cause hyperalgesia. Many variables, such as the circadian rhythm, the general drive state of the animal, and the test being employed would determine the relative roles of O and NO in the final balance. What this would suggest is that a lack of naloxone effect on "baseline pain responsiveness" does not eliminate a role of opioids in pain modulation. It merely points to a well-balanced system striving towards homeostasis. If, on the other hand, we stimulate the O system selectively and powerfully, we could produce analgesia. While the tonic activity of NO may be decreased, the large increase in O would be overpowering and PT would decrease. Such activation of the O system would be completely reversible by naloxone.

Furthermore, if the animal had been previously made tolerant to opiates, the opiate receptor sensitivity would be decreased and the activation of O would become less effective in blocking pain transmission. Thus, a direct activation of the O system would exhibit both naloxone reversibility and cross-tolerance with morphine.

Other events would activate the NO system and produce antinociception which should be resistant to the effects of naloxone. If, however, the O system is still active and is contributing to pain inhibition, then the administration of naloxone would eliminate this component and result in a partial or a subtle blockade of this inhibition.

If both O and NO are simultaneously activated, naloxone may, again, have partial effects. The oscillations between the two systems and the feedback from the comparator circuit are complex enough to make it a difficult situation to predict. The effects of naloxone may vary with time after the induction of antinociception and may be easily modifiable by other variables which determine the delicate balance between the various components.

Finally, analgesia can be brought about by interfering with pain input, somehow decreasing its sensitivity or efficacy (i.e., decreasing the P component). In this case, O and NO are _relatively_ more active, though they have not been directly enhanced. Naloxone would block the O component, thus restoring some of the sensitivity to pain. Under these conditions, naloxone reversal of the analgesic event would not mean that opioid mechanisms caused the analgesia in the first place - but only that opioid systems are critical in the balance which determines pain transmission and responsiveness.

CONCLUSIONS ON THE SIGNIFICANCE OF NALOXONE BLOCKADE

In summary, the following conclusions can be drawn about using naloxone to implicate endogenous opioids in analgesic events:

1. The lack of a naloxone effect in a normal, non-analgesic animal does not mean endogenous opioids are unimportant in pain modulation. It does not even mean that these substances are tonically inactive. Rather, it may simply mean that they are involved in a tightly regulated multicomponent circuit which is difficult to disrupt under some testing conditions.

2. If an analgesic phenomenon is entirely mediated by activation endogenous opioids, it should be completely naloxone reversible. Furthermore, the analgesia should be diminished in a morphine-tolerant animal.

3. Partial reversal by naloxone could occur under three conditions: the first is a situation where both opioid and non-opioid mechanisms are enhanced. The second is when only non-opioid mechanisms are activated, but the opioid mechanisms remain tonically active until naloxone removes their influence. The last is when pain transmission is somehow impaired and the critical balance determining PT is disrupted. Naloxone may restore this balance. A blocker of the NO system would be expected to have a similar effect.

4. It follows from 3 that, if naloxone reverses an analgesic event, we cannot automatically conclude that the analgesia is mediated by an increase in the activity of endogenous opioids but only that they are tonically important in the modulation of pain. The analgesic event itself could be due to activation of non-opioid pain inhibitory mechanisms or to a decrease in pain transmission.

CRITERIA FOR THE OPIOID NATURE OF AN ANALGESIC PHENOMENON

What is, then, a reasonable set of criteria for implicating endogenous opioids in an analgesic phenomenon? While naloxone is necessary, it is obviously not sufficient.

The criterion of cross-tolerance with morphine is a second and important one. While activation of the O system should be clearly less effective in a tolerant animal, what would be the effect of tolerance if NO is being activated? If we assume that tolerance results in a decrease of affinity, capacity, or efficacy of opiate receptors, then the role of the O system would be minimized. However, the NO system could still be activated, and because of the tolerance would escape the inhibitory control by O via OR. Therefore, one could produce an analgesic event via a non-opioid mechanism which would be enhanced rather than diminished in a morphine-tolerant animal. Such a phenomenon has been observed with stress-induced analgesia (9) and with acupuncture analgesia (17).

Thus, it appears that both naloxone and cross-tolerance to morphine would be criteria for stating that an analgesic event is primarily due to opioid mechanisms. Are these two criteria taken together sufficient? Not if we consider the notion of balance between pain input and pain inhibition. Let us say that P is decreased, thus producing analgesia. Pain responsiveness could be restored if the opiate receptor inhibiting PT is made less effective by a history of tolerance. This analgesic phenomenon could therefore appear cross-tolerant to morphine. On the other hand, NO may become more active in that tolerant animal, and no effect or a paradoxical effect of morphine tolerance would be observed. Thus, the complexities of the checks and balances proposed above point to the need for multiple criteria for stating that an analgesic phenomenon is caused by activation of opioids. These would include:

1) Naloxone reversibility of the analgesic event.
2) Diminution of the analgesic event in a morphine-tolerant subject.
3) Demonstration of release of enkephalin, βEP, or other opioids prior to or during the analgesic event.
4) A reasonable correlation between the time course of changes in endogenous opioid levels, release and/or turnover and the time course of pain responsiveness.
5) A decrease of the analgesic event if one or several opioid path ways are destroyed.
6) A potentiation of the analgesic event if the breakdown or metabolism of the opioids in question is decreased.

Some of these criteria need to await better understanding of opioid systems, their anatomy, regulation, turnover, and metabolism. Nonetheless, they should be kept in mind before attributing causation to an analgesic event.

As our understanding of endogenous opioid systems evolves, as we know more about their anatomy, synthesis, metabolism, and receptors, we can hope to devise new and rational methods for pain relief. However, these advances have to progress hand in hand with advances in our understanding of pain mechanisms in general and the role of both opioid and non-opioid mechanisms in pain control in particular.

Acknowledgement. This work was supported in part by the Mental Health Research Institute, University of Michigan and by National Institute of Drug Abuse Grant # DA02265-01 and a grant from the Scottish Rite Schizophrenia Research Foundation. The authors gratefully acknowledge the assistance in the manuscript preparation of C. Criss.

REFERENCES

(1) Akil, H.; Hewlett, W.; Barchas, J.D.; and Li, C.H. Characterization of ^{3}H-β-endorphin binding in rat brain. Life Sci., in press.

(2) Akil, H.; Madden, J.; Patrick, R.; and Barchas, J.D. 1976. Stress-induced increase in endogenous opiate peptides: concurrent analgesia and its partial reversal by naloxone. In Opiates and Endogenous Opioid Peptides, ed. H.W. Kosterlitz, pp. 63-70. Amsterdam: Elsevier/North Holland Press.

(3) Akil, H.; Mayer, D.J.; and Liebeskind, J.C. 1972. Comparaison chez le rat de l'analgesie induite par stimulation de la substance grise et l'analgesie morphinique. C.R. Acad. Sci. Ser. D. 274: 3603-3605.

(4) Akil, H.; Mayer, D.J.; and Liebeskind, J.C. 1976. Antagonism of stimulation-produced analgesia by naloxone, a narcotic antagonist. Science 191: 961-962.

(5) Akil, H.; Richardson, D.E.; and Barchas, J.D. 1979. Pain control by focal brain stimulation in man: relationship to enkephalins and endorphins. In Mechanisms of Pain and Analgesic Compounds, 11th Miles Int. Symposium, eds. R.F. Beers and E.G. Bassett, pp. 239-247. New York: Raven Press.

(6) Akil, H.; Richardson, D.E.; Barchas, J.D.; and Li, C.H. 1978. Appearance of β-endorphin-like immunoreactivity in human ventricular cerebrospinal fluid upon analgesic electrical stimulation. Proc. Natl. Acad. Sci. USA 75: 5170-72.

(7) Akil, H.; Richardson, D.E.; Hughes, J.; and Barchas, J.D. 1978. Enkephalin-like material elevated in ventricular cerebrospinal fluid of pain patients after analgetic focal stimulation. Science 201: 463-465.

(8) Akil, H.; Watson, S.J.; Barchas, J.D.; and Li, C.H. 1979. β-Endorphin immunoreactivity in rat and human blood: Radioimmunoassay, comparative levels and physiological alterations. Life Sci. 24: 1659-1666.

(9) Akil, H.; Watson, S.J.; Berger, P.A.; and Barchas, J.D. 1978. Endorphins, β-LPH, and ACTH: Biochemical, pharmacological and anatomical studies. In The Endorphins: Advances in Biochemical Psychopharmacology, eds. E. Costa and E.M. Trabucchi, vol. 18, pp. 125-139. New York: Raven Press.

(10) Beluzzi, J.D.; Grant, N.; Garsky, V.; Sarantakis, D.; Wise, C.D.; and Stein, L. 1976. Analgesia induced in vivo by central administration of enkephalin in rat. Nature 260: 625-626.

(11) Bernston, G.G., and Walker, J.M. 1977. Effect of opiate receptor blockade on pain sensitivity in the rat. Brain Res. Bull. 2: 157-159.

(12) Bloom, F.E.; Rossier, J.; Battenberg, E.L.F.; Bayon, A.; French, E.; Henricksen, S.J.; Siggins, G.R.; Segal, D.; Browne, R.; Ling, N.; and Guillemin, R. 1978. β-Endorphin: Cellular localization, electrophysiological and behavioral effects. In: The Endorphins: Advances in Biochemical Psychopharmacology, eds. E. Costa and M. Trabucchi, vol. 18, pp. 89-109. New York: Raven Press.

(13) Bodnar, R.J.; Kelly, D.D.; Spiagga, A.; Ehrenberg, C.; and Glusman, M. 1978. Dose-dependent reductions by naloxone of analgesia induced by cold-water stress. Pharmacol. Biochem. and Behav. 3: 667-672.

(14) Bodnar, R.J.; Kelly, D.D.; Steiner, S.S.; and Glusman, M. 1978. Stress-produced analgesia and morphine-produced analgesia: Lack of cross tolerance. Pharmacol. Biochem. and Behav. 8: 661-666.

(15) Bradbury, A.F.; Feldberg, W.F.; Smyth, D.G.; and Snell, C. 1976. Liptotropin C-fragment: An endogenous peptide with potent analgesic activity. In Opiates and Endogenous Opioid Peptides, ed. H.W. Kosterlitz, pp. 9-17. Amsterdam: Elsevier/North Holland.

(16) Buchsbaum, M.S.; Davis, G.C.; and Bunney, W.E. 1977. Naloxone alters pain perception and somatosensory evolved potentials in normal subjects. Nature 270: 620-622.

(17) Cheng, R.; Pomeranz, B.; and Yu, G. 1979. Electro-acupuncture reduces signs of withdrawal in morphine dependent mice and shows no cross-tolerance with morphine. Paper presented at the Meeting of the International Narcotic Research Conf., June, 1979.

(18) Chesher, G.B., and Chan, B. 1977. Footshock-induced analgesia in mice: Its reversal by naloxone and cross-tolerance with morphine. Life Sci. 21: 1569-1574.

(19) Dehen, H.; Willer, J.C.; Prier, S.; Bouran, F.; and Cambier, J. 1978. Congenital insensitivity to pain and the "morphine-like" analgesic system. Pain 5: 351-358.

(20) Eipper, B., and Mains, R. 1978. Existence of a common precursor to ACTH and endorphin in the anterior and intermediate lobes of the rat pituitary. J. Supramolecular Structure 8: 247-262.

(21) Elde, R.; Hokfelt, T.; Johansson, O.; and Terenius, L. 1976. Immunohistochemical studies using antibodies to leucine-enkephalin: Initial observations on the nervous system of the rat. Neuroscience 1: 349-351.

(22) Frederickson, R.C.A.; Burgis, V.; and Edwards, J.D. 1977. Hyperalgesia induced by naloxone follows diurnal rhythm in responsivity to painful stimuli. Science 198: 756-758.

(23) Frederickson, R.C.A.; Wesche, D.L.; and Richter, J.A. 1978. Mouse brain enkephalins: Study of diurnal changes correlated with changes in nociceptive sensitivity. In Developments in Neuroscience, Characteristics and Function of Opioids, eds. J.M. Van Ree and L. Terenius, vol. 4, pp. 169-172. Amsterdam: Elsevier/North Holland.

(24) Goldstein, A., and Hilgard, E.R. 1975. Failure of opiate antagonist naloxone to modify hypnotic analgesia. Proc. Natl. Acad. Sci. USA 72: 2041-2043.

(25) Goldstein, A.; Pryor, G.T.; Otis, L.S.; and Larsen, F. 1976. On the role of endogenous opioid peptides: Failure of naloxone to influence shock threshold in the rat. Life Sci. 18: 599-604.

(26) Grevert, P., and Goldstein, A. 1977. Effects of naloxone on experimentally induced ischemic pain and on mood in human subjects. Proc. Natl. Acad. Sci. USA 74: 1291-1294.

(27) Hayes, R.; Bennett, G.J.; Newlon, P.G.; and Mayer, D.J. 1978. Behavioral and physiological studies of non-narcotic analgesia in the rat, elicited by certain environmental stimuli. Brain Res. 155: 69-90.

(28) Hosobuchi, Y.; Adams, J.E.; and Linchitz, R. 1977. Pain relief by electrical stimulation of the central gray matter in humans and its reversal by naloxone. Science 197: 183-186.

(29) Hosobuchi, Y.; Rossier, J.; Bloom, F.; and Guillemin, R. 1979. Electrical stimulation of periaqueductal grey for pain relief in humans is accompanied by elevation of immunoreactive β-endorphin in ventricular fluid. Science 203: 279-281.

(30) Hughes, J.; Smith, T.W.; Kosterlitz, H.W.; Fothergill, L.A.; Morgan, B.A.; and Morris, H.R. 1975. Identification of two related pentapeptides from the brain with potent opiate agonist activity. Nature 258: 577-579.

(31) Jacob, J.J.; Tremblay, E.C.; and Colombel, M.C. 1974. Facilitation de reactions nociceptives par la naloxone chez la souris et chez le rat. Psychopharmacologia 37: 217-233.

(32) Levine, J.D.; Gordon, N.C.; and Fields, H.L. 1979. Naloxone dose dependently produces analgesia and hyperalgesia in postoperative pain. Nature 278: 740-741.

(33) Levine, J.D.; Gordon, N.C.; Jones, R.T.; and Fields, H.L. 1978. The narcotic antagonist naloxone enhances clinical pain. Nature 272: 826-827.

(34) Li, C.H., and Chung, D. 1976. Isolation and structure of an untriakontapeptide with opiate activity from camel pituitary glands. Proc. Natl. Acad. Sci. USA 73: 1145-1148.

(35) Madden, J.; Akil, H.; Patrick, R.L.; and Barchas, J.D. 1977. Stress-induced parallel changes in central opioid levels and pain responsiveness in the rat. Nature 266: 1358-1360.

(36) Mains, R.E.; Eipper, B.A.; and Ling, N. 1977. Common precursor to corticotropins and endorphins. Proc. Natl. Acad. Sci. USA 74: 3014-3018.

(37) Martin, W.R.; Eades, G.G.; Thompson, J.A.; Huppler, R.E.; and Gilbert, P.E. 1976. The effects of morphine and nalorphine-like drugs in the nondependent and morphine-dependent chronic spinal dog. J. Pharmacol. Exp. Ther. 197: 518-532.

(38) Mayer, D.J., and Hayes, R. 1975. Stimulation-produced analgesia: Development of tolerance and cross-tolerance to morphine. Science 188: 941-943.

(39) Mayer, D.J., and Price, D.D. 1976. Central nervous system mechanisms of analgesia. Pain 2: 379-404.

(40) Mayer, D.J.; Price, D.D.; and Raffi, A. 1977. Antagonism of acupuncture analgesia in man by the narcotic antagonist naloxone. Brain Res. 121: 368-372.

(41) Mayer, D.J.; Wolfle, T.L.; Akil, H.; Carder, B.; and Liebeskind, J.C. 1971. Analgesia resulting from electrical stimulation in the brainstem of the rat. Science 174: 1351-1354.

(42) Melzack, R., and Wall, P.D. 1965. Pain mechanisms: a new theory. Science 150: 971-979.

(43) Pelletier, G. 1979. Ultrastructural localization of neuropeptides with the post-embedment staining method. A paper presented at the annual meeting of the Histochemical Society, April, 1979.

(44) Pomeranz, B., and Chiu, D. 1976. Naloxone blockade of acupuncture analgesia: Endorphine implicated. Life Sci. 19: 1757-1762.

(45) Prieto, G.J.; Giesler, J.G.; and Cannon, T.T. 1979. Evidence for site specificity in naloxone's antagonism of SPA in the rat. Soc. for Neurosciences.

(46) Richardson, D.E., and Akil, H. 1977. Pain reduction by electrical brain stimulation in man: Part 1: Acute administration in periaqueductal and periventricular sites. J. Neurosurg. 47: 178-183.

(47) Richardson, D.E., and Akil, H. 1977. Pain reduction by electrical brain stimulation in man. Part 2: Chronic self-administration in the periventricular gray matter. J. Neurosurg. 47: 184-194.

(48) Terenius, L., and Wahlstrom, A. 1975. Morphine-like ligand for opiate receptors in human C.S.F. Life Sci. 16: 1759-1764.

(49) Von Knorring, L.; Alamay, B.G.L.; Johansson, F.; and Terenius, L. 1978. Pain perception and endorpin levels in cerebrospinal fluid. Pain 5: 359-366.

(50) Watson, S.J. α-MSH in brain β-endorphin neurons, and other neurons as well. Life Sci., in press.

(51) Watson, S.J., and Akil, H. The presence of two α-MSH positive cell groups in rat hypothalamus. Eur. J. Pharmacol., in press.

(52) Watson, S.J.; Akil, H.; Richard, C.W.; and Barchas, J.D. 1978. Evidence for two separate opiate peptide neuronal systems and the coexistence of β-lipotropin, β-endorphin, and ACTH immunoreactivities in the same hypothalamic neurons. Nature 275: 226-228

(53) Watson, S.J.; Akil, H.; Sullivan, S.O.; and Barchas, J.D. 1977. Immunocytochemical localization of methionine-enkephalin: Preliminary observations. Life Sci. 25: 733-738.

(54) Watson, S.J.; Richard, C.W.; and Barchas, J.D. 1978. Adrenocorticotropin in rat brain: Immunocytochemical localization in cells and axons. Science 200: 1180-1182.

(55) Yaksh, T.L.; Yeung, J.C.; and Rudy, T.A. 1976. An inability to antagonize with naloxone the elevated nociceptive thresholds resulting from electrical stimulation of the central gray. Life Sci. 18: 1193-1198.

Pain and Society, eds. H.W. Kosterlitz and L.Y. Terenius, pp. 223-237.
Dahlem Konferenzen 1980. Weinheim: Verlag Chemie GmbH.

Mental Mechanisms in the Control of Pain

B. Finer
Samariterhemmet, Box 609
751 25 Uppsala 1, Sweden

Abstract. In many countries, trance states are part of everyday life and are probably the most striking examples of mental mechanisms in the control of pain. At the same time, the body seems to be protected from damage. In the laboratory and clinic, a suitable method for investigating and utilizing these phenomena is hypnosis, which produces blocks of conditioned pain reflexes and sympathetic pain reflexes to some experimental and clinical pain. Recent observations have reawakened interest in descriptions from the mid-19th century of the protective effect of hypnosis against tissue injury.

INTRODUCTION

In recent years, it has been recognized that severe chronic pain almost always produces psychological changes even in stable individuals (35-37). While somatic methods of treatment can partially and temporarily relieve some of the components of chronic pain, it is usually necessary to use psychological methods to achieve further improvement. Clinically, there are some indications that better results are obtained if somatic and psychological methods can be used at the same time. However, the mental mechanisms in the control of pain are still poorly understood.

CULTURAL OUTLOOK

In many cultures, trance states are part of everyday life,

especially in relation to religious ceremonies. A trance state is any state in which the generalized reality-orientation has faded to relatively nonfunctional unawareness. The usual generalized reality-orientation is a structured frame of reference in the background of attention, which supports, interprets, and gives meaning to all experiences in the usual state of consciousness (33). Trance state is an altered state of consciousness, characterized by a qualitative shift in mental functioning (38). Sometimes, religious devotees undergo procedures in trance which would normally be considered agonizingly painful, with no sign whatsoever of suffering. Indeed, the public taking part in these ceremonies and observing the complete absence of suffering in these participants take these happenings as conclusive evidence "that a spiritual being of vast and undefined powers possesses the body... They go into a trance by autosuggestion, incantation, burning of joss papers and incense, or beating of gongs, and each subject has his or her own way of trance induction. All of them go into a somnambulistic trance with total amnesia" (3). In Singapore, the Chinese Medium has a large spear piercing one cheek, cuts the tongue with a sharp sword, or carries a bundle of flaming joss sticks against his chest wall without experiencing any pain or burn. Also in Singapore, "the trance states observed among the Hindu Devotees carrying the "Kavadi" and fire-walking on Thaipusam Day are induced in a different setting. The Kavadi is a wooden arch on a wooden base decorated with peacock feathers and coloured papers... with the drumming of rhythmic tunes and incantations, 100% of the Devotees go into a somnambulistic trance. The Kavadi is rested on the Devotee's shoulders. Needles, thin steel shafts, connected to the Kavadi, are pierced through the skin. Often, in addition, silver pins are pierced right through the tongue horizontally and vertically, and through the cheeks" (3).

In Bali this year, the author observed a Ketchak Dance of boys and young men, followed by a Fire Dance by one selected subject, a simple peasant from the island. This man danced barefoot for 5 minutes in and out of a heap of red-hot, glowing cinders of coconut shells, kicking and trampling them. At the end of the dance, four men threw themselves on to him, throwing cold water on him to bring him out of trance. Two of my Swedish colleagues and I were allowed to go into the temple with an interpreter and examine the subject before the dance and also in front of the temple after the dance. Before the dance, he appeared completely calm, though he had a heart rate of 100 beats/minute. His feet appeared normal, with soft, uninjured skin. He had danced like this many times before and was one of about eight subjects on the island who danced in this way. After the dance, he sat somewhat dazed on the ground, shiny with sweat, but with a heart rate unchanged at 100 beats/minute and not the least sign of injury to the soles of the feet. In Bali, another religious ceremony involves a Kris Dance. Here, men in trance turn the points of very sharp swords against their chests and press as hard as they can. At the Department of Psychiatry, University of Denpaser, one of the two physicians doing research on trance in Bali, I.G.P. Panteri, has examined these men after trance and told me that they do produce superficial wounds, but never damage the deeper tissues, e.g., lung or heart.

HYPNOSIS, SUGGESTION, PLACEBO AND SELF-REGULATION

Hypnosis is an altered experience of reality, in a trusting relationship, with an increased ability for concentration, detachment, and creativity. The ability to detach from pain is partly a block of conditioned pain reflexes (18) and partly a block of sympathetic pain reflexes (11). Other names for these blocks have been negative hallucination for pain and placebo response, respectively (32). Under some circumstances, pain exists but is denied (21).

Suggestibility is the susceptibility and propensity of persons uncritically to accept and/or automatically to respond to specific statements or non-specific cues. It also refers to the tendency for a person to misperceive or misinterpret stimuli or situations based either on inner fears or wishes (26). Much of the psychological component of chronic pain could thus be due to negative suggestibility following misinterpretation due to inner fears.

Placebo from the classic definition "I will please" (or placate) has been enlarged to include any therapy which cannot be attributed to the specific properties of the treatment (6). In this definition encouragement, literally "giving heart," can be included. The point is that the therapeutic milieu can be manipulated by the people taking care of the patient.

Self-Regulation approaches in the management of chronic pain are based on active participation of the patient during different therapeutic modalities such as hypnosis, biofeedback, placebo, psychotherapy, conditioning, relaxation, and medication (7).

It has been claimed (27) that 50% of the population should be able to develop sufficient hypnotic analgesia to obtain pain relief after upper abdominal operations. In such circumstances, coughing and deep breathing should be easier than in non-hypnotized subjects. This has been put to an experimental test (10). Patients undergoing cholecystectomy were given dynamic lung function tests before and each of the four days following operation. A group trained so that hypnotic analgesia of the abdomen could be produced preoperatively was compared with a control group without this training. Surprisingly, the hypnosis group did no better than the control group, though the former stated that induction of hypnosis in the laboratory reduced the pain. Another group receiving maximal encouragement preoperatively and postoperatively did slightly better, but the difference was not significant. Clinically, it was noticed that the preoperative hypnosis training seemed to make the patient more concentrated on the negative aspects of the coming operation. The experiments were continued with two further groups, one in which no encouragement was given in the beginning, but maximal encouragement at the end, and one in which maximal encouragement was given in the beginning, but not at the end. The differences in lung function between no encouragement and maximal encouragement in these last experiments were significant.

More recently, the effects of alpha-feedback treatment, hypnosis, and a combination of both on chronic pain patients has been analyzed (28). It was concluded that only by a combination of alpha-feedback and hypnosis could the chronic pain be reduced significantly and that the alpha-feedback was a placebo procedure working through distraction of attention, suggestion, relaxation, and sense of control over pain. In the last few years, "a hidden observer" has been implied during hypnosis (21). In experiments with hypnotic subjects, where the non-dominant hand was immersed in ice-cold water, the time of immersion could be significantly prolonged during hypnotic analgesia of the immersed hand. However, automatic writing with the other hand, at the same time, revealed such expressions as "it hurts terribly." The implication was that part of the consciousness is always in touch with reality, however deep the hypnosis.

EXPERIMENTAL APPROACHES TO THE MECHANISMS OF HYPNOSIS

Many years ago, it was postulated (5) that the reflex response to nociceptive stimuli is a generalized, integrated flexor movement. In the cat (16) and in man (17), it has been shown that this flexor reflex does not hold universally. A nociceptive stimulus of skin over the muscle from which EMG recordings were being taken produced an extensor reflex, though such stimuli of all other areas continued to produce a flexor reflex. At about this time, it was shown (19) that midbrain stimulation in the cat could inhibit nociceptive input into the lumbar cord. Soon after, it was found (29) that in puppies some of the seemingly fundamental avoidance responses to pain were learned in early life. It was then shown (20) that the abdominal spinal reflex in man is susceptible to suggestion in the normal waking state and that withdrawal responses to nociceptive stimuli to the lower limb in man varies according to the experimental conditions. When the arousal value of the stimulus was low, a spinal reflex occurred, with a latency of about 60 msec. When the arousal value was increased by fear, the reflex amplitude increased. Some changes could be seen according to suggestions under hypnosis. When the motivation for withdrawal was increased by prolonging the stimulus, a second reflex appeared with latency of about 120 msec., which appeared to be conditioned. It could be taught to change under certain circumstances and seemed to correct mistakes made by the spinal reflexes. These later reflexes were highly susceptible to hypnotic influence. They might well be related to the learned reflexes in the puppies (18).

Among the withdrawal responses of clinical importance in man are the plantar reflexes, abdominal reflexes, pharyngeal reflexes, and eyelash reflexes. When a person under hypnosis is asked to imagine the plantar surfaces of the feet, the abdominal skin, the pharynx, or the eyelids becoming numb, and if the person succeeds, the corresponding reflexes to touch diminish or disappear (18). The hypnotic situation is thus one of trust, in which the subject dares to lend some of the responsibility for self-defense to the hypnotist. Many subjects, who are usually very ticklish under their feet, are surprised that the plantar reflexes are so easily modified. These results cast further interesting light on the religious trance phenomena described above.

Recently, changes in C-fiber activity in human skin nerves during hypnosis have been studied (12). Preliminary results show that during periods of imagined hyperalgesia of the skin, there was a dramatic increase in sympathetic outflow, correlated with pronounced changes in galvanic skin resistance and increases in both respiration and heart rates. By contrast, imagined hypoalgesia was accompanied by a decrease in sympathetic outflow and corresponding decreases in the other parameters. These several results show that hypnosis can affect both central and sympathetic pathways for pain, modulating both the pain sensation and the reaction to pain (2). However, it must be pointed out that these changes were no greater than with corresponding emotional changes without hypnosis.

About 20 years ago, it was noticed that patients with chronic pain in the arm or leg, who gained pain relief with hypnosis, often explained afterwards that as soon as the pain disappeared, they experienced a feeling of pulsating warmth in the extremity. Experiments were begun on blood flow in forearm and calf, which are mostly muscle, and in hand and foot, which are mostly skin, during hypnosis using venous occlusion plethysmography (11). The most profound changes were found during imagined increased pain, where the systolic and diastolic blood pressures and heart rate rose, where muscle blood flow increased, and skin blood flow decreased. These changes were characteristic of stress reactions, usually mediated via the sympathetic nervous system. The changes were counteracted by imagining decreased pain and by some sympathetic blocking agents, such as propranolol; however, placebo was also effective. During an operation for varicose veins in 1972, in which hypnosis was the only premedication, preoperative analgesia, and postmedication, measurements of blood pressure, heart rate, and catecholamines in the urine showed no changes during the operative procedure, except those due to postural reflexes (13).

Studies with naloxone, a pure opiate antagonist, have cast conflicting light on these problems. One report showed that pain following extraction of impacted wisdom teeth was increased by naloxone (24), while another showed that chronic pain is not so affected (25). Several reports have shown that hypnotic analgesia is not counteracted by naloxone (1,15,31), with one showing the opposite (34). One report has shown that placebo analgesia is counteracted by naloxone (23), another that it is not (30).

HYPNOSIS IN MEDICAL CARE

Recently, the use of hypnosis has been described in severe burns within two hours of injury (9). Not only was pain relieved, but the usual inflammatory reaction and the subsequent development of tissue damage was also halted at the second degree stage. Thus, there was little or no infection, no skin necrosis, no need for skin transplantation, and healing occurred without scarring. While ether anesthesia was being

psychiatrist and routine social consultation with our social worker. Patients are given the possibilities of working through their total life situations in individual therapy.

New patients often arrive with their own and even referring colleagues magical expectations that hypnosis can definitely cure their pain for good with no demands on them personally. At the very first meeting, it is pointed out that no promise can be made of pain relief. On the other hand, attempts are made to help the patient live a richer life in spite of the pain. Of course, one is happy if the pain is less, but no guarantees can be given. The cotherapist meets the new patients first, putting into their hands a little brochure she has written, describing what they can expect of us. She points out that it is essential that what is said in the group stays in the group. On the first day, a routine history and examination are carried out by a medical colleague and the patient may be referred to, e.g., a gynecologist.

Every day, usually between 2:00-3:00 p.m., when the routine anesthetic work has quieted down somewhat, the patients, cotherapist, and I meet, possibly also a preregistration doctor, training in anesthesia with me, who might be interested. The first part of the treatment is directed to hypnosis training, with the emphasis on autohypnosis. The patients are encouraged and exhorted to imagine, in a realistic manner, the ability to reduce symptoms, diminish worrying, stress, and pain, increase self-confidence, and be able to cope better with life in society later. The patients are encouraged to record the hypnosis program on tape, so that they can listen when they are tense and alone. This possibility gives the patients added security and independence. After the end of the group autohypnosis, the patients are given the possibility, together with others who understand, of expressing former helplessness, disappointment, aggressiveness, and sorrow. At the same time, they are given support and company during these painful moments. By this means, we hope to motivate the patients to be able to create another life, in which pain is not the main point, but where physical and mental activity also have their place. It is hoped that this can lead to an increased joy in life. At the same time, little interest is shown in long, drawn-out, repeated descriptions of the martyrish small details of pain. In this way, attempts are made to treat both psychodynamically and behaviorally at the same time. The aim is to help the patients abandon their former passivity, with constant hopes of magical cures, and instead take responsibility for a realistic development of their lives, even if the pain itself does not change. The patients' frequent attempts at bargaining for sympathy are counteracted by the therapists and the other patients, who remind them of the possibility of an active life in spite of their handicap.

When the patients return home, they know that they may return for two weeks twice a year, and this knowledge gives them very great security. This makes it easier for them to leave the protective atmosphere of the hospital and be able to cope with everyday life at home. Once a week a staff round is organized. Apart from the psychiatrist, social worker, cotherapist, and myself, there are the physiotherapist, the ward doctors, the chief nurse, assistant nurses and orderlies, ward secretary and admissions secretary, as well as the possible preregistration doctor. I present the changes during the past week and the others come freely with comments, points of view, criticism, etc. Since the patients talk with all kinds of staff and can arouse anxiety and worry in them, it is vital that the whole staff discuss with each other differing points of view about treatment and at the same time get support for their respective contributions.

Once a month, the psychiatrist, social worker, cotherapist, and I meet for a supervisory round table discussion. It is necessary to discuss the technical side of therapy and also possible difficulties which we experience in the therapy situations. We have begun to assess the results of treatment by interview questionnaire and we go to these supervisory meetings with suggestions for improvement.

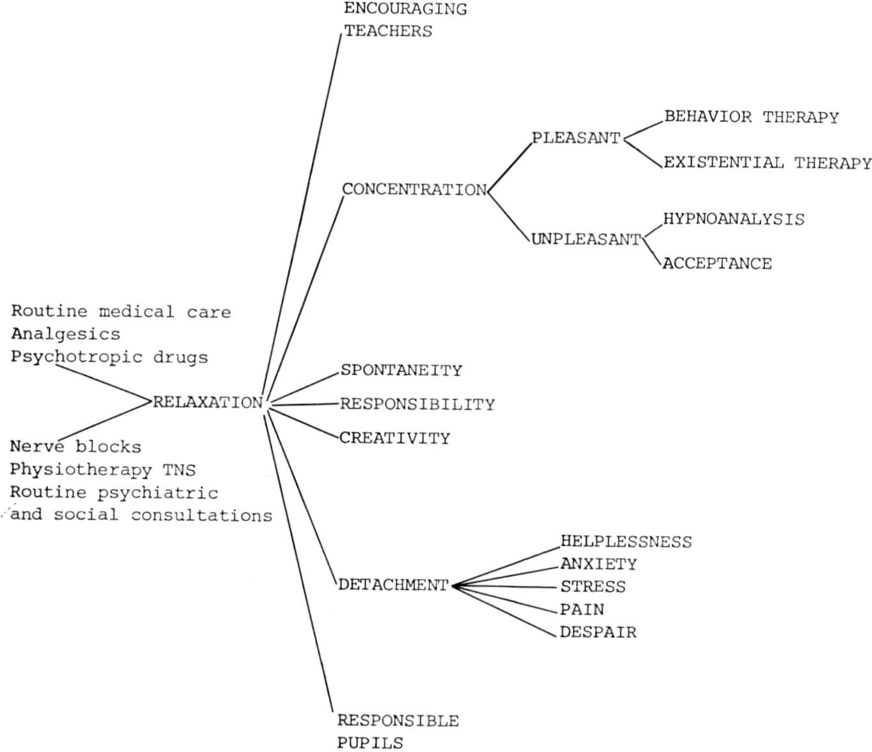

USE OF HYPNOSIS IN PAIN

REFERENCES

(1) Barber, J., and Mayer, D. 1977. Evaluation of the efficacy and neural mechanism of a hypnotic analgesia procedure in experimental and clinical dental pain. Pain 4: 41-48.

(2) Beecher, H.K. 1959. Measurement of Subjective Responses. New York: Oxford University Press.

(3) Chong, T.M. 1975. The Truth about Hypnosis. Singapore: T.M. Chong.

(4) Crasilneck, H.B.; Stirman, J.A.; and Wilson, B.J. 1955. Use of hypnosis in the management of patients with burns. JAMA 158: 103-106.

(5) Creed, R.S.; Denny-Brown, D.; Eccles, J.C.; Liddell, E.G.T.; and Sherrington, C.S. 1932. Reflex Activity of the Spinal Cord. London: Oxford University Press.

(6) Egbert, L.D. 1967. Psychological support for surgical patients. In Psychological Aspects of Surgery, ed. H.S. Abram, pp. 37-51. Boston: Little, Brown.

(7) Elton, D.; Burrows, G.D.; and Stanley, G.V. 1979. Hypnosis in the management of chronic pain. In Hypnosis 1979, eds. G.D. Burrows, D.R. Collison, and L. Dennerstein, pp. 113-120. Amsterdam: Elsevier/North-Holland Biomedical Press.

(8) Esdaile, J. 1957. Hypnosis in Medicine and Surgery. New York: Julian Press. (Original date 1850).

(9) Ewin, D. 1979. Hypnosis in burn therapy. In Hypnosis 1979, eds. G.D. Burrows, D.R. Collison, and L. Dennerstein, pp. 269-275. Amsterdam: Elsevier.

(10) Finer, B. 1970. Studies of the variability in expiratory efforts before and after cholecystectomy. Acta Anaesth. Scand. suppl. 38.

(11) Finer, B., and Graf, K. 1968. Mechanisms of circulatory changes accompanying hypnotic imagination of hyperalgesia and hypoalgesia in causalgic limbs. Z. ges. exp. Med. 148: 1-21.

(12) Finer, B.; Hallin, R.; and Torebjörk, E. 1978. Sympathetic outflow in human skin nerves during hypnosis. Pain abstracts, p. 33. Second World Congress on Pain, Montreal, Canada.

(13) Finer, B.; Jonzon, A.; Sedin, G.; and Sjöstrand, U. 1973. Some physiological changes during minor surgery under hypnotic analgesia. Acta Anaesth. Scand. suppl. 53: 94-96.

(14) Finer, B., and Nylén, B. 1961. Cardiac arrest in the treatment of burns, and report on hypnosis as a substitute for anaesthesia. Plast. Reconstr. Surg. 27: 49-55.

(15) Goldstein, A., and Hilgard, E.H. 1975. Failure of the opiate antagonist naloxone to modify hypnotic analgesia. Proc. Nat. Acad. Sci. USA 72: 2041-2043.

(16) Hagbarth, K.E. 1952. Excitatory and inhibitory skin areas for flexor and extensor motoneurones. Acta Physiol. Scand. suppl. 94.

(17) Hagbarth, K.E. 1960. Spinal withdrawal reflexes in the human lower limbs. J. Neurol. Neurosurg. Psychiat. 23: 222-227.

(18) Hagbarth, K.E., and Finer, B. 1963. The plasticity of human withdrawal reflexes to noxious skin stimuli in lower limbs. Progr. Brain Res. (Amst.) 1: 65-78.

(19) Hagbarth, K.E., and Kerr, D.I.B. 1954. Central influences on spinal afferent conduction. J. Neurophysiol. 17: 295.

(20) Hagbarth, K.E., and Kugelberg, E. 1958. Plasticity of the human abdominal skin reflex. Brain 81: 305-318.

(21) Hilgard, E.R. 1978. Hypnosis and pain. In The Psychology of Pain, ed. R.A. Sternbach, pp. 219-240. New York: Raven Press.

(22) Khatami, M., and Rush, A.J. 1978. A pilot study of the treatment of outpatients with chronic pain: symptom control, stimulus control and social system intervention. Pain 5: 163-172.

(23) Levine, J.D.; Gordon, N.C.; and Fields, H.L. 1978. The mechanism of placebo analgesia. Lancet ii: 654-657.

(24) Levine, J.D.; Gordon, N.C.; Jones, R.T.; and Fields, H.L. 1978. The narcotic antagonist naloxone enhances clinical pain. Nature 272: 826-827.

(25) Lindblom, U., and Tegnér, R. 1979. Are the endorphins active in clinical pain states? Narcotic antagonism in chronic pain patients. Pain 7: 65-68.

(26) Ludwig, A.M. 1966. Altered states of consciousness. Arch. gen. Psychiat. 15: 225-234.

(27) Mason, A.A. 1961. The problem of postoperative pain. In Simpson, B.R.J., and Parkhouse, J. Brit. J. Anaesth. 33: 336-344.

(28) Melzack, R., and Perry, C. 1975. Self-regulation of pain: the use of alpha-feedback and hypnotic training for the control of chronic pain. Exp. Neurol. 46: 452-469.

(29) Melzack, R, and Scott, T.H. 1957. The effects of early experience on the response to pain. J. comp. physiol. Psychol. 50: 155-161.

(30) Mihic, D., and Binkert, E. 1978. Is placebo analgesia mediated by endorphins? Pain abstracts, p. 19. Second World Congress on Pain, Montreal, Canada.

(31) Nasrallah, H.A.; Holley, T.; and Janowsky, D.S. 1979. Opiate antagonism fails to reverse hypnotic-induced analgesia. Lancet ii: 1355.

(32) Orne, M. 1974. Pain suppression by hypnosis and related phenomena. In Advances in Neurology, ed. J.J. Bonica, vol. 4, pp. 563-572. New York: Raven Press.

(33) Shor, R.E. 1959. Hypnosis and the concept of the generalized reality-orientation. Amer. J. Psychotherapy 13: 582-602.

(34) Stephenson, J.B.P. 1978. Reversal of hypnosis-induced analgesia by naloxone. Lancet ii: 991-992.

(35) Sternbach, R.A. 1968. Pain: A Psychophysiological Analysis. New York: Academic Press.

(36) Sternbach, R.A. 1974. Pain Patients: Traits and Treatment. New York: Academic Press.

(37) Sternbach, R.A. 1978. The Psychology of Pain. New York: Raven Press.

(38) Tart, C.T. 1969. Altered States of Consciousness. New York: Doubleday Anchor.

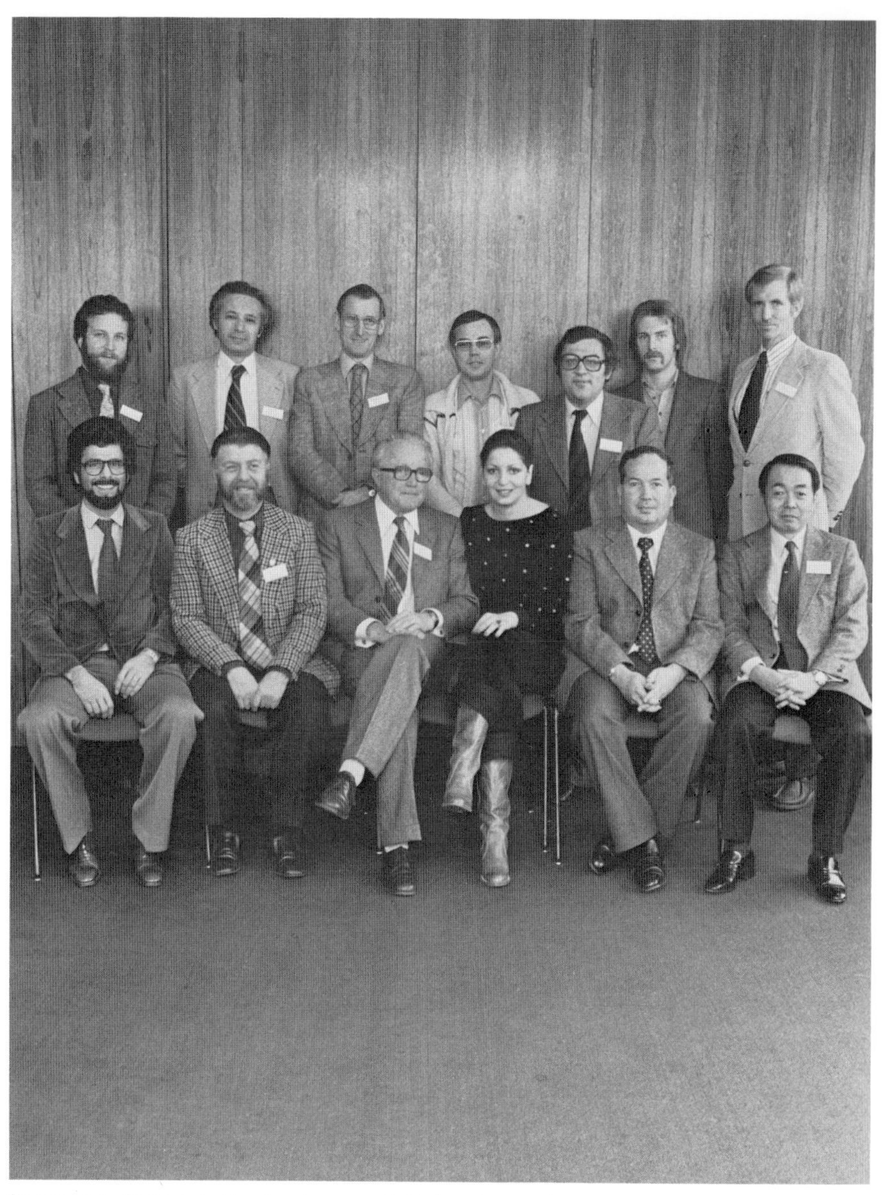

Group on Central Mechanisms of Pain Control: Seated, left to right: Walter Zieglgänsberger, Basil Finer, Albert Herz, Huda Akil, Bill Willis, Hiroshi Takagi. Standing: Allan Basbaum, Jack Fishmar Ainsley Iggo, Volker Höllt, Jean-Marie Besson, Earl Carstens, Ken Casey.

Pain and Society, eds. H.W. Kosterlitz and L.Y. Terenius, pp. 239-262.
Dahlem Konferenzen 1980. Weinheim: Verlag Chemie GmbH.

Central Mechanisms of Pain Control Group Report

W. D. Willis, Rapporteur
H. Akil, A. I. Basbaum, J.-M. R. Besson, E. Carstens,
K. L. Casey, B. L. Finer, J. Fishman, A. Herz, V. Höllt,
A. Iggo, H. Takagi, W. Zieglgänsberger

INTRODUCTION

It is clear from studies done during the past decade that not only are there central nervous system mechanisms that can be engaged experimentally to modulate nociceptive responses in animals, but that such mechanisms are likely to occur in man and to be accessible to therapeutic interventions for the control of pain. For this reason, it is important that we learn as much as possible about the anatomy, physiology, and pharmacology underlying these control systems in animal models and to see how far such systems can account for the results of currently used therapeutic procedures, such as transcutaneous nerve stimulation, acupuncture, dorsal column stimulation, depth electrode stimulation, the administration of centrally acting analgesics, and hypnosis. A better understanding of these control systems could well lead to improvements of such therapeutic procedures or even to new and more effective measures for the relief of pain.

HOW DOES ONE RECOGNIZE NEURONS INVOLVED IN NOCICEPTION?

A basic approach to the study of central nervous system mechanisms for the control of pain includes the identification of mechanisms within the nervous system that can be engaged by electrical or chemical stimuli with a resultant reduction of behavioral responses to tissue threatening or damaging stimuli. Such stimuli were termed "noxious" by Sherrington (9). A behavioral change of this kind is often called "analgesia," although it must be recognized that the very existence of pain in animals is a controversial topic because of the impossibility of proving the existence of any psychological phenomenon in animal subjects. The reduction in responses to noxious stimuli due to electrical stimulation of nervous tissue is generally called "stimulation produced analgesia," abbreviated SPA. Other forms of "analgesia" in animals include that due to opiate drugs, like morphine, and those due to other causes, such as stress. A useful working hypothesis is that procedures which reduce the responses of animals to noxious stimuli will also result in analgesia in man.

Progress in analyzing the neural mechanisms involved in "analgesia" may derive from recordings of changes in the activity of central neurons during procedures that result in "analgesia." However, it is important that such recordings be from neurons that are likely to be involved in some aspects of nociception. This gives rise to the question of how one can recognize a nociceptive neuron.

Tests of nociceptive function should involve stimuli known to cause pain in man. In animal experiments, it is possible to find neurons that have thresholds similar to the threshold for human pain in psychophysical tests. Actually, there are at least two different kinds of neurons in the dorsal horn that respond to noxious stimuli, in addition to a mechanoreceptive type (Iggo, this volume). One type of nociceptive dorsal horn neuron is activated just be nociceptor afferents. The other type is activated to some extent by weak mechanical stimuli that would cause a sensation of touch in man, but also by noxious stimuli. Such neurons have a convergent input from sensitive mechanoreceptors and nociceptors.

It is difficult to say at the present time whether both types of nociceptor neuron contribute to pain sensation or whether they have more or less separate functions. A further complication is that the response properties of dorsal horn neurons can be changed through the operation of pathways descending from the brain. An argument in favor of the participation of both types of neuron in nociception is that cells belonging to the spinothalamic tract can be found that have either response property. Whereas one can be fairly confident that the (high threshold) neurons (responding just to noxious stimuli) are nociceptive, there is no compelling reason to rule out the participation of the "wide dynamic range" cells, especially in view of the ability of the brain to alter their responses preferentially either to innocuous or to noxious stimuli.

Cells having similar response properties will no doubt be found at levels of the neuraxis other than the spinal cord. Caution is advisable in interpreting the responses of such neurons. Some may contribute to sensory experiences relating to the noxious stimulus, others may be involved in the somatic motor or autonomic reactions to such stimuli, and still others may participate in feedback circuits that may modulate the nociceptive response. It is also possible that neurons having nothing to do with nociception will respond to noxious stimuli, especially in reduced preparations in which normal responsiveness is altered by such factors as anesthesia.

Open Questions

a. What is the relative contribution of class 3 (high threshold or nociceptive specific) and class 2 (wide dynamic range) neurons to nociception? Which are involved in hyperesthesia?

b. To what extent are the properties of dorsal horn neurons dependent on descending control systems in intact freely behaving animals?

c. How effective are cold blocks in preventing transmission in descending pathways, especially those with fine axons?

d. Can selected groups of neurons be eliminated, e.g., chemically, to determine the effect of their loss on nociception?

e. Given the responses of individual dorsal horn neurons, what additional information is encoded in the population response to noxious stimuli?

f. What is the role of inhibition of noxious stimuli in the processing of nociceptive information?

g. What proportion of the neurons in a particular lamina, such as lamina I, are class 3?

h. To what extent are the responses of dendrites or axons being misinterpreted as cell body responses in studies of dorsal horn neurons?

i. How do convergent inputs get sorted out in order for the brain to distinguish between noxious stimuli to the skin, muscle, or viscera?

j. What is more critical for information processing by a dorsal horn neuron, the location of the cell body or the location of the dendrites?

k. Is pain created in the central nervous system?

Trends for Future Research

a. Recordings from nociceptive neurons in trained, freely behaving animals.

b. Development of ways to remove selected populations of neurons.

c. Statistical treatment of population responses to noxious stimuli, including excitation and inhibition.

MORPHOLOGY AND FUNCTION OF THE DORSAL HORN

The structure of the dorsal horn is generally described in terms of the cell layers, called by Rexed laminae I-VI (Basbaum, this volume). However, the various layers are sometimes indistinct in Nissl stained material, especially in adult animals, and so criteria are needed to help distinguish between layers on grounds other than just the pattern of cell bodies. The boundaries of laminae I and II and of II and III are clear, but it is more difficult to distinguish laminae III and IV. Perhaps histochemical criteria and the presence of particular types of afferent terminals will help in making such distinctions.

There are several cell types in each of the laminae of the dorsal horn. For example, there are Waldeyer cells (large, flat neurons) and small neurons within lamina I, and there are limiting (or stalk) cells and central (or islet) cells as well as other cell types in the substantia gelatinosa (=lamina II). Some of these neurons are tract cells, but many are interneurons. Progress is rapidly being made in characterizing the response properties of neurons in laminae I and II, despite the fact that such recordings were unavailable just 10 years ago (Iggo, this volume). Somewhat slower progress is being made in correlating functional properties with particular morphological types of dorsal horn neurons. Such correlations require intracellular staining after recording the activity of the cell and then histological reconstruction of the shape of the cell. No clear correlations have as yet been described between function and morphology. It may turn out that the best correlations exist between the pattern of connectivity to postsynaptic neurons and morphological types rather than between response properties and morphological types. There is also good progress in the investigation of the pattern of termination of various types of myelinated afferent fibers within the dorsal horn, again by recordings followed by intracellular injections of marker into the afferents. More attention is needed to the distribution of nociceptive afferents having conduction velocities over 20 m/s, and techniques are needed for tracing the terminals of identified C fibers.

Work is already in progress in which single afferent fibers and single postsynaptic neurons are marked intracellularly and their synaptic connections observed morphologically. More needs to be done in the dorsal horn with this approach, which is perhaps more readily applied to group Ia fibers from muscle spindles and motoneurons.

Another useful approach to the analysis of the circuitry of the dorsal horn is the reconstruction of marked and functionally identified interneurons in electron micrographs. It has already been possible to identify some of the components of the glomeruli in the dorsal horn found in association with certain types of afferent endings. An extension of such studies in the near future will be double marking experiments in which both pre- and postsynaptic elements are labelled and identified by their projections and also by their content of an active substance such as a transmitter or modulator or an enzyme.

Little is known about the details of development of specific types of dorsal horn neuron, but it is conceivable that such an analysis might help in the development of strategies for the selective elimination of particular sorts of neurons. Alternatively, the application of immunological techniques, specific toxins, or the selection of special genetic strains of animals might provide such a selective elimination of dorsal horn neurons. Experiments of this type might simplify the circuitry of the dorsal horn to permit a better analysis or might cause functional alterations that might lead to better hypotheses about the function of particular neuronal populations.

Open Questions

a. Exactly where do different categories of Aδ and C afferent fibers project in the dorsal horn?

b. Are there differences in the projections of myelinated nociceptors having conduction velocities above and below 20 m/s?

c. By what criteria can one distinguish between Rexed's laminae III and IV?

d. Are particular types of interneuron in the substantia gelatinosa, such as the limiting (stalk) cell or the central (islet) cell identifiable as excitatory or inhibitory?

e. Are the response properties of dorsal horn neurons correlated with their morphology?

f. Can degeneration time give a clear differentiation in the distribution of terminals of large vs. small afferents, of Aδ vs. C afferents?

g. Can the afferent input to particular dorsal horn neurons be completely explained in terms of direct and interneuronal connections?

h. Can a study of the development, immunology, or chemistry of different neuronal types in the dorsal horn provide a rationale for selective elimination of particular populations?

i. What is the role of the cells in the substantia gelatinosa that have responses inverse in sign to those of cells in neighboring laminae?

j. What is the effect of stimulation of axons in Lissauer's tract that arise from interneurons as compared with the effects of the number of such axons that are primary afferents?

k. What is the functional significance of the background discharges of substantia gelatinosa neurons?

l. Would it be possible to breed "pain-free" animals?

Trends for Future Research

a. Detailed analysis of dorsal horn circuitry, using new techniques or combinations of techniques.

b. Efforts to determine synaptic actions of morphological classes of cells.

c. Determination of possible correlations between morphology and functional classes of cells.

d. Development of means to destroy selected populations of dorsal horn neurons.

ROLE OF NON-NOCICEPTOR AFFERENTS IN DETERMINING THE QUALITY OF PAIN SENSATION

Although it is tempting to think of pain sensations as being produced by the activation of nociceptors, this is clearly an oversimplification. Noxious stimuli will of course activate nociceptors, but in addition they will often activate non-nociceptor afferents (Iggo, this volume). Experiments have demonstrated that the responses of central nociceptive neurons can be altered by the interaction of afferent volleys in nociceptor and non-nociceptor afferents and also between nociceptor afferents arising from within and outside of the excitatory receptive field of the cell.

Such interactions undoubtedly contribute to the quality of the sensory experience and perhaps also to some of the discriminative aspects of pain perception. In addition, advantage can be taken of inhibitory interaction in therapeutic interventions, such as transcutaneous nerve stimulation.

In addition to interactions at the level of spinal cord neurons, there are likely to be interactions between volleys in various ascending pathways. For example, it is possible that volleys carried in the dorsal column pathway interact with volleys in the spinothalamic tract at the level of the ventral posterior lateral nucleus of the thalamus. Such interactions are poorly understood, but could be important as mechanisms for pain relief and also for an explanation of central pain states that result from lesions at rostral levels of the neuraxis.

Some of the inhibitory effects of peripheral stimulation may not be due to segmental mechanisms but rather to activation of descending control systems.

Open Questions

a. What are the interactions between inputs from the various sensory receptors in determining the discharges of dorsal horn neurons?

b. What is the relative significance of interactions at various levels of the somatosensory pathways?

c. Does inhibitory convergence provide a mechanism for sharpening contrast?

d. To what extent are excitatory receptive fields altered by stimulating inhibitory receptive fields?

e. Could non-nociceptive afferents contribute to a feature detection role of nociceptive neurons?

Trends for Future Research

a. Detailed study of interactions between specific kinds of inputs from sensory receptor.

b. Evaluation of interactions at levels of the neuraxis other than the spinal cord (e.g., in the thalamus).

c. Development of models for effects of inhibition in nociceptive pathways.

WHERE IS PAIN?

Pain undoubtedly results from the activity of large numbers of neurons distributed throughout the nervous system. It is thus a function of a population of neurons and not localized in a particular place. In fact, it is an inappropriate question to ask for a position in space of a psychological phenomenon. What can be asked is what specific brain structures are engaged during nociception and perhaps during pain and what structures are not engaged. Such methods as the 2-deoxyglucose technique or the equivalent using positron emission tomography may help to answer such a question. However, it will be difficult to distinguish between neuronal activity related to sensation and that related to the motivational-affective, motor, and autonomic components of the pain response. Nevertheless, it would be of interest to know if particular cortical areas or thalamic nuclei are activated by noxious stimuli.

Open Questions

a. Which regions of the neuraxis are and which are not involved in nociception?

b. Is pain a state of the nervous system comparable to sleep?

c. Which are the highest levels of the nervous system that are involved in nociception?

Trend for Future Research

Mapping of nociceptive neurons, perhaps using new techniques like 2-deoxyglucose labelling.

TO WHAT EXTENT IS THE PAIN SYSTEM SIMILAR TO OTHER SENSORY SYSTEMS?

There appear to be a number of similarities and a number of differences between the pain system and other sensory pathways. For this discussion, pain will be considered to involve an internal experience that is aversive in addition to tissue damage and its recognition (Casey, this volume). Features of the pain response that resemble aspects of other sensory systems include the possibility of making psychophysical measurements of at least selected aspects of the experience, the presence of specific sets of neurons that convey a particular kind of information, and possibly a set of specific chemical substances utilized by neurons in this sensory system for synaptic transmission and modulation. Aspects of the pain response that appear to differ from those typical of other sensory systems include the fact that pain is never affectively neutral, and there is a nondiscriminative set of neurons that contribute to the motivational-affective component of pain. It is, of course, possible to demonstrate that other sensory systems can also produce an affective response, but this seems to be always so in pain but only sometimes in other sensations. The division between sensory-discriminative and motivational-affective components of pain can be manipulated independently by surgical interventions (like frontal lobotomy or cingulumotomy) or by drugs (centrally acting analgesics).

There has been disagreement about the role of the cerebral cortex in pain (Basbaum, this volume). However, a number of lines of evidence suggest a role of the somatosensory cortex, perhaps including several regions (SI, SII, retroinsular) in the sensory-discriminative aspects of pain and of the frontal cortex and limbic cortex in the motivational-affective aspects.

A major involvement of the reticular formation in pain responses is likely. The reticular formation may not be designed for a sensory-discriminative role but rather for setting a behavioral mode (Casey, this volume). In addition to influences on the motivational-affective aspect of pain, the reticular formation seems to be involved in the motor and autonomic output and also in sensory filtering. The latter function makes the reticular formation one of the pain modulating systems.

Open Questions

a. To what extent is the psychophysics of pain comparable to the psychophysics of other sensations?

b. How different is the emotional content of pain experiences from that of other sensory experiences?

c. How well can the sensory-discriminative component of pain be separated from the motivational-affective component by surgical or pharmacological interactions?

d. What are the similarities and differences in the neural pathways involved in nociception and in other sensations?

e. Is there a special role of the reticular formation in establishing a behavioral state related to pain?

Trends for Future Research

a. Determine more clearly if the sensory-discriminative and motivational-affective components of pain can be distinguished by psychophysics or by interventions.

b. Develop models of how the reticular formation may contribute to pain and to other sensations.

MULTIPLICITY OF MODULATING SYSTEMS

A number of pathways descending from the brain into the spinal cord have already been shown to modulate the responses of spinal cord neurons to noxious stimuli or to produce behavioral evidence of "analgesia." Some of these pathways originate in the midbrain, others in the pons and medulla. Particular attention has been directed to the periaqueductal gray, the midbrain reticular formation, the nucleus raphe magnus, and the nucleus reticularis gigantocellaris, but other structures that may also be involved are the locus coeruleus, the nucleus reticularis paragigantocellularis, and others (Basbaum, Besson, this volume).

Experiments on particular descending pathways have shown that the mechanisms by which modulation is accomplished can vary and that a number of different chemical substances are used as transmitters or modulators.

Parallels are often drawn between the effectiveness of stimulation within a particular region of the brain and inhibition of responses of dorsal horn neurons to noxious stimuli. However, it is not clear what dorsal horn neurons must be inhibited to produce "analgesia," especially if this term is alternatively defined by a spinal reflex or by a reduced sensation of pain, nor is it clear that the absence of "analgesia" implies that none of the neurons in a stimulated area produce "analgesia."

Open Questions

a. What are the various descending pathways involved in the control of nociception?

b. What alternative mechanisms are employed by particular pathways in modulating nociceptive responses?

c. Does the absence of "analgesia" during stimulation at a particular site rule out participation of neurons of that site in "analgesia"?

d. What neurons must have their activity modulated in order for "analgesia" to result?

e. To what extent are descending controls operating specifically on nociceptive as opposed to non-nociceptive responses?

f. Are descending inhibitory effects best explained by pre- or postsynaptic inhibition?

g. What are the presynaptic effects of descending pathways on C fibers of different types?

Trends for Future Research

a. Detailed analysis of various descending pathways and their effects on dorsal horn neurons.

b. Analysis of mechanisms of descending control.

MONOAMINERGIC MECHANISMS IN PAIN CONTROL

There is considerable evidence that 5-hydroxytryptamine is involved in both stimulation produced analgesia and in morphine analgesia (Basbaum, Besson, this volume). However, the observation that neurons containing 5-hydroxytryptamine may also contain substance P raises questions about the effects of activation of serotonergic neurons. What is the role of the substance P? Furthermore, experiments in which 5-hydroxytryptamine is depleted by para-chlorophenylalanine are complicated by the fact that the animals are sleep deprived and have disturbed circadian rhythms.

In addition to serotonergic neurons, it is likely that noradrenergic neurons contribute to the modulation of nociceptive responses in the dorsal horn. This can be shown pharmacologically and may relate to descending projections from the A1 group of neurons in the medulla or possibly to the locus coeruleus.

One complicating factor in studies of the actions of monoamine pathways is that there are species differences in the anatomical distribution of monoaminergic neurons in the brain stem.

Open Questions

a. What is the role of the multiple active substances shown by histochemistry in certain neurons (e.g., 5-hydroxytryptamine and substance P in neurons of the raphe)?

b. How do "analgesia," sleep deprivation, and alterations in circadian rhythmicity interact?

c. How appropriate are the various tests for "analgesia" in animals?

d. When stimuli are applied at a particular site in the brain stem, how can one establish what pathways are activated to produce descending modulation of dorsal horn cells?

e. What difficulties in the analysis of monoamine pathways (or other pathways) result from species differences?

f. Do descending serotonergic and noradrenergic axons end on the same or different dorsal horn neurons?

g. What are the functional differences in the descending controls mediated by terminals containing 5-hydroxytryptamine versus norepinephrine?

Trends for Future Research

a. Analysis of effects of neurons releasing more than one transmitt

b. Detailed analysis of anatomy and pharmacology of descending pathways.

c. Evaluation of behavioral significance of various control systems. For example, does modification of the serotonin system have different behavioral consequences than modification of the norepinephrine system.

ROLE OF MULTIPLE OPIOID SYSTEMS IN ANALGESIA

There are multiple opioid systems in terms of several different variables (Akil and Watson, this volume). There are two enkephalins in addition to β-endorphin in brain and pituitary. There are also other opiate-like compounds in the nervous system that have been less well characterized. Furthermore, there are several types of opiate receptor.

If the opiate-like compounds are transmitters or modulators, they could have various effects at different levels of the nervous system, much like acetylcholine has. The lack of specificity of acetylcholine for a particular behavior may have a parallel in the numerous effects of opiates injected systemically This difficulty results from the fact that opiates administered systemically can act at opiate receptors throughout the nervous system, yet the endogenous release of opiate-like substances would be discrete.

Experiments utilizing the blocking effects of naloxone may be hard to interpret if negative, because naloxone is more effective in blocking some opiate receptors than others.

There is no particular reason to assume that the endogenous opiate-like compounds are there to counteract pain. These substances may be involved in a variety of functions, one being pain modulation.

More needs to be learned about the mechanism of action of the opiates on particular kinds of neurons. Many neurons are depressed by opiates, others seem to be excited. Are these truely different actions, or are the excited neurons actually being disinhibited?

Stimulation produced analgesia is being tried clinically at several centers. It will be useful to know how consistently effective this therapeutic approach proves to be. Detailed examination of sensory changes in the patients will be of interest. In addition to more thorough evaluation of the neurological status of such patients during brain stimulation, it will be important to have better pre-operative testing and also investigations of other changes (e.g., in endocrine function).

Open Questions

a. What are the other opioid substances in nervous tissue in addition to the enkephalins and β-endorphin?

b. Can antagonists be developed which preferentially interact with each type of opiate receptor?

c. What are the mechanisms of interaction if several active substances are co-released from a given neuron?

d. How can pharmacologic effects of exogenous opiates be distinguished from the actions of endogenous compounds?

e. What functions other than pain control are subserved by the endogenous opioid compounds?

f. What can be deduced from the changes seen in CSF levels of opioids?

g. Do opiates excite or disinhibit, as well as depress activity?

h. How consistently effective is stimulation produced analgesia in patients?

i. What neurologic changes can be demonstrated in patients undergoing stimulus produced analgesia?

Trends for Future Research

a. Isolation and characterization of endogenous opioids.

b. Development of suitable drugs that interact specifically with different receptor types.

c. Detailed study of pharmacology of opioids, with emphasis on drug interactions.

d. Analysis of the mechanisms of release and turn-over of opioids from nervous tissue.

e. Determination of the neurophysiologic actions of opioids on specific neurons.

f. Demonstration of the usefulness of stimulation-produced analgesia in patients.

g. Development of agents that specifically affect synthesis or release of particular endogenous opioids.

SPINAL VERSUS SUPRASPINAL SITES OF MORPHINE ACTION

There is evidence for a spinal action of morphine, in addition to an action at the level of the brain stem. This is particularly evident when morphine is administered intrathecally. It will be important to evaluate the efficacy of this approach, since it may be possible to avoid many of the side effects of morphine by such a route of administration. Of theoretical interest is the relative effect of morphine in systemic injections on spinal and supraspinal structures and to what extent such actions are synergistic.

Open Question

Is the action of systemically administered morphine primarily on the brain stem, the spinal cord, or both?

Trend for Future Research

To what extent will intrathecal administration of morphine prove to be a useful therapeutic maneuver?

PEPTIDES IN THE DORSAL HORN

In experiments on spinal neurons, it is possible to demonstrate that enkephalins affect the responses of postsynaptic cells to excitatory transmitter without any sign of a change in membrane potential of conductance (Zieglgänsberger, this volume). Possibly, the enkephalin action is due to alteration of the responsiveness of sodium channels to the excitatory transmitter. In addition, enkephalins probably have a presynaptic action, causing a reduction in transmitter release, perhaps by a change in the calcium influx required for excitation-secretion coupling.

Enkephalin-containing neurons are found in the dorsal horn. It can be suggested that these serve as interneurons that modulate transmission from nociceptive afferents to dorsal horn neurons. It is also possible that the enkephalin-containing neurons are involved in the interactions between large and small fiber inputs. However, at the present time these suggestions are speculative.

In addition to enkephalins, the dorsal horn contains other peptides, such as neurotensin, and other substances, such as gamma aminobutyric acid. These are likely to play a significant role in the functioning of the dorsal horn circuits. The known axo-axonal synapses appear to be GABAergic.

Substance P is another dorsal horn peptide. Substance P is found in certain afferent fibers; it is not at present certain that these are the nociceptors, but this seems likely. Iontophoretic application of substance P within the dorsal horn excites neurons that respond to non-noxious stimuli as well as neurons that signal noxious events. Thus it is possible that small afferents from non-nociceptors may also utilize substance P as a transmitter or modulator.

The action of substance P is long-lasting and does not appear to involve a conductance change, although the neurons are depolarized. The long action may reflect a continued action of the peptide far beyond the time of action of ordinary transmitters. Since repeated noxious stimuli will cause a build-up in the discharges of dorsal horn neurons, a process known as "wind-up," it may be speculated that wind-up may result from a progressive increment in substance P.

Open Questions

a. What are the mechanisms of the pre- and postsynaptic actions of opioid substances?

b. How do enkephalin-containing neurons fit into the dorsal horn circuits?

c. Do small afferents inhibit and large afferents excite enkephalin-containing neurons?

d. Do enkephalin-containing neurons have tonic discharges?

e. What is the basis for the long-lasting effect of morphine on neurons when morphine is applied iontophoretically within the substantia gelatinosa?

f. What are the functions of different classes of neurons in the substantia gelatinosa?

g. What is the role of substantia gelatinosa neurons that contain active substances other than enkephalin, such as gamma aminobutyric acid, neurotensin, etc.?

h. Are the neurons of lamina I that contain enkephalin projection neurons, local circuit neurons, or both?

i. Could enkephalin be released from the soma or from presynaptic dendrites and act as a local hormone?

j. Does enkephalin act on neurons that release it?

k. What neurons in the dorsal horn have opiate receptors?

l. Is substance P acting as a neuromodulator in the sense of producing a postsynaptic effect by a mechanism other than a conductance change?

m. Is the long-lasting action of substance P responsible for the increment in discharge of dorsal horn neurons with repeated stimulation ("wind-up")?

Trends for Future Research

a. Detailed analysis of mode of action of opioids.

b. Functional characterization of neurons containing opioids and other peptides.

c. Double labelling of neurons of dorsal horn to identify both the axonal projection and the presence in the neuron of a specific active substance.

d. Demonstration of possible spread of substances like enkephalin through the extracellular space of the dorsal horn.

e. Specific activation of afferents containing substance P and correlation of release with synaptic effects, such as "wind-up."

THE PITUITARY AND PAIN

Not much is known about the role of the pituitary in pain. The presence of a large amount of β-endorphin in the pituitary leads to the speculation that this may play some part in analgesia (Akil and Watson, this volume). However a correlation between the release of pituitary β-endorphin and analgesia is not yet established. In fact, removal of the pituitary has been reported to result in pain relief. It has been proposed that this occurs not only in patients suffering from endocrine-dependent cancers but also others. The mechanism of this phenomenon is obscure. One possibility is that there may be algesic factors in the pituitary. By contrast, in experimental work stress-induced analgesia is counteracted by hypophysectomy.

Open Questions

a. Does pituitary endorphin have anything to do with analgesia?

b. Do ACTH or other pituitary hormones affect pain?

c. What is the mechanism causing the analgesia found after removal of the pituitary?

Trend for Future Research

Try to establish mechanism of analgesia resulting from pituitary removal by further investigation of effects of endocrine changes.

MECHANISMS OF ACUPUNCTURE

The acupuncture used in surgery in China may well have a basis different from that underlying experimental acupuncture. The effects are stronger, and there may be no particular or necessary relationship between the presence of analgesia and the location of the needles. In acupuncture-like transcutaneous nerve stimulation, the effects are less profound and the stimulus is best placed in the appropriate segment. The acupuncture produced by needling trigger points may involve still another mechanism.

It is proposed that the acupuncture used for surgery may resemble hypnosis. Evidence for this is the similarity in patient selection for this form of acupuncture and for hypnosis.

One important point with regard to acupuncture for surgery may be the fact that it appears not to be widely used in children. This observation may be helpful in assigning a mechanism.

Open Questions

a. Are there several different mechanisms of acupuncture?

b. Is the acupuncture used during surgery in China more similar to hypnosis than to experimental acupuncture?

c. What is the mechanism of acupuncture involving needling of trigger points?

d. Can acupuncture be used widely for surgery in cultures other than Chinese?

e. Can acupuncture for surgery be used in children or animals?

f. Does experimental acupuncture (e.g., low frequency, high intensity transcutaneous nerve stimulation) work as well in children as in adults?

Trends for Future Research

a. Compare the effects of acupuncture for surgery and hypnosis in the same individuals.

b. Determine if acupuncture for surgery is dependent on an opiate mechanism.

c. Learn more about acupuncture in children.

MECHANISMS OF HYPNOTIC MANIPULATION

Hypnosis should be regarded as the therapeutic application of normal psychological mechanisms (Finer, this volume). These include concentration and detachment. During hypnosis induced in certain ways, it appears possible to prevent reflexogenic or autonomic responses to noxious stimuli, although such changes are not prevented when hypnosis is induced in other ways. The details of the mechanisms involved in hypnosis are still obscure.

Open Questions

a. How close is hypnosis to such normal psychological phenomenon as concentration and detachment?

b. Can hypnosis interfer with reflex and autonomic function?

c. What pain control nechanisms are involved in hypnotic analgesia

Trends for Future Research

a. Further studies in which somatic and autonomic function are monitored during noxious stimulation under hypnosis.

b. Additional experiments on alterations in hypnotic analgesia by interventions that disrupt particular control systems as these become better understood.

c. Investigation of hypnotic analgesia in children and comparison with acupuncture and analgesia due to transcutaneous nerve stimulation.

d. Study of the changes in endogenous opioid levels in the cerebrospinal fluid during hypnotic hyperalgesia and hypoalgesia.

e. Are the effects of acupuncture, transcutaneous nerve stimulation and hypnosis analgesia additive (experimentally and clinically)?

GIVEN THE EXPERIMENTAL EVIDENCE FOR NEURAL SYSTEMS THAT CAN MODULATE NOCICEPTIVE RESPONSES, WHAT EVIDENCE IS THERE FOR AN ENDOGENOUS SYSTEM THAT IS NORMALLY USED TO CONTROL PAIN?

Several lines of evidence can be used to support the notion that there are neural mechanisms that can control pain. These fall into at least the following categories: behavioral evidence, lesions, electrical stimulation, and chemical stimulation. The behavioral evidence includes the observation of analgesia during such maneuvers as hypnosis and acupuncture and also during spontaneous events like warwounds, etc. Lesions of the nervous system can produce changes in either direction in pain responses. Stimulation of certain areas of the brain and of peripheral nerves can modulate pain, as can administration of certain drugs. The presence of endogenous opiate-like substances that have similar effects to morphine lends credence to this proposition.

Despite these statements, it is still not at all clear that there is an endogenous system designed specifically for the control of pain. It is perhaps more likely that the systems that are used in experimental or therapeutic interventions, are normally involved in a variety of functions. It is nevertheless possible and perhaps testable that when pain occurs, such systems are of importance in pain control.

REFERENCES

(1) Beaumont, A., and Hughes, J. 1979. Biology of opioid peptides. Ann. Rev. Pharm. Tox. 19: 245-267.

(2) Bowsher, D. 1976. Role of the reticular formation in responses to noxious stimulation. Pain 2: 361-378.

(3) Fields, H.L., and Basbaum, A. 1978. Brain controls of spinal pain transmission neurones. Ann. Rev. Physiol. 40: 193-221.

(4) Fishman, J., ed. 1978. The Bases of Addiction. Berlin: Dahlem Konferenzen.

(5) Herz, A., ed. 1978. Developments of Opiate Research. New York: Dekker.

(6) Iggo, A., ed. 1973. Handbook of Sensory Physiology, vol. II. Berlin: Springer.

(7) Kerr, F.W.L., and Casey, K.L. 1978. Pain. Neurosci. Res. Prog. 16: MIT Press.

(8) Mayer, D.J., and Price, D.D. 1976. Central nervous system mechanisms of analgesia. Pain 2: 379-404.

(9) Sherrington, C.S. 1906 (reprinted in 1947). The Integrative Action of the Nervous System. New Haven: Yale University Press.

(10) Terenius, L. 1978. Endogenous peptides and analgesia. Ann. Rev. Pharm. Tox. 18: 189-204.

(11) Yaksh, T.L., and Rudy, T.A. 1978. Narcotic analgesics: CNS sites and mechanisms of action as revealed by intracerebral injection techniques. Pain 4: 299-380.

Pain and Society, eds. H.W. Kosterlitz and L.Y. Terenius, pp. 263-282.
Dahlem Konferenzen 1980. Weinheim: Verlag Chemie GmbH.

Deep and Visceral Pain

F. Cervero
Department of Physiology, University of Edinburgh
Medical School, Edinburgh EH8 9AG, Scotland

Abstract. Pain of deep and visceral origin is the most common form of pain produced by diseases. In contrast to the well-localized and generally acute cutaneous pain, deep and visceral pain are aching, ill-localized and of chronic evolution. There is still no agreement on whether visceral pain is referred to the surface of the body or is simply vaguely localized by the higher centers of the nervous system. Some viscera are insensitive to noxious stimuli whereas others are extremely sensitive to them. The phenomenon of referred pain has been attributed to the convergence of visceral and somatic afferent fibers onto the same pool of sensory neurons in the spinal cord and subsequent cutaneous localization by the upper centers of the brain. There is no electrophysiological evidence of the existence of specific visceral nociceptors. Some visceral afferent fibers enter the spinal cord via the ventral roots. Studies in the spinal cord have shown convergence of visceral and cutaneous afferent fibers onto interneurons and neurons projecting through several sensory ascending pathways including the spinothalamic tract. No pure visceral pathway has so far been found in the spinal cord. Data on the central nervous system representation of visceral information is scarce and inconclusive.

INTRODUCTION

Pain arising from deep somatic structures or from viscera accounts for a substantial proportion of recurrent and persistent pain syndromes. In fact, pain of deep or visceral origin is the chief, if not the only, reason for most patients to seek medical attention. Yet, our knowledge of the mechanisms of deep pain is very limited whereas research efforts concentrate more on pain of cutaneous origin. From a social point of view, deep and visceral pain receive less attention than they deserve.

There is a reason, and a very strong reason indeed, for this apparent lack of research interest in visceral pain. The dichotomy between "la douleur maladie" and "la douleur laboratoire" so vividly pictured by Leriche (11) has its roots in the inability of reproducing visceral pain for the purpose of research analysis. If deep and visceral pains are by nature ill-defined, dull, vague, and referred, it is not surprising that a proper rigorous analysis of their mechanisms is lacking. This failure in bringing the limits of deep and visceral pain within a rigorous framework has led to wide speculations and ambiguities on the definition of the problem as well as on the very existence of visceral pain as such. It is not only the particular neurophysiological mechanisms of deep and visceral pain that are the subject of controversy, it is also the conceptual approach to the problem that is at stake.

When trying to prepare an overview of the current status of the subject, it is therefore useful to separate those problems which can be classified as conceptual from those aspects of the topic which correspond to precise physiological problems. This background paper intends to reflect our current ideas on the qualities of visceral pain as well as the present status of some aspects of the neurophysiology of visceral pain.

CONCEPTUAL ASPECTS OF DEEP AND VISCERAL PAIN

Classes of Deep and Visceral Pain

The general view currently held is that there are two basic forms of pain: (a) a bright and well-localized superficial pain and (b) a dull, aching, and ill-localized deep pain. The first class is normally described as cutaneous pain whereas the second is divided into pain from visceral structures, either hollow or parenchymatous (visceral pain) and pain from somatic structures beneath the skin, such as muscles, ligaments, bones, and joints (deep pain). It is important to emphasize at this point that the distinction between superficial and deep pain is only based on their differences in qualities and not on any other anatomical or physiological considerations. To bear this observation in mind is important in order to understand the sometimes radically opposite views on the origins and mechanisms of visceral pain. Leriche (11) considered that pain is of two main classes: (a) the consistent type, corresponding to the peripheral distribution of a cerebro-spinal nerve and responding to division of the pain pathways and (b) the badly-localized, diffuse, and somewhat "illogical" pain that does not disappear by sections along the cerebro-spinal system and is of sympathetic origin. Needless to say, visceral and deep pains were included by Leriche in the second category. The leading role that Leriche attributed to the sympathetic nervous system in many painful conditions was later questioned but the division between superficial and deep pains based on terms of quality has survived. Lewis (12) stated that there are basically two classes of pain, each of them with a different representation in the central nervous system: The superficial and the deep pains. To Lewis, pain derived from deep-lying somatic structures was similar in character to that to which "visceral disturbances give rise."

Grouping pain of deep somatic origin with visceral pain requires the assumption that both sets of structures involved share the same representation in the central nervous system. This was considered to be a controversial view since it would mean that organs innervated by somatic nerves (muscles, joints, bones) would have more in common with organs innervated by sympathetic nerves (viscera) than with organs innervated by other somatic nerves (skin and mucous membranes). On the other hand, pain of deep somatic origin and visceral pain, although having many properties in common, cannot be considered similar in every respect. Rather than trying to classify pain by the division of the nervous system which subserves the innervation of the organ, it would be perhaps more appropriate to consider the embryological aspects of the problem. This was already suggested by

Lewis and could be the basis of a new approach to the question. In this sense, there would be pain of ectodermal origin (skin and mucous membranes) characterized by its good localization and brightness, pain of mesodermal origin corresponding to our present concept of deep pain, and pain of endodermal origin (alimentary canal) which would be the visceral pain. The degree of ill-localization and dullness would be greater in pain of endodermal origin than in that of mesodermal origin.

Site of Origin of Deep and Visceral Pain

That pain of mesodermal origin (muscles, joints, ligaments, parietal membranes) arises from the diseased or injured structures seems to be a view held without disagreement (12). Deep somatic pain has generally been attributed to direct stimulation of "pain receptors" within the organs in which pain is elicited. As far as visceral pain is concerned, the situation is however quite different. Observations made on patients undergoing abdominal surgery under local anesthesia or on human volunteers receiving localized injections of hypertonic saline have produced contradictory results on the sensitivity of viscera. Based on his surgical experience, Lennander (see ref. (12)) stated that viscera were insensitive and Mackenzie (14) strongly supported this view with his own observations. However, whereas Lennander believed that viscera lacked innervation, Mackenzie thought that pain in visceral disease arises from the viscus itself via afferent impulses not related to pain, and Morely (16) stated that visceral pain is due only to the action of the diseased viscus on the parietal wall or on branches of somatic nerves, thus supporting the lack of innervation of visceral structures proposed by Lennander.

It is true that some viscera, particularly the parenchymatous organs (liver, kidney), are insensitive and that certain inflammatory conditions, such as some forms of cholecystitis, only become painful when the parietal membranes are affected. But it is also true that visceral pain can easily be evoked from some viscera. The whole argument of the sensitivity or insensitivity of viscera to noxious stimuli rests on the lack of agreement on what forms of stimuli can be considered to be noxious to a particular viscus. Moreover, the sensory innervation of many viscera has not yet been properly studied and the results so far available are contradictory as to whether or not viscera possess specific "visceral nociceptors." This point will be dealt with in more detail later in this paper as it is one of the key points in the controversy regarding the sensitivity of viscera.

A different approach has also been taken to the question of visceral noxious stimuli. Rather than defining what stimuli are noxious and then looking for responses to such stimulation, some authors have decided to term as noxious all such stimuli which will evoke pain or discomfort, no matter whether they are of general or local nature. This is an extension of the "adequate stimulus" approach to cutaneous sensibility.

In 1937 Ayala (1) listed the following as adequate stimulations to evoke visceral pain: (a) spasm of the smooth muscle in hollow viscera, (b) distension of hollow viscera, (c) ischemia, (d) inflammatory states, (e) chemical stimuli, and (f) traction, compression, or twisting of mesentery. Although in general this list is still valid, it is important to point out that the stimulations listed above are far from being general ways of evoking visceral pain as not all viscera will respond to all of those stimuli.

Qualities of Deep and Visceral Pain

Cutaneous pain has an element of usefulness: to avoid injury. Good localization is thus a prime qualitiy to achieve its goal. Deep somatic pain, though dull and aching, is sufficiently well circumscribed to provoke defense reactions suitable for the avoidance of further damage to the muscles, joints, or bones involved. These protective mechanisms are also triggered by other forms of pain of mesodermal origin, such as cardiac pain in coronary artery disease.

Some forms of visceral pain are, however, useless to the organism. Extensive damage to some organs (liver, lungs) does not evoke pain whereas relative minor injuries or situations which cannot be improved by any form of natural therapy are extremely painful (renal and bile calculi). Leriche (11) strongly supported the view of the uselessness of pain in some diseases: "Pain is always a baleful gift, which reduces the subject of it and makes him more ill than he would be without it." The two major qualities of visceral pain: ill-localization and reference to superficial areas have been claimed to be the consequence of this lack of useful purpose of some forms of visceral pain (11).

In 1893, Head first used the term "referred pain" to point out the reference of pain to the skin when the lesion affects an internal organ. Head, who did not deny the existence of pain of visceral origin and localization, divided visceral pain into that localized vaguely inside the body (dull visceral pain) and that referred to the skin surface (aching referred pain). He assumed that the reference was due to convergence of visceral and skin nerves onto the same spinal cord structures and a subsequent "psychical error" of localization. The concept of referred pain has suffered a long series of modifications after Head's first proposal and the modern use of the term "referred" is largely a matter of convention. Three different modern interpretations of the concept of referred pain are: (a) faulty localization, (b) poor localization, spread beyond the point of origin, or (c) localization in a remote part from the point of origin.

There seems to be two contradictory views on the problems of localization of visceral pain. To some, visceral pain is purely referred to the skin surface, to others, visceral pain is simply ill-localized. Mackenzie (14), who was the major defender of the reference hypothesis, did not deny that stimuli from viscera produce pain. He maintained that the location of such pain is in the viscus but its localization is achieved by an "irritable focus" in the spinal cord; this, in turn, is responsible for the reference of pain to the corresponding skin areas, the muscular spasm, the vascular changes, and the secretory changes.

On the other hand, reference of visceral pain to the skin surface was emphatically denied by Leriche (11) who vigorously put forward the idea of ill-localization, a view also held by Lewis (12). Leriche attacks the "mistaken doctrine" of referred pain as an idea of "English origin" and criticizes Head and Mackenzie. He suggests that visceral pains are felt in the viscera but that they are imperfectly appreciated because visceral sensibility is not normally conscious and therefore when brought to conscience produces an indefinite type of sensation: visceral pain. Lewis, in spite of being an "Englishman," expressed views more in line with those of Leriche. To him visceral pain is purely a central phenomenon due to the lack of detailed central representation of visceral structures. Viscera have a mass representation in the central nervous system which results in only very coarse sensations being awakened by their stimulation.

Both interpretations of the basic mechanisms of visceral pain, ill-localization, and reference contain large elements of objective observation. True reference exists, such as in anginal pain, but it is also common experience that some types of abdominal pain are felt "inside" the body in a vague manner. Whether it is possible to present visceral pain as a function which can be reduced to a simple general law is a completely different matter.

A number of theories have been proposed to account for the phenomena of referred pain. All of them are based on the presence of convergence between visceral and somatic information along the neuraxis and subsequently faulty interpretation. The current theory is the "convergence-projection" theory of Ruch (22): "Some visceral afferents converge with cutaneous pain afferents to end upon the same neuron at some point in the sensory pathway. The first oppurtunity for this is in the spinothalamic tract. The resulting impulses, upon reaching the brain, are interpreted as having come from the skin, an interpretation which has been learned from previous experiences in which the same tract fiber was stimulated by cutaneous afferents." The essence of this theory had already been stated by Ross in 1888 and by Head in 1893.

A clinical phenomenon often associated with referred pain is hyperalgesia (hyperaesthesia in Noordenbos (19) nomenclature) of the skin area where pain is referred to. That this hyperalgesia is not of intrinsic cutaneous origin seems to be well established by the observations of abnormal reference of pain to a phantom left arm in attacks of angina pectoris. The "convergence-projection" theory of Ruch accounts for the hyperalgesia as a result of facilitation of cutaneous nerve impulses onto spinothalamic tract neurons already highly excitable by the barrage of visceral impulses. This and similar earlier interpretations led to the view that local anesthesia of the cutaneous hyperalgesic area would result in an amelioration of the visceral pain. Clinical tests of this hypothesis produced contradictory results, and the lack of a unifying nomenclature prevents rigorous analysis of the available literature. The only point of agreement is that cutaneous hyperalgesia is not necessarily a symptom always associated with referred pain. Whereas referred pain appears to be a quality of visceral pain, hyperalgesia of the referred area seems to be an additional phenomenon in some cases of visceral pain.

NEUROPHYSIOLOGICAL CORRELATES OF DEEP AND VISCERAL PAIN

Deep and Visceral Nociceptors

There seems to be little doubt that specific nociceptors are widely distributed in deep somatic structures. In contrast, no definite electrophysiological or histological evidence of specific visceral nociceptors exists.

Deep nociceptors. Muscle nerves contain a large amount of small myelinated and unmyelinated afferent fibers that do not originate from proprioceptors. Both Aδ and C afferent fibers generate from free nerve endings associated with muscle fibers, capsules of spindles and tendon organs, tendon tissue, vessels, fat cells, and connective tissue (23). These small afferent fibers respond to high intensity mechanical and thermal stimuli as well as to the administration of algogenic substances (9,15). They are considered nociceptors. Recordings from unmyelinated muscle afferents have yielded some responses interpreted as produced by "ergoceptors" (receptors responding to muscle contractions). Nevertheless, the borderline between nociceptors and ergoceptors is not sharp.

Free nerve endings originating from unmyelinated or small myelinated afferent fibers have also been described in other deep somatic tissues such as tendons, ligaments, fat pads, articular capsules, and periosteum. Electrophysiological studies have only been carried out on small myelinated fibers arising from joints and claims have been made of their nociceptive nature. Further electrophysiological studies are needed to analyze different kinds of deep nociceptors in several structures, but the principle of the existence of specific nociceptors in deep tissues seems to be firmly established.

Visceral nociceptors. Pain impulses arising within the abdominal and thoracic cavities may reach the central nervous system by three channels: (a) the parasympathetic nerves (i.e., pelvic and vagus nerves), (b) the sympathetic nerves (i.e., splanchnic nerves), and (c) somatic nerves innervating the body wall and the diaphragm (i.e., phrenic nerve). The relative importance of these pathways in conveying visceral pain is, however, quite heterogeneous, with the sympathetic nerve carrying the major share of visceral impulses.

Over the past twenty years a number of careful studies on visceral sensory receptors have yielded a comprehensive view of the different types of receptors present in the internal organs and a useful clarification of their mechanisms of activation. Yet, in all these studies no clear electrophysiological evidence has emerged as to the existence of specific visceral nociceptors.

The open question of the peripheral origin of visceral pain can thus be approached from at least three different points of view: (a) Receptors responsible for the sensations of visceral pain are the same population of visceral receptors responding to innocuous stimuli and responsible for visceral reflex actions. These receptors would respond with higher frequencies of firing to noxious stimuli. This approach is essentially based on the intensity theory of pain mechanisms. (b) Receptors responsible for the sensations of visceral pain are a different population of visceral receptors which respond to the same stimuli that evoke visceral reflex actions but with different thresholds. This view is an extension to viscera of the current ideas on cutaneous nociceptors. (c) Receptors responsible for the sensations of visceral pain are a different population of visceral receptors which respond to the same stimuli that evoke visceral reflex actions but by different mechanisms (i.e., release of chemicals, presence of irritants). This is a view based on the existence of specific visceral nociceptors, but it also would account for some of the mechanisms peculiar to the eliciting of visceral pain (inflammation, ischemia).

None of these three interpretations has been wholly proved or disproved. The observation that some forms of visceral pain can be relieved by section of the splanchnic nerves without affecting visceral reflexes, which are mediated by the vagus nerves, seems to strengthen the opinion that some form of specific visceral nociceptors may exist. Based on the well documented algogenic properties of bradykinin when injected in the mesenteric arteries and on the existence of numerous free nerve endings associated with small intestinal vessels, Lim (13) proposes that the fibers originating perivascular receptors constitute the visceral division of the spinal nerves and are responsible for evoking the sensation of visceral pain. According to Lim these specific visceral nociceptors are most effective when stimulated by chemical agents such as may be formed during inflammation, i.e., bradykinin. This generalizing view received a severe blow when it was shown that bradykinin is a non-specific depolarizing agent which not only causes the activation of sensitive mechanoreceptors but also produces contractions in smooth muscle which in their turn will further excite visceral receptors.

The current approach to the study of visceral nociceptors is to link particular visceral conditions known to evoke pain with the receptors likely to be activated under these circumstances. This is the best approximation to the concept of an adequate stimulus although it has not yet yielded a distinct type of "pure" visceral nociceptor.

Unpleasant respiratory sensations such as dyspnea, tightness in the chest produced by inhalation of irritant chemicals, and burning pain evoked by mechanical stimulation of endotracheal and endobronchial mucosae are thought to be provoked by the activation of "irritant receptors" connected to $A\delta$ vagal afferent fibers (6). Other types of pulmonary receptors, such as the juxta-pulmonary capillary receptors (J-receptors) from which vagal C-afferents arise, have been implicated in the generation of pain in pulmonary edema and lung embolism (20). The pain of angina pectoris has been attributed to the activation of cardiac receptors which respond to ischemia due to coronary occlusion. These receptors are connected to $A\delta$ and C afferent fibers which reach the upper thoracic dorsal roots via sympathetic cardiac branches. Some crucial questions, such as the chemical sensitivity of these receptors and their differentiation from other types of cardiac receptors involved in cardio-vascular reflexes, have still to be answered adequately.

Pain arising from the alimentary canal has been attributed to the activation of the in-series tension receptors located in the muscular walls of hollow viscera (9). Most of the conditions that give rise to sensations of abdominal visceral pain also evoke discharges in this type of receptor. Passive distensions of a viscus, isometric contractions, impactions, and constrictions produce vigorous discharges in the in-series tension receptors of the visceral walls (10). Most of these receptors are connected to unmyelinated afferent fibers which join the parasympathetic vagus and pelvic nerves. This observation suggests that the sensations of pain from abdominal organs must be mediated by another set of receptors since in animals most of the pseudoaffective responses to noxious visceral stimuli are abolished by section of the sympathetic splanchnic nerves but not by section of the parasympathetic pelvic and vagus nerves.

Morrison (17) has described splanchnic afferents whose receptive fields contain up to eight punctate mechanosensitive sites distributed along the superior mesenteric artery and the vessels in the mesentery and the walls of the viscera. These serosal receptors, connected to Aδ and C afferent fibers respond with a slowly adapting discharge not only to light mechanical stimuli but also to tension applied to the mesentery and visceral peritoneum, to smooth muscle contractions and to visceral distensions. Morrison (17) suggests that they are directly involved in the mechanisms of visceral pain since they respond to stimuli known to evoke pain sensations and follow the pathways of the sympathetic nerves. Their lack of specificity to noxious stimuli is a puzzling factor which underlies the conflicting views on the existence of visceral nociceptors and seems to favor the opinion that visceral pain is associated with maximal discharges of unspecific visceral receptors.

Visceral and Deep Afferent Fibers in the Ventral Roots

The so-called "Bell-Magendie Law" has met a considerable amount of opposition since it was first formulated. Magendie himself had to explain the pain reactions evoked in animals when the ventral roots were stimulated as a consequence of "recurrent" afferent fibers from the dorsal roots. In 1894 Sherrington described a few small myelinated "recurrent" fibers in the ventral roots. In 1942 Lewis (12) reviewed past and current criticisms and concluded that the ventral roots could only be considered subsidiary channels for the conduction of pain.

Recently a number of studies carried out by Coggeshall and his associates (see (24) for references) have attempted to quantify the afferent component of the ventral roots at different levels of the cord in several species, including man. The conclusion is that many ventral roots contain a large number of sensory axons (up to 30%), the vast majority of which (up to 99%) are unmyelinated.

When electrophysiological experiments were conducted to establich the nature of these afferent fibers in the ventral root, it was reported that about one third of them came from cutaneous and deep nociceptors and that the other two thirds were of visceral origin (see references in (24)). These findings have led to a reconsideration of earlier proposals that the sensations of deep and visceral pain are always mediated via the ventral roots (see (12)). Such an opinion cannot be upheld in view of the numerous studies of visceral afferents on the dorsal roots, but the fact that most of the ventral root afferent fibers seem to come from deep and visceral structures strengthens Lewis' view that the ventral roots can act as subsidiary channels for the conduction of pain.

Viscero-Somatic Convergence in the Spinal Cord

It has been mentioned before that all interpretations of the ill-localization and referred qualities of deep and visceral pain have been based on the postulate that afferent fibers from deep and visceral structures converge onto spinal cord neurons that also have a cutaneous receptive field. Although there is some experimental evidence that such a convergence exists, detailed studies on the precise anatomical and physiological organization of viscero-somatic interactions in the spinal cord are needed.

In order to study the distribution of visceral afferent fibers in the spinal cord, microelectrode searches of the dorsal horn were carried out while electrical stimuli were delivered to visceral and cutaneous nerves. These initial studies yielded the first indications of viscero-somatic convergence in the spinal cord (i.e., (21)). Stimulation of the skin and distensions of hollow viscera were later employed and resulted in more information on the characteristics of the interactions between cutaneous and visceral afferents in the spinal cord (i.e., (5)).

It has been established that most of the spinal cord neurons showing viscero-somatic convergence are located in lamina V to VIII. The majority of neurons in lamina V are monosynaptically driven by small myelinated visceral afferents, which, according to field potential studies, seem to end exclusively in this region of the cord. Convergence of visceral afferents appears to occur only onto those neurons responding to both noxious and non-noxious stimulation of their cutaneous receptive fields (class 2 neurons). Neurons responding only to light mechanical stimulation of the skin (class 1 neurons) are unaffected by visceral afferents, whereas the experimental evidence of viscero-somatic convergence onto the specific nociceptor-driven cells of lamina I (class 3 neurons) is scarce and inconclusive.

There are no reports of neurons in the spinal cord driven exclusively by deep or visceral afferent fibers. It must be mentioned, however, that no studies have been reported in which there was a deliberate search for these cells. Therefore, it is possible that "specific visceral-driven" neurons may exist. Projections of thin afferent fibers from muscle (groups III and IV) to spinal cord neurons have been studied; again it seems that class 2 dorsal horn neurons take the major share in the proportion of cells showing musculo-cutaneous convergence. Some specific nociceptor-driven neurons in the lamina I are also excited by Aδ and C muscle afferents (3), but not all of them. Foreman et al. (7) have proposed that class 3 neurons without convergence from high threshold muscle afferents mediate cutaneous pain, whereas class 3 neurons that do receive an input from muscle afferents as well as class 2 neurons signal the poorly localized, aching deep pain. It would be desirable to have such proposals stimulate the interest of neurophysiologists in the subject and lead to investigations on viscero-somatic convergence in the spinal cord.

There is, however, one aspect of the problem that remains to be tackled. There are no anatomical studies on the distribution and endings of visceral afferents in the spinal cord. Such studies would help greatly to localize the neurons that receive visceral information. It is now well established that the substantia gelatinosa of the dorsal horn is the major site at which peripheral unmyelinated afferent fibers terminate. Since most of the visceral and deep receptors are connected to unmyelinated fibers, it is evident that the substantia gelatinosa must play a role in the mechanisms of visceral pain. Perhaps some of the most obscure and enigmatic characteristics of visceral pain outlined in the first part of this paper may be clarified when the recently revived interest on the anatomy and physiology of the substantia gelatinosa produces a more comprehensive picture of its functional organization.

Pathways for Deep and Visceral Pain in the Spinal Cord

The "convergence-projection" theory of Ruch (22) postulates that the main carrier of viscero-somatic convergence in the spinal cord is the spinothalamic tract (the traditional "pain pathway"). However, electrophysiological studies on spinal cord pathways activated by visceral impulses have produced a less clear-cut picture. It has been demonstrated that the dorsal columns contain a significant number of visceral afferent fibers which are mainly made up of the fastest Aβ visceral afferents and are not presumed to be involved in the sensations of pain.

Small myelinated and unmyelinated visceral fibers activate spinal cord neurons that project mainly through the ventrolateral quadrant of the cord. Convergence from visceral and deep afferent fibers has been described onto neurons projecting via the spinothalamic and spinoreticular tracts, both of which course in the ventrolateral quadrant. However, pathways located in the dorsolateral funiculus have also been shown to carry visceral and deep information.

Spino-cervical tract neurons respond to muscle groups III and IV afferent fibers, but not to activation of visceral afferents (2). Other pathways in the dorsolateral funiculus can be activated by visceral stimulation (see (24)). On the other hand, lesions of various pathways in the spinal cord white matter in animals fail to abolish pseudoaffective reflexes evoked by visceral noxious stimulation. This had been invoked as a proof (4) that visceral impulses are transmitted via a polysynaptic spinal system through the central gray matter.

The current evidence has, therefore, to be described as incomplete. The "convergence-projection" theory still stands as the most satisfactory explanation for the data available; however, our knowledge of the spinal cord mechanisms involved in the transmission of visceral pain can be improved only when basic problems such as the specificity of visceral nociceptors or the existence of pure visceral channels within the cord will be solved.

Visceral Representation in the Upper Centers of the Nervous System

A crucial physiological problem of deep and visceral pain relates to the mechanisms underlying ill-localization. Whether or not there is viscero-somatic convergence at the lower levels of the spinal cord, the subjective qualities of deep and visceral pain need to be analyzed by the study of the representation of visceral information in the upper levels of the nervous system. Projections of visceral impulses have been described as leading to the brain stem, the cerebellum, the thalamic nuclei, the hypothalamus, and the somatosensory and frontal areas of the cerebral cortex (see (18)). Yet all this information is incomlete.

It would be desirable to apply sophisticated techniques, developed for the study of higher functions of the nervous system, such as kinaesthesia, vision, audition or tactile recognition, to the study of visceral localization. It is not difficult to imagine situations where awake animals or human beings in acute or chronic visceral pain are assessed for their ability to localize the source of stimulation and/or interfere with it. Would it be possible to study the "visceral sense" as the sixth sense? After all, the colloquial "sixth sense" is generally associated with emotional and intuitive aspects of behavior.

REFERENCES

(1) Ayala, M. 1937. Douleur sympathique et douleur viscerale. Rev. Neurol. 68: 222-242.

(2) Cervero, F., and Iggo, A. 1978. Natural stimulation or urinary bladder afferents does not affect transmission through lumbosacral spinocervical tract neurones in the cat. Brain Res. 156: 375-379.

(3) Cervero, F.; Iggo, A.; and Ogawa, H. 1976. Nociceptor-driven dorsal horn neurones in the lumbar spinal cord of the cat. Pain 2: 5-24.

(4) Davis, L.; Hart, J.T.; and Crain, R.C. 1929. The pathway for visceral afferent impulses within the spinal cord. Surg. Gynecol. and Obst. 48: 647-651.

(5) Fields, H.L.; Partridge, L.D.; and Winter, D.L. 1970. Somatic and visceral receptive field properties of fibres in ventral quadrant white matter of the cat spinal cord. J. Neurophysiol. 33: 827-837.

(6) Fillenz, M., and Widdicombe, J.G. 1972. Receptors of the lungs and airways. In Handbook of Sensory Physiology Vol. III, ed. E. Neil, pp. 81-112. Heidelberg: Springer-Verlag.

(7) Foreman, R.D.; Schmidt, R.F.; and Willis, W.D. 1979. Effects of mechanical and chemical stimulation of fine muscle afferents upon primate spinothalamic tract cells. J. Physiol. 286: 215-231.

(8) Head, H. 1893. On disturbances of sensation with special reference to the pain of visceral disease. Brain 16: 1-133.

(9) Iggo, A. 1962. Non-myelinated visceral, muscular and cutaneous afferent fibres and pain. In The Assessment of Pain in Man and Animals, eds. C.A. Keele and R. Smith, pp. 74-87. Edinburgh: Livingstone.

(10) Leek, B.F. 1977. Abdominal and pelvic visceral receptors. Br. Med. Bull. 33: 163-168.

(11) Leriche, R. 1939. The Surgery of Pain. London: Bailliere, Tindal and Cox.

(12) Lewis, T. 1942. Pain. New York: MacMillan.

(13) Lim, R.K.S. 1960. Visceral receptors and visceral pain. Ann. N.Y. Acad. Sci. 86: 73-89.

(14) Mackenzie, J. 1909. Symptoms and Their Interpretation. London: Shaw and Sons.

(15) Mense, S. 1977. Muscular nociceptors. J. Physiol. (Paris) 73: 233-240.

(16) Morley, J.A. 1931. Abdominal Pain. Edinburgh: E. and S. Livingstone.

(17) Morrison, J.F.B. 1977. The afferent innervation of the gastro-intestinal tract. In Nerves and the Gut, eds. F.P. Brooks and P.W. Evers, pp. 297-326. New York: CBS inc.

(18) Newman, P.P. Visceral Afferent Functions of the Nervous System. London: E. Arnold Ltd.

(19) Noordenbos, W. 1959. Pain. Amsterdam: Elsevier & Co.

(20) Paintal, A.S. 1973. Vagal sensory receptors and their effects. Physiol. Rev. 53: 159-227.

(21) Pomeranz, B.; Wall, P.D.; and Weber, W.V. 1968. Cord cells responding to fine myelinated afferents from viscera, muscle and skin. J. Physiol. 199: 511-532.

(22) Ruch, T.C. 1946. Visceral sensation and referred pain. In Howell's Textbook of Physiology, 15th edition, ed. J.F. Fulton, pp. 385-401. Philadelphia: Saunders.

(23) Stacey, M.J. 1969. Free nerve endings in skeletal muscle of the cat. J. Anat. 105: 231-254.

(24) Willis, W.D., and Coggeshall, R.E. 1978. Sensory mechanisms of the spinal cord. New York: Plenum Press.

Pain and Society, eds. H.W. Kosterlitz and L.Y. Terenius, pp. 283-298.
Dahlem Konferenzen 1980. Weinheim: Verlag Chemie GmbH.

Physiological Mechanisms of Chronic Pain

M. Zimmermann
II. Physiologisches Institut, Universität Heidelberg
6900 Heidelberg, F. R. Germany

Abstract. Chronic pain is different from acute pain produced, e.g., by an experimental stimulus. It may result from the following mechanisms: a) increase in sensitivity of nerve axons to mechanical stimuli, after long-term mechanical irritation, b) excitation of nociceptors by endogenous algesic substances released, e.g., during inflammation, c) ongoing discharges originating from nerve sprouts in a neuroma, d) increased excitability of nociceptors regenerated following nerve lesions, e) positive feedback via motor and sympathetic reflexes, f) release from tonic inhibition of neurons in the central nervous system, and g) long-term changes such as supersensitivity of synapses following partial deafferentation of central neurons.

INTRODUCTION

The present knowledge of the physiological mechanisms of pain has been deduced predominantly from experimental studies on animals and humans using acute noxious stimuli (e.g., radiant heat to the skin). Since stimuli of this kind usually can be quickly terminated in every day life by an appropriate behavioral response (escape, avoidance), they do not result in a chronic pain state. However, it is its persistence which makes chronic pain a most urgent problem in medicine. As to the origin of chronic pain, it is clear that it can arise at the level of nociceptors and the nociceptive afferent fibers as well as within the central nervous system. A survey of some fundamental mechanisms will be given here. A detailed compilation of literature can be found elsewhere (19).

COMPRESSION OF NERVES

Excitation of nerves not only takes place at the nociceptor, nerve impulses can also be elicited anywhere along the sensory fiber in the nerve trunk, e.g., by local mechanical distortion. In normal nerve fibers acute mechanical stimuli applied anywhere along the axon have been shown to evoke a rapidly adapting discharge at the onset of the stimulus (Fig. 1), which is not sufficient to explain pain arising in mechanically irritated nerves in patients. However, ongoing discharges lasting up to 25 minutes are produced when a mechanical stimulus, even of short duration, acts on the spinal ganglion cell or on nerve or dorsal root fibers in which a chronic injury has been produced experimentally, e.g., by placing a chromic gut ligature around the dorsal roots some weeks before (11).

Mechanosensitivity of afferent nerves
according to Howe,Loeser and Calvin,77

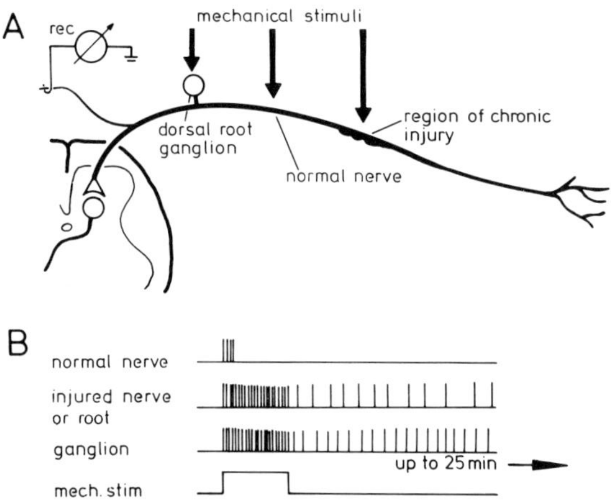

FIG.1 - Responses of afferent fibers of a cat's nerve to mechanical irritation (11). A: Experimental situation. B: Typical responses to a mechanical stimulus acting on intact nerve, injured dorsal root or nerve, and spinal ganglion. Reproduced from (19).

It is conceivable that such ongoing discharges, which can occur in all types of nerve fibers, produce paresthesia and pain when nerves or roots are distorted repeatedly or chronically (e.g., by vertebral discs or carpal ligaments). These sensations are localized by the patient to the innervation territory of that nerve.

A long-lasting compression, which might also produce some local ischemia of the nerve, can eventually result in a conduction block which is preferential for Aβ-fibers, as has been shown in experiments in man and on animals (16). The persistence of ongoing activity in nociceptive afferents and the absence of concomitant discharges in tactile afferents have been suggested to be the reason why the resulting pain is particularly disagreeable in these cases. However, histological investigation of nerves in patients with neuropathies of various types and the characteristics of their pain do not support this general assumption (9).

CHEMICAL INFLUENCES ON NOCICEPTORS AND THEIR AFFERENTS

Pathological conditions of the skin and viscera as produced by trauma, inflammation, or muscle ischemia are accompanied by release or enhanced production of substances such as KCl, serotonin, bradykinin, and prostaglandin E. Each of these can either excite or sensitize a nociceptor, depending on its local concentration and may therefore be called algesic substances (see H.O. Handwerker, this volume). Since their actions will persist during the whole pathological process, they may be causes of chronic pain.

It has been recently claimed that excitation by algesic substances of the axons in the nerve trunk is a basic mechanism in pain (12). We have tested this question directly by recording from single A- and C-fibers when the desheated sural nerve of the cat was exposed to some of the algesic chemicals (Klumpp and Zimmermann, unpublished observations). Bradykinin, serotonin, acetylcholine, histamine, and prostaglandin E all failed to excite the fibers even at concentrations 1000 times those known to excite the nociceptors. Only KCl produced a transient discharge, and eventually blocked conduction. Thus, our findings do not support the hypothesis that algesic substances activate axons of afferent fibers in producing pain. We do, however, not yet know whether excitation by chemicals can occur after a long lasting irritation of the nerve trunk.

REGENERATING NERVES

Nerve transections by trauma, amputation, or neurosurgical operation strongly induce the fibers of the proximal stump to regenerate. Such sites are often sources of severe pain, particularly when a neuroma has developed. Can this pain arise from the sprouts of the regenerating fibers? Experiments on rats have recently been conducted in which a neuroma was induced by placing the proximal stump of the cut sciatic nerve into a plastic cap (6,17).

In such preparations, ongoing impulse activity, initiated at the fiber sprouts in the neuroma, was found in Aδ- and C-fibers (Fig. 2), while no such activity occurred in Aβ-fibers. Also, ongoing discharges were observed to arise from spinal ganglion cells following injury to the peripheral axon. Since many of the spontaneously active Aδ- and C-fibers previously had nociceptive endings, it is tempting to consider that the impulse flow in these fibers could be interpreted by the central nervous system as being due to a noxious stimulus.

Two additional results of importance emerged from these investigations on experimental neuroma: a) The ongoing impulse discharges were enhanced by intravenous administration of noradrenaline (Fig. 2B), an effect which was prevented by simultaneous injection of the α-blocker phentolamine. This is indirect evidence that sympathetic efferents might exert some stimulatory action on nociceptive fibers in the neuroma. Such a mechanism has been claimed to operate in causalgia, a pain

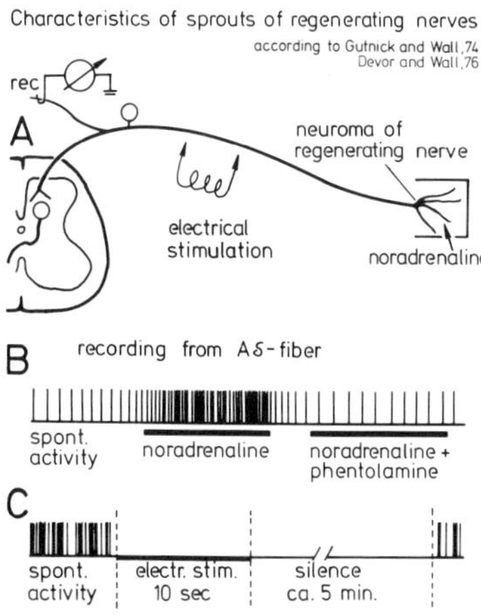

FIG. 2 - Properties of nerve sprouts in an experimental neuroma (6,17). A: A neuroma was induced in transected rat sciatic nerve by putting a plastic cap over the proximal stump. When a neuroma had formed, the nerve was prepared for stimulation and recording. B: Discharge frequency in Aδ-fibers increased by intravenous noradrenaline, an effect which was prevented by the α-blocking agent phentolamine. C: Spontaneous activity in Aδ-fibers arising in the neuroma was blocked for a long time by a short period of repetitive electrical nerve stimulation. Reproduced from (19).

syndrome that often occurs in patients having a neuroma caused by partial lesions of a nerve. b) A short period (e.g., 10 s) of repetitive electrical stimulation of the nerve at a strength above threshold for the single fiber under study completely stopped the ongoing discharge for several minutes (Fig. 2C). This may be a possible model for the pain relief produced by peripheral nerve stimulation in amputees which, apart from a peripheral suppressive action, may activate inhibitory processes in the central nervous system.

When a regenerating nerve reaches its peripheral innervation territory, such as in the skin, hyperpathia can be observed in patients (15). This situation has been simulated in animal experiments (8). When the sprouting fibers reached the skin, nociceptors having functional characteristics similar to those in normal skin immediately develop (Fig. 3). However, in a sample of regenerated C-nociceptors, the average threshold to noxious skin heating was significantly reduced by about 4°C when compared to normal conditions in control animals. This finding may explain the hyperpathia to thermal stimuli in patients with regenerated nerves.

Redevelopment of C-nociceptors in regenerating nerve

Dickhaus, Zimmermann and Zotterman, 76

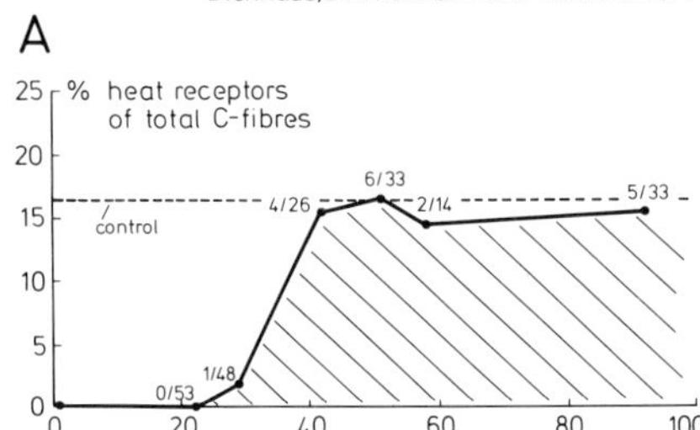

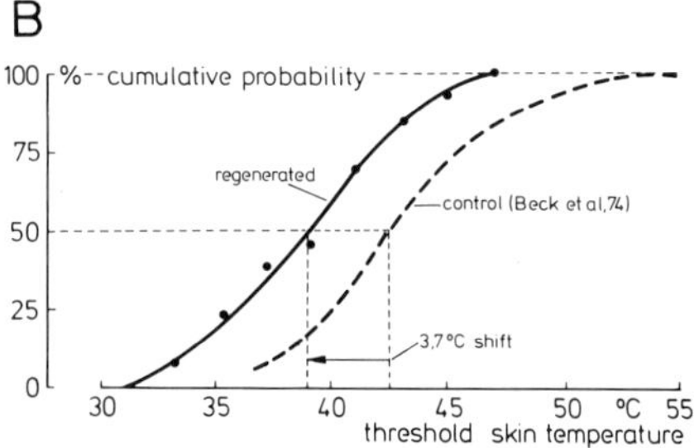

FIG. 3 - Regenerating C-nociceptors in the cat's skin (8). A: Time course of regeneration of heat sensitive C-nociceptors after nerve crush. The ordinate gives the percentage of heat receptors relative to the total number of C-fibers which were identified by electrical stimulation of the plantar nerves at a site proximal to the crush. Numerals at the points indicate number of heat nociceptors versus total number of C-fibers tested for responsiveness to skin heating. Each point contains data from one or two experiments. B: Temperature thresholds of regenerated C-nociceptors. The continuous curve shows the proportion of fibers (ordinate) excited at the temperature given (abscissa) in a population of 13 regenerated C-nociceptors; the threshold criterion was the generation of at least one spike during a heat stimulus of 10 s duration. Control values in A and B are from experiments performed on normal nerves under identical conditions of thermal stimulation (2).

INVOLVEMENT OF MOTOR AND SYMPATHETIC REFLEXES IN CHRONIC PAIN

Motor and sympathetic reflexes to noxious stimuli usually serve to counteract the algesic effect; they can be considered as negative feedback mechanisms to protect the organism from injury. However, such reflexes sometimes have a positive feedback role, i.e., they increase rather than decrease the effect of a noxious stimulus (Fig. 4).

Positive feedback by motor (A) and sympathetic (B) reflexes might produce or facilitate sustained nociceptor excitation

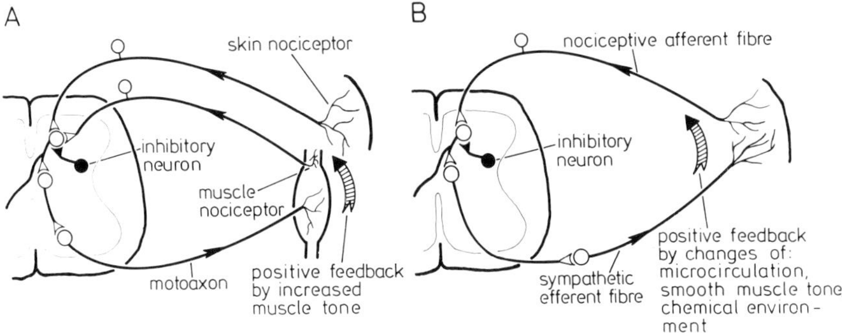

FIG. 4 - Hypothetical mechanisms of self-excitation of nociceptors by spinal reflexes. A: Motor reflex induced by skin or muscle nociceptors, the contraction acting as stimulus on muscle nociceptors. B: Sympathetic reflex evoked by nociceptors; various sympathetic effector mechanisms are indicated which can enhance the excitability of the nociceptors. Reproduced from (19).

For example, a motor reflex initiated by a cutaneous or visceral nociceptive stimulus may lead to activity in muscle or tendon nociceptors by contraction of the muscle (Fig. 4A). This, in turn, can increase the motor reflex which will eventually lead to a self-sustained reflex muscle hypertonia and, concomitantly, to ongoing pain. Such a mechanism might occur via the γ-loop (10) since chemical activation of muscle nociceptors produces excitation of γ-motoneurons in both flexor and extensor muscles.

In the intact animal, this would lead to increased muscle tone via the stretch reflex.

Such a vicious circle is also possible in the case of sympathetic reflexes (Fig. 4B). Positive feedback mechanisms may be considered as causative in the clinically well-known syndromes of sympathetic reflex dystrophy (see Nathan, this volume). The sympathetic effector thus enhances rather than decreases the level of excitation of the nociceptors. Several mechanisms could account for such a deleterious effect: vasoconstriction and ischemia; vasodilatation and increase in vascular permeability, thus changing the extracellular fluid environment of the nociceptor; contraction of smooth muscle surrounding the nociceptor; and direct action on the nociceptor of locally released neurotransmitters, neuromodulators, and algesic agents such as noradrenaline, serotonin, bradykinin, prostaglandin E, and substance P. These adverse effects of sympathetic efferent activity, although apparent from many clinical observations still lack a physiological foundation. A systematic investigation of these problems is highly desirable.

Therapeutic actions should be aimed at interrupting the positive feedback or self-excitatory loop by a conduction block in either the afferent or efferent branch of the reflex loop. Local anesthesia of the afferent nerve yields pain relief which often outlasts, by days or even weeks, the duration of the local nerve block. This enduring pain relief lends support to the view that the pain was really of the self-sustaining type. Another method of interrupting the positive feedback loop is to activate neuronal inhibition in the spinal cord (Willis et al., this volume).

TONIC INHIBITORY CONTROL OF PAIN INFORMATION

It has been established that sensory information on painful events is modulated in the CNS. Failure of a tonic inhibitory system to operate properly might be a cause of chronic pain. For example, in the spinal dorsal horn, several systems descending from the brain stem exert inhibitory control onto the afferent inflow at the first synaptic relay.

Descending systems, suppressing nociceptive signals in dorsal horn neurons have been reported to originate a) in the mesencephalic periaqueductal gray, b) in some of the raphe nuclei which contain serotonergic neurons, c) in the locus coeruleus with noradrenergic neurons, and d) in the reticular formation. They are reviewed in detail by Besson (this volume). Examples of brain stem control mechanisms are given in Fig. 5. Spinal neuronal responses to noxious skin heating at varying intensities have been measured. In Fig. 5A, at each temperature of skin heating, measurements were performed before and during repetitive electrical stimulation in the midbrain of either the periaqueductal gray (PAG) or the lateral reticular formation (LRF). The sites of stimulation are shown in Fig. 5B. A major feature of PAG inhibition was that the discharge frequency increased more slowly with increasing skin temperature, while the threshold remained the same. LRF stimulation affects the intensity coding in a different manner (Fig. 5A); the response line shifted in a practically parallel fashion to lower discharge rates and higher thresholds. The inhibitory system arising in the PAG may thus be interpreted as controlling the efficacy or gain of nociceptive transmission in the spinal dorsal horn (5), whereas inhibition from LRF is operating to adjust the set point of spinal transmission.

The existence of tonically active descending inhibition is evident from experiments in which a block of spinal conduction was performed (Fig. 5C, D). The characteristics of heat intensity coding displayed a parallel shift to lower temperatures. By comparison with Fig. 5A, this result suggests that the tonic inhibition removed by the spinal cold block was that originating in the LRF.

The descending brain stem systems have also been characterized by neurochemical and pharmacological means. Thus, serotonin has been found to play a role as an inhibitory neurotransmitter or neuromodulator in at least one of these systems. Endogenous opiates have also been suggested as being involved in pain

Two systems of descending inhibition from midbrain

Carstens, Klumpp and Zimmermann, 80

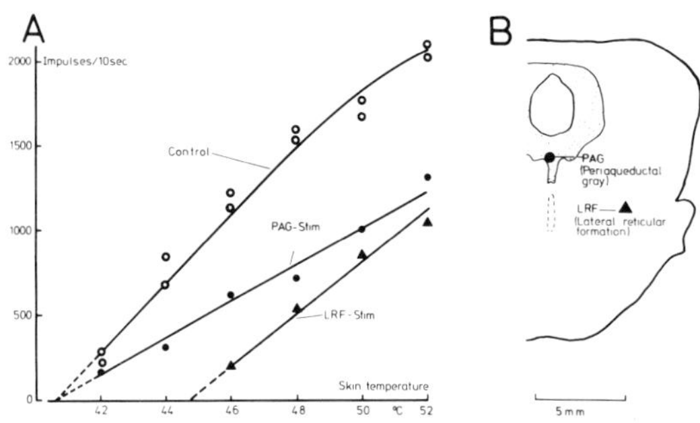

Tonic descending inhibition

Dickhaus, Pauser and Zimmermann, 78

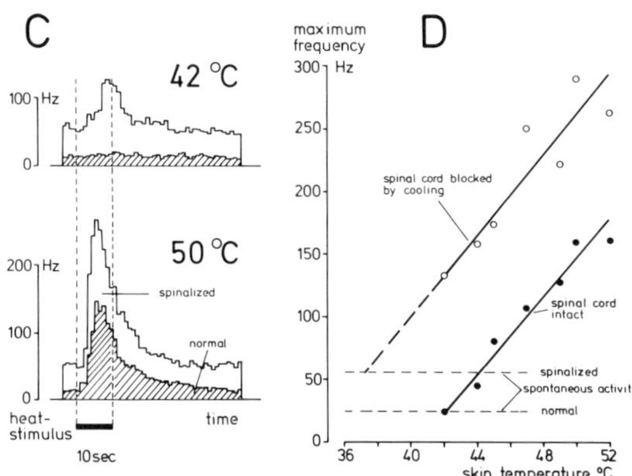

FIG. 5 - Multiple systems of descending inhibition in the cat's dorsal horn. A: The encoding of intensity of noxious skin heating in a single dorsal horn neuron as affected by stimulation in the periaqueductal gray (PAG) and the lateral reticular formation (LRF) of the midbrain. B: Location of stimulation sites in the midbrain. C: Discharges of a dorsal horn neuron upon noxious skin heating to 42°C and 50°C, before and during reversible conduction block by cooling of descending pathways at spinal L_1 level. D: Intensity characteristics (maximum frequency of discharge plotted versus skin temperature) of the same unit as in C before (●) and during (o) spinal blockade. Data in A, B are from (4), those in C, D from (7).

inhibition at spinal and supraspinal sites (see Akil and Watson, and Zieglgänsberger, this volume). Accordingly, the tonic inhibitory control of pain might be impaired by a deficiency of either serotonin or endogenous opiates (see Terenius, this volume), which have been proposed as being a mechanism of chronic pain.

PAIN ORIGINATING FROM DEAFFERENTATION OF NERVE CELLS

Sometimes pain is not related to the activation of nociceptors and their afferent fibers; rather, it must be assumed to be of central origin. The most convincing evidence for this contention is the occurrence of phantom limb pain in several patients with spinal transections, the completeness of which had been surgically verified (14). Since all sensory nerves from the phantom region entered the spinal cord far below the site of transection, the authors have postulated that deafferented neurons above the transection may produce abnormal spontaneous discharges in the absence of afferent synaptic drive. Such ongoing discharges in neurons related to ascending pain pathways would eventually be perceived as pain localized to the previous receptive fields of these neurons.

How could such abnormal behavior develop? The neurons which are partially deafferented by the spinal lesion are positioned critically, since it is known that nerve cells will undergo several types of changes upon loss of presynaptic terminals. These changes may be described by the terms "neuronal plasticity" and "supersensitivity" and are thought to play roles in, e.g., ontogenetic development of the nervous system, learning and memory, restitution of function after brain lesions, and abnormal neuronal behavior. Functional and morphological alterations that have been observed or postulated to occur in the synaptic connectivity of neurons following partial deafferentation are compiled in Fig. 6. Previously ineffective synapses can be switched on (B), the efficiency of the persisting synapses may be increased (C), new aberrant nerve connections can develop by contact with sprouts from foreign axons (D), and supersensitivity of the neuron to neurotransmitters and neuromodulatory substances can develop (E). All of these mechanisms of action have been extensively investigated in the "model synapses" of the neuromuscular junction and of the parasympathetic cardiac ganglion cells.

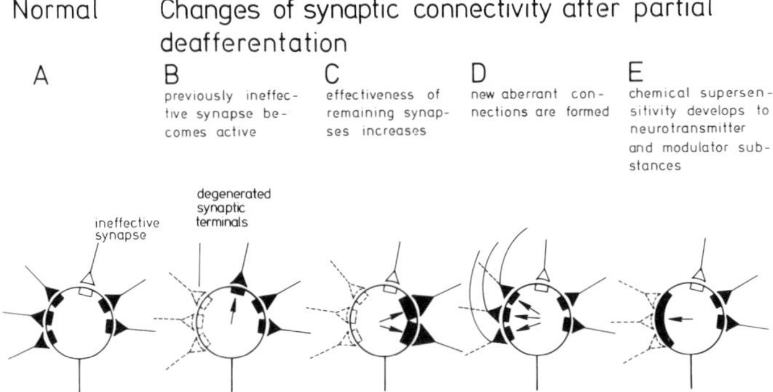

FIG. 6 - Schematic survey of possible long-term effects of partial deafferentation of a nerve cell. Arrows indicate the sites of the effects as explained in the text. Reproduced from (19).

These chronic changes in synaptic connectivity have been suggested as being involved in pain of central origin, such as the phantom pain in paraplegic patients reported above, phantom limb pain recurring after rhizotomy of all relevant dorsal roots, thalamic pain after local cerebrovascular infarction, analgesia dolorosa sometimes developing after neurosurgical operations, dermatome border hyperalgesia after dorsal root lesions, and recurrence of pain after temporary relief by cordotomy. Neurophysiological observations in the CNS supporting such pain mechanisms have been reported from experiments in the spinal cord and the thalamus, where units have been observed showing a high level of ongoing activity as well as erratic behavior after chronic deafferentation. A spatial spread of excitatory connections from intact roots into deafferented cord segments has been reported by some authors (1) but not by others (3).

It is tempting to hypothesize that the states of pain mentioned above are due to denervation supersensitivity, sprouting of aberrant nerve connections, and derepression or unmasking of ineffective synapses. Are there means to prevent these processes? I would like to speculate that perhaps activation of the deafferented neurons, e.g., by electrical stimulation of the remaining afferents or of the neurons directly, may interfere with the development of plastic changes. Experiments on synapses, in the neuromuscular junction, indeed revealed that both extra-junctional supersensitivity to acetylcholine and development of synapses with a foreign nerve were prevented by electrical stimulation of the silent presynaptic afferents or of the post-synaptic muscle elements. Assuming that analogous mechanisms operate in deafferented central neurons, one could predict that the development of pain states after central lesions might be prevented, e.g., by the implantation of an electrical stimulator at the time of, or immediately after, the lesion.

The relationship of the experimental findings to pain is to date still conjectural. It would be highly desirable to intensify research on the problem of these presumed pain mechanisms.

REFERENCES

(1) Basbaum, A.I., and Wall, P.D. 1976. Chronic changes in the response of cells in adult cat dorsal horn following partial deafferentation: the appearance of responding cells in a previously non-responsive region. Brain Res. 116: 181-204.

(2) Beck, P.W.; Handwerker, H.O.; and Zimmermann, M. 1974. Nervous outflow from the cat's foot during noxious radiant heat stimulation. Brain Res. 67: 373-386.

(3) Brinkhus, H., and Zimmermann, M. 1978. Influence of partial deafferentation on spinal neurons in the cat. Pflügers Arch.-Eur. J. Physiol. 373: suppl. R 90.

(4) Carstens, E.; Klumpp, D.; and Zimmermann, M. 1980. Differential inhibitory effects of medial and lateral mid-brain stimulation on spinal neuronal discharges to noxious skin heating in the cat. J. Neurophysiol. 43: 332-343.

(5) Carstens, E.; Yokota, T.; and Zimmermann, M. 1979. Inhibition of spinal neuronal responses to noxious skin heating by stimulation of the mesencephalic periaqueductal gray in the cat. J. Neurophysiol. 42: 558-568.

(6) Devor, M., and Wall, P.D. 1976. Type of sensory fiber sprouting to form a neuroma. Nature 262: 705-708.

(7) Dickhaus, H.; Pauser, G.; and Zimmermann, M. 1978. Hemmung im Rückenmark, ein neurophysiologischer Wirkungsmechanismus bei der Hypalgesie durch Stimulationsakupunktur. Wiener klinische Wochenschrift 90: 59-64.

(8) Dickhaus, H.; Zimmermann, M.; and Zotterman, Y. 1976. The development in regenerating cutaneous nerves of C-fiber receptors responding to noxious heating of the skin. In Sensory Functions of the Skin in Primates, ed. Y. Zotterman, pp. 415-425. Oxford, New York, Toronto, Sydney, Paris, Frankfurt: Pergamon Press.

(9) Dyck, P.J.; Lambert, E.H.; and O'Brien, B.C. 1976. Pain in peripheral neuropathy related to rate and kind of fiber degeneration. Neurology 26: 466-471.

(10) Hong, S.K.; Kniffki, K.-D.; and Schmidt, R.F. 1978. Reflex discharges of extensor and flexor gamma motoneurones by chemically induced muscle pain. Pain Abstracts, vol. 1, p. 58. 2nd World Congress Pain, Montreal.

(11) Howe, J.F.; Loeser, J.D.; and Calvin, W.H. 1977. Mechanosensitivity of dorsal root ganglia and chronically injured axons: a physiological basis for the radicular pain of nerve root compression. Pain 3: 25-41.

(12) Khayutin, V.M.; Baraz, L.A.; Lukoshkova, E.V.; Sonina, R.S.; and Chernilovskaya, P.E. 1976. Chemosensitive spinal afferents: thresholds of specific and nociceptive reflexes as compared with thresholds of excitation for receptors and axons. In Progress in Brain Research 43: Somatosensory and Visceral Receptor Mechanisms, ed. A. Iggo and O.B. Ilyinski, pp. 293-306. Amsterdam: Elsevier.

(13) Lynn, B. 1977. Cutaneous hyperalgesia. Brit. Med. Bull. 33: 103-108.

(14) Melzack, R., and Loeser, J.D. 1978. Phantom body pain in paraplegics: evidence for a central "pattern generating mechanism" for pain. Pain 4: 195-210.

(15) Sunderland, S. 1978. Nerves and nerve injuries. 2nd ed. Edinburgh and London: Livingstone.

(16) Torebjörk, H.E., and Hallin, R.G. 1973. Perceptual changes accompanying controlled preferential blocking of A and C fiber responses in intact human skin nerves. Exp. Brain res. 16: 321-332.

(17) Wall, P.D., and Gutnick, M. 1974. Ongoing activity in peripheral nerves: the physiology and pharmacology of impulses originating from neuroma. Exptl. Neurol. 43: 580-593.

(18) Zimmermann, M. 1977. Encoding in dorsal horn interneurons receiving noxious and non-noxious afferents. J. Physiol. (Paris) 73: 221-232.

(19) Zimmermann, M. 1979. Peripheral and central nervous mechanisms of nociception, pain and pain therapy: facts and hypotheses. In Advances in Pain Research and Therapy 3, eds. J.J. Bonica et al., pp. 3-32. New York: Raven Press.

Pain and Society, eds. H.W. Kosterlitz and L.Y. Terenius, pp. 299-310.
Dahlem Konferenzen 1980. Weinheim: Verlag Chemie GmbH.

Animal Models for Chronic Pain

D. G. Albe-Fessard and M. C. Lombard
Laboratoire de Physiologie des Centres Nerveux
Université P. et M. Curie, 75230 Paris, France

Abstract. - Two types of pain can be recognized in man: pain associated with an increase in impulse activity in afferent pathways and pain associated with lesions of nervous tissue. The different animal models to study pain can be classified under these same two headings.

The majority of the classical animal models, particularly those used by pharmacologists and neurophysiologists, are of the first type and their limitations are discussed.

Animals with lesions of their nervous tissue have been studied rarely until 10 years ago. Since then, central epileptic foci, lesions of nerves, and lesions of dorsal roots have been used to induce pain-like behaviors in rats and cats. These three sorts of animal models will be described. The characteristics of animals with dorsal root lesions, as used by the authors, have been reviewed extensively.

NEED FOR NEW ANIMAL MODELS

It has become obvious in recent years that we urgently need to develop new animal models for the study of chronic pain (21). The major reason is that while pain, as represented in man, can be schematically separated into two large groups as a function of its underlying lesion, the existing animal models mimic only one of the groups of pain syndromes. By way of simplification, we will group these two types of pain observed in the human under the following headings.

1) Pain associated with increase in impulse activity in afferent pathways. In these cases the nervous system is intact. The stimuli differ from those provoking normal defensive reactions only in their intensity and overall duration. For example, in experimental toothache while short stimulation is easily tolerated, a longer train of stimuli of the same intensity is unbearable (3). It is certain that most types of nociceptive weak stimuli become unbearable when prolonged. Such pain is relatively easy to treat; because of the peripheral origin of the painful stimulation, it may be removed through surgery or blocked by drugs having peripheral action, e.g., aspirin and analogues.

2) Pain associated with lesions of nervous tissue. This is due to trauma of the central or peripheral nervous system produced by external or internal mechanisms. Section of nerves or central pathways, destruction of central areas due to circulatory disturbances, or destructive disease (tabes dorsalis, tumor, sclerosis, etc...) result in erratically localized pain apparently originating in those areas deprived of central connections by the disease. Thus the central area of projection deprived of afferent impulses seems to be able to create a new event, an abnormal pattern of excitation.

As a general rule, these pains are difficult to treat with classical methods. There is no possibility to suppress the afferent pathways of the noxious stimulus because they are already suppressed by the disease. Peripherally acting drugs cannot be effective for the same reason, and addictive drugs cannot be used due to the long duration of these diseases. Thus it is necessary to search for a specific treatment for these pain patients who, according to Sternbach (21), represent 40% of the cases in a pain clinic. However, the majority of pharmacological as well as neurophysiological research is performed on models with increased afferent input, in spite of the fact that there is no evidence showing that pain in the two groups can activate the same central mechanisms or in fact be treated with the same analgesic methods.

ANIMAL MODELS WITH AN INCREASE OF AFFERENT INPUT AND THEIR LIMITATIONS

In the majority of these models, pain is evoked by peripheral stimuli at intensities which activate mechanical or thermic nociceptors. The effects of these stimulations are observed with behavioral, neurochemical or electrophysiological techniques, and methods for suppressing these effects are needed.

The first difficulty which arises is that it is always hard to stimulate nociceptors without stimulating receptors for other modalities. This is especially the case where mechanoceptors are concerned and different techniques have been proposed to avoid this difficulty (see review and bibliography in (22)).

Heat as a painful stimulus has the advantage that it can be applied without stimulating mechanoceptors. It has become a widely used method for producing pain in man and animals (8).

Electrical stimulation of peripheral nerves has also been used in the search for a selective blockade of "pain fibers." Nerve fibers in the Aδ and C group are said to be the only ones connected with nociceptors. Thus, procedures that block conduction selectively in these two types of fibers or block the result of their stimulation, as the flexor reflex, are frequently considered to produce analgesia. These techniques do not take into account the facts that not only noxious but also tactile messages are conducted in Aδ fibers and that Aβ fibers can also conduct noxious messages in man when temporal or spatial convergences are applied (25).

The fact that pain is the sensation commonly recognized by patients when their tooth pulp is manipulated has led to the use of tooth pulp stimulation to activate nociceptive afferents exclusively. There is, however, no consensus that tooth stimulation will activate nociceptive fibers only, because the results are affected by the way the stimulation is applied. It is evident that when stimulation is applied externally to the tooth without appropriate and strict precautions, there is great danger that stimuli will spread to other tissues and excite periodontal terminals or fibers. However, if dentine bipolar electrode are implanted, evidence obtained in man shows that a truly painful experience succeeds a prepain when the stimulus is increased in intensity or duration. This stimulation is only painful when local spatial or temporal convergence is produced (25). For instance, the jaw opening reflex obtained in chronic cats with a low threshold dentine stimulation cannot be taken as a truly nociceptive reflex, since these animals do not seem affected otherwise, (personal results and (22)). It is only with an increase in duration of the stimulation that the animal is disturbed and thus for deontological reasons such stimulation cannot be applied. In conclusion, the techniques which suppress either the jaw opening reflex or the central projection of tooth pulp afferents obtained with threshold stimulation, cannot be considered to lead to analgesia unless we accept that these threshold behaviors or projections use the same pathways as those activated when long trains of stimuli are applied to the tooth pulp.

Chemical agents producing pain in man are also widely used, for instance, acetylcholine, KCl, histamine, 5HT, bradykinin, and formalin. They are applied at the periphery either directly to the skin, to deeper regions, or to blisters as it was done in man (9). As bradykinin was found to evoke pain in man and an intense nociceptive reaction in animals (12), its intraarterial administration was used to study the central neuronal mechanisms of nociception. A unique action on nociceptors by these drugs is questionable.

Recently, production in animals of articular diseases mimicking the syndromes observed in man has been proposed.

All the techniques we have quoted above increase the nociceptive afferent traffic and thus mimic the first type of pain. However, each of these procedures is subject to the same criticism, namely, that the activity they provoke is not purely nociceptive. When performed in animals all these techniques are confronted, however with other difficulties:

a) If the animal is anesthetized, it is difficult to know whether in non-anesthetized animals or man the activation of nociceptive afferents has similar reflex effects or brain distribution.

b) If the animal is totally awake, then, for deontologic reasons, the intensity of the stimuli have to be maintained at a relatively low level of intensity and duration. We have to accept that a light, short noxious stimulus has the same central distribution as a strong, long one, a hypothesis that has not yet been demonstrated.

ANIMAL MODELS OF PAIN DUE TO LESION OF NERVOUS TISSUE

Compared to the large number of pain models mentioned above, only a few pain models exist where lesions of nervous tissue have been used; these were developed only during the last 10 years. They tend to mimic three major neurological diseases: a) anesthesia dolorosa which follows section of peripheral nerves, b) trigeminal neuralgias, and c) central pain due to dorsal root lesions.

Nerve Lesions

Nerve lesions were performed (23) in the inferior limbs of rats. Sciatic and saphenous nerves were sectioned and regeneration of the peripheral end prevented so that the animal had a totally anesthetic foot. After about a week self-amputation or autotomy of the anesthetic foot is observed; this behavior is suppressed by pharmacologic treatment which prevents fiber sprouting in the neuroma. This fact suggests that the autotomy was due to anesthesia dolorosa caused by the generation of impulses in sproutings of the central stump of the peripheral nerves.

Thus, this model of anesthesia dolorosa has a peripheral origin in the neuroma. It is observed after nerve section and it is not very different from the somatic models we have already described in the previous section. The pain is due to the neuroma causing an increased and prolonged distortion of the peripheral message rather than to a new event appearing in the brain.

Trigeminal Neuralgia

Two types of models were developed:

a) The first one is based on the following two observations. In a patient having trigeminal neuralgia, epileptic activities were observed at the mesencephalic level (19). The majority of tic douloureux patients are relieved by anti-epileptic drugs. Black (5) created an experimental epileptic focus, using alumina gel within the spinal fifth nucleus in cats. Krishanowsky (11) produced identical effects by injecting tetanus toxin at the same level; similar effects were obtained with the same techniques at the spinal cord level. In the Black model the animals had a way of protecting their ipsilateral face which mimics the behavior of tic douloureux patients.

b) The second model was based on the observation that partial deafferentation triggers epileptic discharges in central cells (24). Partial hemideafferentation was performed in cats through a nerve lesion or the destruction of the gasserian ganglion. Such deafferentation resulted in epileptic activity at the ipsilateral spinal trigeminal level (2). This model takes into account the fact that some trigeminal neuralgia patients present either a lack of, or a change in, discriminative sensations of a part of the face.

Deafferentation Syndrome by Root Sections

Deafferentation hyperpathia occurs in man after a traumatic root avulsion of the brachial plexus. This chronic pain is described as burning, crushing, or tearing in nature, and when it appears it usually lasts for the lifetime of the patient. That is to say such pain is difficult to relieve through known drugs or analgesic maneuvers. The dorsal root pain is felt in regions which have lost a part of their sensations through deafferentation, as in face neuralgia. This fact may allow a comparison of this syndrome with anesthesia dolorosa due to nerve section.

However, it is only an analogy because the lesion in this case is central to the ganglion, and if sprouting occurs it will be at the distal and not the central stump. It is thus worthwhile to try to create an animal model of dorsal root avulsion which will help in an understanding of the mechanisms of the disease and in the search for effective treatment. Early work was done in cats (14), but behavioral studies of this model were largely performed in rats. Effects of dorsal root lesions were studied in this species by four groups (4,7,6,15,16,17). After lesions of the dorsal roots, three abnormal behaviors can appear in the rat: a) The animal scratches the ipsilateral side of the lesion and in some cases the contralateral loci. This scratching behavior results in wounds that can momentarily heal, but will always return. b) The animal chews the ipsilateral forelimb and produces self-amputation. c) The animal presents hyper-reaction to light touch.

This last behavior is interesting but difficult to measure and was observed only episodically. The first two behaviors, however, were studied extensively. The production of scratching wounds were essentially studied by our group, while the self-mutilation was studied by all of the research groups.

A comparison of the locations where wound scratching occurred with dermatomes has shown that they appear in zones of only partial deafferentation. However, self-amputation requires the total deafferentation of the area. It is difficult to decide with this observation whether self-amputation corresponds to the ablation of an anesthetic area or is due to the fact that analgesia dolorosa has developed at this level - analgesia dolorosa which in this case cannot be attributed to a neuroma. In favor of an analgesia dolorosa syndrome are the observations that chewing and self-amputation are suppressed by lesions of anterolateral ascending pathways (4) and by hydantoin treatment (7). The fact that self-amputation occurs only at a certain moment of the nycthemeral cycle (7) or during the induction phase of anesthesia (1) implies that chewing and self-amputation are responses to an active, sensitive process and not just the disposal of a totally analgesic zone. The number of roots which have to be sectioned to observe the complete behavior consisting of self-amputation and scratching wounds, was also determined (6,15,17). Sections of at least four contiguous roots on one side are necessary at the brachial plexus level, between C5 and Th1, whereas at the posterior limb level the behavior is difficult to produce with restricted lesions. The delays in appearance of the different components of the behavior were also studied.

In this model, there has been so far only a relatively small amount of research on the possible treatment of the syndrome. However, as we have said before, it was shown that section of ascending pathways in the cord (4) and hydantoin treatment (7) can suppress the chewing. In our group (1), the animals were subjected daily to peripheral electrical stimulation (similar to that used in pain patients) of the intact side of the body. Using an evaluation scale for both self-amputation and scratching wounds, it was shown that the delay of onset and development of both behaviors is increased by the electrical stimulation, this effect being more important for scratching. In cats, after dorsal root sections at the brachial plexus level, wound provoking scratching develops as in the rat. However, in those animals, after a few weeks the wounds healed and totally disappeared. The cats never developed self-amputation after lesioning the five contiguous roots.

RECORDINGS OF CENTRAL NEURONS OF ANIMALS WITH SECTIONED DORSAL ROOTS

Until now these models have mainly been used in attempt to understand the central abnormalities which correspond to this type of anesthesia dolorosa. Recordings were performed at spinal, bulbar and thalamic levels of animals having undergone dorsal root sections. Different results were obtained in rats and cats.

In rats, at the level of the cord, cells presenting epileptic-like rhythmic bursts are present in the cervical dorsal horn not only on the side of the lesion but also on the contralateral side. The bursts appear after 24 hours and seem to decrease in number after a few weeks. In rats having five roots lesioned, rhythmic bursts were recorded from cells at a specific thalamic level (VP) in the representation region of the deafferented zone and its contralateral homologue. But this abnormal activity appears after a longer delay of 6 months. In the thalamus contralateral to the lesion, the bursts involve a great number of cells which are frequently totally deprived of peripheral fields.

In similarly lesioned cats, cells with rhythmic epileptic-like bursts were first described at the spinal cord level (14) and later at the bulbar level (10). The abnormal spinal cells were present on the 14th day after the section. At the thalamic level we recently recorded from cats one year after scratching wounds had disappeared. If a few epileptic-like cell activities appeared, they were the exception as were the cells without a peripheral field. The results are thus very different from those obtained in rats.

In cats with dorsal root sections we have also found a distorted thalamic map, the zone adjacent to the peripherally deafferented area being more fully represented than in the normal cat. This distortion was described in rats for other partial deafferentations (18), but we have not been able to confirm this finding in animals with five dorsal roots sectioned.

In order to explain the behavior produced by root lesions it is proposed that scratching and chewing behavior occur in rats because of the epileptic-like cell spiking. This spiking appears in the cord or thalamic zones of specific representation and are projected to cortical areas, where by an error of localization they are felt to originate in the peripheral area to which these zones normally project. The long lasting duration of the epileptic-like phenomena in the rat explains why there can be no healing of the wounds in these animals. However, in cats, spiking began to appear but progressively disappeared thus allowing the self-inflicted wounds to heal.

If this hypothesis is true, then what is needed for an understanding of central pain is the knowledge of the mechanisms which lead to the development of the rhythmic activity and its progressive disappearance. The fact that epileptic spiking disappears in cats and that in this species the number of thalamic deafferented cells is small compared to those in the rat with the same cord lesion, leads to the proposition that a certain quantity of totally deafferented cells is required to trigger epileptic spiking. This must be the case in the early period after lesioning of both rats and cats and persists only in the rat, because in the cat other afferents take over and the cells, again activated, return to normal spiking. The suggestions that the reinnervation could be due to the presence of previously ineffective synapses (23) or to sprouting coming from an intact fiber system (13) are to be discussed and subjected to more experiments (20).

REFERENCES

(1) Albe-Fessard, D.; Nashold, B.S., Jr.; Lombard, M.C.; Yamaguchi, Y.; and Boureau, F. 1979. Rat after dorsal rhizotomy. A possible animal model for chronic pain. In Advances in Pain Research and Therapy, eds. J.J. Bonica et al., vol. 3. New York: Raven Press.

(2) Anderson, L.S.; Black, R.G.; Abraham, J.; and Ward, A.A. 1971. Neuronal hyperactivity in experimental trigeminal deafferentation. J. Neurosurgery 35: 444-452.

(3) Azerad, J., and Woda, A. 1977. Sensation evoked by bipolar intrapulpal stimulation in man. Pain 4: 145-152.

(4) Basbaum, A.I. 1974. Effects of central lesions on disorders produced by multiple dorsal rhizotomy in rats. Experimental Neurology 42: 490-501.

(5) Black, R.G. 1974. A laboratory model for trigeminal neuralgia. In International Symposium on Pain. Advances in Neurology, ed. J.J. Bonica, vol. 4, pp. 651-658. New York: Raven Press.

(6) Dennis, S.G., and Melzack, R. 1978. Forelimb chewing behavior in rhizotomized rats. Factors that contribute to its onset and latency. In Pain abstracts, Second World Congress on Pain, vol. 1, p. 56, Seattle.

(7) Dukrow, R.B., and Taub, A. 1977. The effect of diphenylhydantoin on self-mutilation in Rats produced by unilateral multiple dorsal rhizotomy. Exp. Neurology 54: 33-41.

(8) Hardy, J.D.; Wolff, H.G.; and Goodell, H. 1940. Studies on pain. A new method for measuring pain threshold, observations on spatial summation of pain. J. Clin. Investig. 19: 649-657.

(9) Keele, C.A., and Armstrong, D. 1969. Substances producing pain and itch. In Monographs of the Physiological Society, pp. 339. London: Edward Arnold.

(10) Kjerulf, T.D., and Loeser, J.D. 1973. Neuronal hyperactivity following deafferentation of the lateral cuneate nucleus. Exp. Neurol. 39: 70-85.

(11) Kryzhanovsky, G.N. 1976. Experimental central pain and itch syndromes: modeling and general theory. In Advances in Pain Research and Therapy, eds. J.J. Bonica and D. Albe-Fessard, vol. 1, pp. 225-230. New York: Raven Press.

(12) Lim, R.K.S. 1970. Pain. Ann. Rev. Physiol. 32: 269.

(13) Liu, C.N., and Chambers, W.W. 1958. Intraspinal sprouting of dorsal root axons. Arch. Neurol. Psychiat. 79: 46-61.

(14) Loeser, J.D., and Ward, A.A. 1967. Some effects of deafferentation on neurons of the cat spinal cord. Arch. Neurol. 17: 629-636.

(15) Lombard, M.C.; Nashold, B.S., Jr.; and Albe-Fessard, D. 1979. Deafferentation hypersensitivity in the rat after dorsal rhizotomy. A possible animal model for chronic pain. Pain 6: 163.

(16) Lombard, M.C.; Nashold, B.S., Jr.; and Pelissier, T. 1979. Thalamic recordings in rats with hyperalgesia. In Advances in Pain Research and Therapy, eds. J.J. Bonica et al., vol. 3. New York: Raven Press.

(17) Lombard, M.C.; Sakr, C.; Salman, N.; and Nashold, B.S., Jr. 1977. Hyperesthesies chroniques provoquées chez le rat par la lésion de racines dorsales du plexus brachial. C.R. Acad. Sc., Paris 284: 2369-2372.

(18) Merrill, E.G., and Wall, P.D. 1978. Plasticity of connection in the adult nervous system. In Neuronal Plasticity, ed. C.N. Cotman. New York: Raven Press.

(19) Nashold, B.S., Jr., and Wilson, W.P. 1966. Central pain observations in Man with chronic implanted electrodes in the midbrain tegmentum. Second Symp. Stereoencephalotomy Vienna, Conf. Neurol. 27: 30-44.

(20) Nelson, S.G., and Mendell, L.M. 1979. Enhancement in Ia-Motoneuron synaptic transmission caudal to chronic spinal cord transection. J. of Neurophysiol. 42 (3): 642-654.

(21) Sternbach, R.A. 1976. The need for an animal model of chronic pain. Pain 2: 2-4.

(22) Vicklicky, L. 1979. Techniques for the study of pain in animals. In Advances in Pain Research and Therapy, eds. J.J. Bonica, J.C. Liebeskind, and D. Albe-Fessard, pp. 727-747. New York: Raven Press.

(23) Wall, P.D.; Scadding, J.W.; and Tomkiewicz, M.M. 1979. The production and prevention of experimental anaesthesia dolorosa. Pain 6 (2): 175.

(24) Ward, A.A., Jr. 1966. The hyperexcitable neuron Epilepsy. In Nerve as a Tissue, ed. Rodahl, p. 379-411. Boston: Little, Brown & Company.

(25) Willer, J.C.; Boureau, F.; and Albe-Fessard, D. 1978. Role of large diameter cutaneous afferents in transmission of nociceptive messages: electrophysiological study in man. Brain Res. 152: 358-364.

Pain and Society, eds. H.W. Kosterlitz and L.Y. Terenius, pp. 311-324.
Dahlem Konferenzen 1980. Weinheim: Verlag Chemie GmbH.

Involvement of the Sympathetic Nervous System in Pain

P. W. Nathan
Medical Research Council
National Hospital for Nervous Diseases
London WC1N 3BG, England

Abstract. The aspect of pain and the sympathetic system that is considered are cases of sympathetic algodystrophy that follow traumatic lesions of peripheral nerves and lesions in the spinal cord. Sympathetic blocks relieve those cases in which there is hyperpathia; these patients usually have burning pain. Three propositions arising from this effect are considered: whether the sympathetic system has the normal role of influencing receptors; whether sympathetic nerves influence conduction throughout the length of the somatic nerves that they accompany; whether sprouting nerve fibers at the site of an injury are abnormally excited by various transmitters, including noradrenalin. It is concluded that in some cases afferent fibers become abnormal in certain specified ways and that they cause an abnormal central state, and that this abnormal state spreads within the central nervous system. It is also concluded that this can occur the other way round: an abnormal central state can induce an abnormal state in the afferent fibers entering this region of the gray matter.

INTRODUCTION

That there is some relationship between the sympathetic system and pain is shown by certain clinical states. Anatomists, physiologists, and pharmacologists have taken no interest in this relationship. Drug companies do not advertize alpha- and beta-blockers for the relief of pain.

SYMPATHETIC ALGODYSTROPHY

Mainly since the first World War, clinicians have tended to group together certain cases in which a traumatic lesion is followed by constant pain much increased by stimulation and where the pain and tenderness are relieved by blocking the sympathetic nerves to the region. This syndrome is often called reflex sympathetic dystrophy: dystrophy, because all tissues of the region, including muscle and bone, eventually waste, and because there are abnormal features of growth, such as ridging of the nails or hyperkeratosis of the skin; sympathetic, because there are features indicating abnormal sympathetic control, such as inappropriate sweating, vasodilatation or constriction, because the condition responds to sympathetic blocks, and because it is thought that the condition spreads within a sympathetic system distribution; reflex, because the condition appears to spread from the lesion into the spinal cord and out via sympathetic nerves.

There are various causes of the condition such as myocardial infarction, sprains, superficial thrombophlebitis, and fractures of small bones, such as those of the wrist or foot. The examples of this syndrome that neurologists see are those where it follows a lesion of a peripheral nerve or, more rarely, a lesion of the central nervous system - in which case they do not recognize it.

The conception of grouping together those cases which are relieved by sympathectomy comes from Leriche. It was based on his experience in treating causalgia and related cases in the first World War. The influence of Leriche made French clinicians interested in all states in which the sympathetic system appeared to play a part. For these various clinical states, they proposed the name 'sympathetic algodystrophy'; now called by them simply 'algodystrophies.'

Until we understand more about these conditions, I think it is helpful to group together all cases in which the condition is relieved by sympathetic blocks. This means relief during the time of the block; we are not at present thinking of therapy. This criterion of the effect of sympathetic block is useful for the clinician as he knows how to approach the case, and to pharmacologists and physiologists as they have a common starting point in investigating these states.

In cases of algodystrophy due to a lesion of a peripheral nerve, there is typically hyperpathia* and allodynia* within the territory of the damaged nerve. This is obvious in the skin; it is present, though less obvious, in the deeper tissues, including muscle and bone. Sympathetic blocks relieve the state of hypersensitivity to stimulation and the accompanying pain.

The relationship between the effectiveness of sympathetic blocks and the presence of hyperpathia and allodynia is shown in Table 1, from Loh and Nathan (5).

TABLE 1 - Effect of sympathetic block on pain in hyperpathic and non-hyperpathic states.

Effect on constant pain	Patients with hyperpathia	Patients without hyperpathia	Total
Relieved	21	2	23
Partially relieved	2	0	2
Unrelieved	8	13	21
Total	31	15	46

From this Table, one deduces that there is a relation between hyperpathia and sympathetic activity. Most of these patients had allodynia, which was also removed by sympathetic block. Whatever other pains accompany hyperpathia and allodynia, one pain is burning pain, which is particularly relieved when hyperpathia is relieved.

*These are the terms recommended by the International Association for the Study of Pain. Hyperpathia is "a painful syndrome, characterized by delay, over-reaction and after-sensation to a stimulus, especially a repetitive stimulus." Allodynia is "pain due to a non-noxious stimulus to normal skin." This word is now used to describe the state where a very light stimulus, such as touch or stroking with cotton-wool causes particularly unpleasant pain.

The pain and hyperpathia can be removed by blocking the sympathetic chain and ganglia with local anesthetics and also by stopping the release of noradrenalin by giving guanethidine into the limb. The circulation is occluded and guanethidine is injected intravenously below the cuff, a method of giving local anesthetic introduced by Bier in 1908 and forgotten until recently. This way of blocking the sympathetic nerve fibers with guanethidine shows that the pain and hyperpathia are being maintained by the release of noradrenalin in the periphery.

What Role does the Sympathetic System Play in Sympathetic Algodystrophy?

The immediate relief of hyperpathia and pain by blocking the sympathetic nerve supply to the affected region suggests the following questions:

(a) Does the sympathetic system normally influence receptors?
(b) Do sympathetic nerves influence conduction in somatic nerves?
(c) In sympathetic algodystrophy, do nerve fibers damaged by a lesion acquire abnormal characteristics so that they become excited by transmitters, such as noradrenalin?

(a) The suggestion that the sympathetic system controls, alters, or has some influence on receptors comes from some physiological experiments. More notice would be taken of these investigators if the results were consistent; but, as we shall see, they are not.

Loewenstein (6) first reported that "stimulation of the sympathetic nerve supply to an isolated frog's skin or the application of adrenalin or noradrenalin" lowered the threshold of mechanoreceptors so much that they eventually fired spontaneously. This was not found by physiologists who tried it out in the cat. Perhaps Loewenstein also failed to find it in the cat, for his next paper concerns the cat's Pacinian corpuscles in the mesentery with no mention of receptors of the skin. Working with Altamirano-Orrego (7), he reported that stimulating sympathetic nerves or applying adrenalin or noradrenalin to the Pacinian corpuscle increased its firing rate. Others have obtained the same results in the frog and have added gustatory receptors to mechanoreceptors.

In mammals, some large cutaneous receptors are accompanied by a very small nerve fiber. For the case of the Pacinian corpuscle, Santini (10) produced evidence that this is a sympathetic efferent fiber. Fuxe and Nilsson (4) had already examined the Pacinian corpuscles with the Falck-Hillarp fluorescence technique. They found no adrenergic terminals in the Pacinian corpuscles of the cat's mesentery. "Adrenergic fibers lay scattered in the surrounding adipose tissue without making any close contact with the corpuscles, and a sympathetic influence on these corpuscles through released catecholamines is thus not likely."

Santini also disagreed with Loewenstein and his colleagues. He repeated their experiments and got the opposite results. He found that stimulating the sympathetic chain or applying noradrenalin or adrenalin decreased the firing of Pacinian corpuscles. He therefore thinks that the sympathetic system inhibits receptors.

The opposite results are obtained on stimulation of sympathetic fibers to the tooth pulp. Matthews (8) reported an "increase of up to 30-fold in the discharge" caused by applying a solution of sodium chloride to the dentine; this solution causes pain in man. The same effect was obtained by applying adrenalin and noradrenalin; and it was prevented by alpha-, but not beta-, blockers.

These experiments have clearly given more inconsistent results. Santini emphasizes that posterior root ganglia have a very rich sympathetic supply, and that this is distributed in two ways. A part of it supplies the blood vessels, and a part supplies the axonal bifurcation of large afferent neurons. As he says, this supply and the actual arrangement of the supply must be there for some purpose. At present we know nothing about it.

Leaving aside these inconsistent observations on other species and turning to man, we find the evidence unsatisfactory. Many people have looked for changes in sensibility in man after sympathectomy (done for non-neural conditions such as angina pectoris or vascular pathology) and not found any. In conditions of sympathetic over-activity as with phaeochromocytomata or under-activity as hypothyroidism, there are no changes in sensibility.

But Procacci et al. (9) did find slight changes in the threshold of heat pain in normals given stellate blocks. Later (10) he and his colleagues investigated patients with sympathetic dystrophy and reported that the heat-pain threshold was different in the affected and the opposite limb - a difference that does not occur in normal people. After sympathetic blocks, lasting for at least 48 hours, the difference in the threshold between the two limbs had gone. They concluded that the cutaneous pain threshold was under the control of the sympathetic system. They later (11) reported that in patients with severe sympathetic algodystrophy there were lower sensory thresholds in the affected limb.

One of the difficulties one has in coming to a conclusion is that the changes observed were slight in comparison with the extreme change in threshold, pain, hyperpathia, and allodynia that characterize most cases of causalgia.

(b) As far as I know, there is only one piece of work showing that conduction in peripheral nerve is altered by sympathetic activity. Bülbring and Whitteridge (1) found that the intrarterial injection of adrenalin increased the size of the action potential of the sciatic nerve in the cat. The alpha-beta spike was increased up to 100% regularly, and sometimes to 300%. This effect was more marked in fatigued nerve. I have never seen this work referred to, which is strange.

One knows that sympathetic fibers release noradrenalin throughout their course. Dismukes (3) has calculated that there are 330,000 varicosities in a noradrenergic nerve per cu.mm. Thus peripheral nerves accompanied by sympathetic nerves will be bathed in a solution of noradrenalin whenever there is sympathetic activity.

(c) It is apparent that in cases of sympathetic dystrophy in which there is a lesion of a peripheral nerve, some or all afferent somatic nerve fibers have acquired certain abnormal features. One of these is that sprouting myelinated fibers are excited by noradrenalin. If one prevents noradrenalin acting on these fibers, their other abnormal features are removed.

The actual lesion does not have to be included in the noradrenergic block in order to render the entire nerve fiber normal again. The reasons for stating this are these. In many of our cases, we block the sympathetic supply by giving guanethidine intravenously by Bier's block. In some of these cases, the lesion may be above the cuff and so the guanethidine never reaches the lesion and yet the whole abnormal state is relieved. In others, the lesion is in the central nervous system and yet a sympathetic block with guanethidine relieves the abnormal state in the region peripheral to the block. Furthermore, if guanethidine is given by iontophoresis into a small area of skin within the affected region, this treated region will lose its abnormal features, regardless of where the lesion is that is causing the abnormal state.

As blocking the release of noradrenalin in the neighborhood of the afferent fibers of the peripheral nerves stops the pain and hyperpathia, we must conclude that the entire posterior root neuron has become sensitive to noradrenalin, and that when this neuron is sensitive to noradrenalin there is spontaneous burning pain, hyperpathia, and allodynia. One must stress, too, that this peripheral neuron is abnormal in the same way when the lesion is in the spinal cord or brain.

I wrote at the beginning of this paper that we know various facts and that we cannot yet put them together to make a satisfactory whole. We know that sprouting nerve fibers have special properties, including sensitivity to some neurotransmitters. When they rejoin their normal targets or their normal environment, they lose these properties. The evidence that outgrowing somatic afferent fibers are sensitive to acetylcholine, noradrenalin, and adrenalin is now given.

Diamond (2) showed that regenerating nerves in the sural nerve of the rabbit are abnormally sensitive to acetylcholine and nicotine; this was so for the nerves in a crush injury and the nerves in a neuroma following cutting the nerve. This sensitivity was in afferent and not in motor nerves. It was present within 3 days of making the lesion and sometimes may have been present by 12 hours. Diamond also asked the question whether causalgia was due to the release of acetylcholine. In his experiments, it was only the regenerating, outgrowing nerve fibers that showed this abnormal sensitivity.

Wall and Gutnick (11, 12) also examined the behavior of nerve fibers within a neuroma. They encouraged neuroma formation in the rat's sciatic nerve by placing the cut end in a polythene tube. After a certain time, constant spontaneous firing developed in small afferent myelinated fibers but not in motor fibers; non-myelinated fibers were not examined. Noradrenalin (11) activated these nerve fibers when they were not firing and it increased their firing rate when they were. This was all stopped by alpha-blockers. Later (12) they found that adrenalin had the same effect. Scadding (personal communication), working in Wall's laboratory, has repeated the work in mice and confirmed that the outgrowing fibers are also sensitive to adrenalin, and he found that the beta-blocker, propranolol, stops their firing. Wall then asked the question whether the same thing occurred when a lesion did not divide the whole nerve but when the nerve was merely crushed. The answer is - yes: sprouting nerve fibers within a minor lesion of a peripheral nerve show the sensitivity to catecholamines.

If nerve fibers regenerating within a lesion are abnormally excited by neurotransmitters, including noradrenalin, then one may propose that the emission of noradrenalin by the varicosities on sympathetic fibers accompanying somatic afferent fibers fires these fibers and that this causes burning pain, hyperpathia, and allodynia. It is probable that the afferent fibers concerned are myelinated fibers, because allodynia occurs with stimulation too light to excite non-myelinated fibers.

Damaged nerves or out-growing nerve fibers have certain other features. They are unduly excited by mechanical stimulation, and this abnormal activity is soon stopped by ischemia. Wall and Gutnick also showed that the spontaneous activity of the small outgrowing nerve fibers was quickly stopped by ischemia.

Therapy used for over fifty years for cases of sympathetic algodystrophy due to damaged peripheral nerves fits in well with the findings of Wall and Gutnick. The main treatment consists of sympathetic blocks. Many years ago, I found that even short periods of ischemia may remove the pain and sensitivity for longer periods. I have treated patients with painful peripheral nerve lesions by giving them sphygmomanometer cuffs so that they could occlude the circulation. Occluding the circulation for 10 mins may remove the state for an hour or more. Sometimes occlusion several times a day for weeks improves the condition permanently. Another treatment is strong vibration on, or hammering, the neuroma; this probably removes the sensitivity of the outgrowing nerve fibers, if it does not actually remove the fibers.

If the axonal sprouts have the properties we have been discussing in the peripheral nervous system, it may well be the same in the central nervous system. Anywhere on the edge of a lesion, such as plaques in multiple sclerosis, there may be axonal sprouts. Although there are no accompanying sympathetic fibers in the central nervous system, there are many transmitters around, including acetylcholine, noradrenalin, and adrenalin, which could fire off fibers growing out from the region where they have been divided by a lesion.

One of the problems with this and most other theories of causalgia and of reflex algodystrophy is that it explains too much; most injuries do not go on to the state of reflex dystrophy; most nerve lesions do not become causalgic.

The time of onset of pain in some algodystrophic conditions with nerve lesions must be mentioned. The severe burning pain of causalgia can start at the moment of injury. Yet axonal sprouts do not appear immediately. Wall and his colleagues find actively firing nerve fiber sprouts and sensitivity to adrenalin and noradrenalin coming on within 36 to 48 hours of making a lesion of a peripheral nerve. But even this early start is too late to explain the immediate onset of causalgia.

The duration of pain and hyperpathia does not fit with the duration of abnormal firing and sensitivity found by Wall and his colleagues. In the clinical cases, the abnormality lasts for 2 years or more. In the experimental crush injuries in rats and mice, it lasts for months or less.

We must now summarize the facts we have been considering and then propose a hypothesis.

Abnormal Afferent Fibers Cause an Abnormal Central State

Those who first described cases of sympathetic algodystrophy, for instance, Weir Mitchell, Morehouse, and Keen's description of causalgia, included the spread of the dystrophic state from the original region to neighboring regions. For example, the abnormal state due to a partial lesion of a median nerve spreads beyond the median nerve territory to the rest of the hand and eventually may advance up the forearm, even involving the whole forequarter of the body. This can only mean that an abnormal state is spreading within the central nervous system.

It appears to be spreading locally in the spinal cord to the region contiguous to the site of entry of the damaged fibers. In Figure 1, the spread of the abnormal state is shown by the arrows. When the abnormal central state spreads from the segment of entrance of the damaged and sprouting nerve fibers, then the afferent fibers coming to this neighboring region also come to take on the abnormal state. The neighboring fibers rendered abnormal are not only those of neighboring nerve roots. For in cases of partial peripheral nerve lesions, the neighboring nerve are those of the damaged peripheral nerve itself that have not been divided by the lesion.

A further reason for suggesting an abnormal state within the posterior horns is the nature of allodynia. It can hardly be

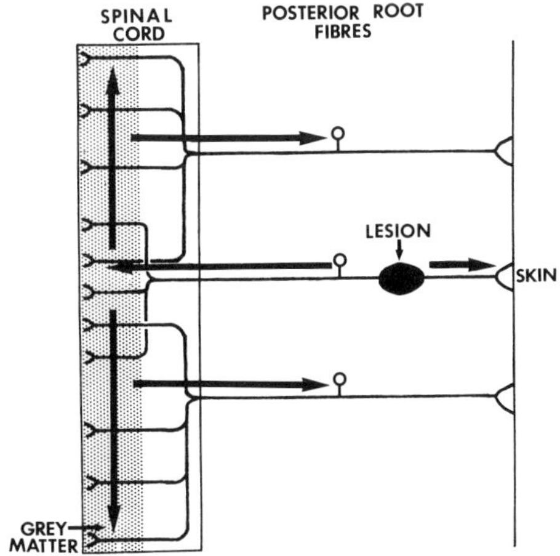

FIG. 1 - The arrows show spread of an abnormal state from a lesion of a peripheral nerve throughout the affected neurons into the posterior horns, to neighboring regions of the posterior horns, and out along afferent nerves that end in the neighboring posterior horns.

that light tactile stimuli, which excite only mechanoreceptors, cause pain by some change in the peripheral nerve fibers or receptors. The first place where this change could occur would be in the posterior horns; this is probably at neurons onto which mechanoreceptors and nociceptors converge.

An Abnormal Central State Causes an Abnormal State of Afferent Fibers

Lesions of the central nervous system can cause the same abnormal state. In this case, the lesion affects the afferent fibers coming into the abnormal region of the gray matter.

Figure 2 illustrates the case of a lesion in the posterior horns. The afferent fibers connected to this region acquire an abnormal state; this then spreads along these primary afferent neurons, as shown by the arrows.

My colleagues and I have had one case with a lesion in the thalamus and another with a lesion in the lower midbrain with the same ab-

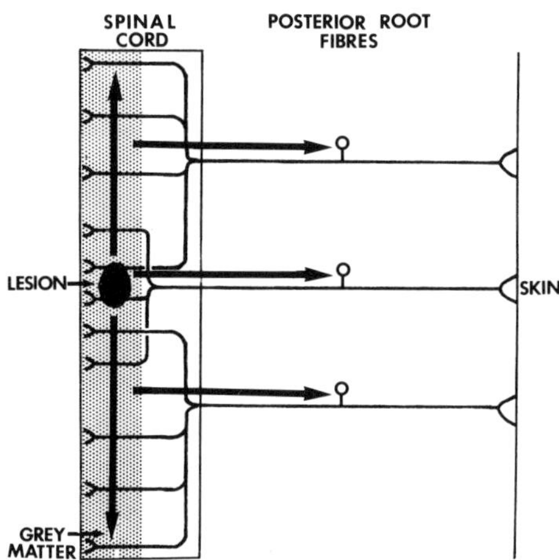

FIG. 2 - The arrows show spread of an abnormal state from a lesion in the posterior horns to neighboring regions of posterior horns, and out along afferent nerves that end in the affected posterior horns.

normal state of the relevant peripheral nerves. It was removed by the infusion of guanethidine distal to a cuff on the affected limb. In the cases with lesions of the central nervous system, the abnormality is within an afferent tract in the brain. This lesion causes neurons that are in functional connection with the damaged tract to become abnormal. Finally, this abnormality spreads to involve the posterior root neurons.

The total abnormal state is relieved by blocking the sympathetic fibers to the nerves that connect to the central neurons affected by a lesion. It is difficult to understand how a central lesion produces a sensitive peripheral state that is relieved by sympathetic blocks; yet it is so.

A Hypothesis

We are seeing a spreading state of abnormality affecting a chain of afferent neurons. If it starts in the thalamus, it ends in the peripheral neuron. If it starts in the peripheral neuron, it may end in the thalamus. Moreover, as soon as the peripheral neuron's state of sensitivity to noradrenalin has been removed, the abnormal state of the connected neurons is also removed.

The hypothesis is that in cases of sympathetic dystrophy of neural origin there is an abnormal state spreading along a chain of neurons that are functionally connected together. This abnormal state is likely to be due to changes in the flow of constituents that occurs in both directions along axons. The flow of these constituents provides various trophic substances to the neurons and to tissues supplied by the neurons. An upset of this flow causes a dystrophic state.

REFERENCES

(1) Bülbring, E., and Whitteridge, D. 1941. The effect of adrenaline on nerve action potentials. J. Physiol. 99: 201-207.

(2) Diamond, J. 1959. The effects of injecting acetylcholine into normal and regenerating nerves. J. Physiol. 145: 611-629.

(3) Dismukes, K. 1977. New look at the aminergic nervous system. Nature 269: 557-558.

(4) Fuxe, K., and Nilsson, B.Y. 1965. Mechanoreceptors and adrenergic nerve terminals. Experientia 21: 641-642.

(5) Loh, L., and Nathan, P.W. 1978. Painful peripheral states and sympathetic blocks. J. Neurol. Neurosurg. Psychiat. 41: 664-671.

(6) Loewenstein, W.R. 1956. Modulation of mechanoreceptors by sympathetic stimulation. J. Physiol. 136: 40-60.

(7) Loewenstein, W.R., and Altamirano-Orrego, R. 1956. Enhancement of activity in a Pacinian corpuscle by sympathomimetic agents. Nature 178: 1292-1293.

(8) Matthews, B. 1976. Effects of stimulation on the response of intradental nerves to chemical stimulation of dentine. In Advances in Pain Research and Therapy, eds. J.J. Bonica and D. Albe-Fessard, vol. 1, pp. 195-203. New York: Raven Press.

(9) Procacci, P.; Marchetti, G.; Buzzelli, G.; and Rocchi, P. 1963. Effetti del blocco farmacologico del ganglio stellato sulla sensibilita dolorifica cutanea nell' individuo sano. Arch. Fisiol. 62: 332-342.

(10) Procacci, P.; Francini, F.; Zoppi, M.; and Maresca, M. 1975. Cutaneous pain threshold changes after sympathetic blocks in reflex dystrophies. Pain 1: 167-175.

(11) Procacci, P.; Francini, F.; Maresca, M.; and Zoppi, M. 1979. Skin potential and EMG changes induced by cutaneous electrical stimulation. II. Subjects with reflex sympathetic dystrophies. Appl. Neurophysiol. 42: 125-134.

(12) Santini, M. 1976. Towards a theory of sympathetic sensory coupling: the primary sensory neuron as a feedback target of the sympathetic terminal. In Sensory Functions of the Skin in Primates, ed. Y. Zotterman, pp. 15-35. Oxford: Pergamon Press.

(13) Wall, P.D., and Gutnick, M. 1974. Properties of afferent nerve impulses originating from a neuroma. Nature 248: 740-743.

(14) Wall, P.D., and Gutnick, M. 1974. Ongoing activity in peripheral nerves: the physiology and pharmacology of impulses originating from a neuroma. Exp. Neurol. 43: 580-593.

Pain and Society, eds. H.W. Kosterlitz and L.Y. Terenius, pp. 325-338.
Dahlem Konferenzen 1980. Weinheim: Verlag Chemie GmbH.

Pain Producing Substances

H. O. Handwerker
II. Physiologisches Institut, Universität Heidelberg
6900 Heidelberg, F. R. Germany

Abstract. The relevance of the research on chemical algogenic substances for the study of pain mechanisms is discussed under three main headings:

1. Are endogenous agents released from inflamed tissue a key to nociceptor mechanisms?
2. Are endogenous pain producing substances relevant to clinical pain states?
3. What are the advantages and disadvantages of chemical as compared with physical stimuli in experimental pain research?

It is shown that especially the first two questions can be answered only to a very limited extent because of our lack of knowledge of membrane mechanisms of nociceptors.

INTRODUCTION

Substances producing pain are of considerable interest in pain research, especially those substances which originate in the body itself in the course of pathophysiological processes. There are several comprehensive reviews of the endogenous chemical agents which might produce pain (14,25). Most frequently studied have been: peptides such as bradykinin (BK), amines such as serotonin (5-HT) and histamine (HIS), and prostaglandin E.

This paper intends to give a short review of some of the work done in this field. Its primary aim, however, is to point out the limits of our present knowledge.

When categorizing the literature on pain producing substances according to the intention of the study, one might separate reports roughly into three groups:

1. Studies on nociceptor mechanisms.
2. Studies which test the hypothesis that endogenous chemical substances are instrumental in clinical pain, e.g., in inflammation or in migraine.
3. Studies using chemical stimuli as a means of producing an experimental nociceptive input to the CNS.

These three aspects shall be discussed separately.

PAIN PRODUCING SUBSTANCES AS MEANS FOR THE STUDY OF NOCICEPTOR MECHANISMS

Some Historical Notes

Von Frey (28), using "Stachelborsten" to produce pain sensations in experimental subjects, noted that the latency of these sensations was much longer than the latency of touch sensations evoked by stimulation with hairs. He concluded that nociceptors are excited by physical stimuli only through release of a chemical substance. This hypothesis was abandoned for a time when C-fibers were discovered, the slower conduction velocity of which was taken to explain the longer latency of the pain compared to touch sensation. However, in 1968 Lim (20) made the following statement: "The pain receptor is chemoceptive and not nociceptive and may be stimulated by a variety of algesic agents (H^+, K^+ions, some amines and peptides), a specific structure is evidently not required for stimulation."

The blister base technique introduced by Keele and Armstrong (14) was perhaps the most powerful tool to study the endogenous pain producing substances. Bradykinin, 5-HT, and some other substances evoke pain at very low concentrations when applied to the blister base. On the other hand, they are mediators of inflammatory reactions mainly by their powerful action on the permeability of small vessels. Physical and/or chemical influences producing pain in man at the same time usually induce inflammatory processes. Hence these substances are qualified as candidates for physiological pain producing substances.

Because of their double action on microcirculation and on nociceptors, it is useful to list these substances under the heading "vaso-neuroactive agents."

The hypothesis that vaso-neuroactive substances are the unique cause of the excitation of nociceptors was further supported by pharmacological studies on the mechanisms of action of aspirin and aspirin-like nonsteroid antiinflammatory drugs. The currently most popular concept is based on the pioneer work of Vane and co-workers who found that these drugs inhibit biosynthesis of prostaglandins E (24). Though prostaglandins are not potent algogenic substances themselves (9,13,19,24), they can elicit and/or intensify the symptoms of inflammation and potentiate the action of bradykinin on nociceptors. On the other hand, bradykinin is one of the agents contributing to the release of prostaglandins. If inhibition of the release of prostaglandins explains both the antiphlogistic and the antinociceptive actions of aspirin-like drugs, these actions support the supposition that vaso-neuroactive substances are involved in both inflammation and pain.

It has to be noted, however, that alternative mechanisms of the antinociceptive action of aspirin-like drugs are also discussed in the literature (3).

Are Endogenous Vaso-neuroactive Substances Specific Stimulants of Nociceptors?

The action of vaso-neuroactive substances on cutaneous receptors has been studied by recording from single nerve fibers and injecting the respective substance intraarterially close to the receptive field of the receptor under study. It has been found that injection of, for example, 5μg bradykinin or of 5-50 μg 5-HT evokes action potentials in Aδ and C-fibers which were classified as nociceptors according to their responses to physical noxious stimuli such as heating the skin or squeezing skin folds. Some types of cutaneous afferents, however, which respond vigorously are definitely not nociceptive according to their excitability by physical stimuli, especially the slowly adapting mechanoreceptors (SA-receptors) with Aβ afferents (2,5). On the other hand, rapidly adapting-(RA-), hair follicle-, and Vater-Pacinian receptors with Aβ afferents are usually not excited (2). Most receptors excited by one substance out of this group react to others as well; no receptor class reacts to only one substance.

Excitability spectrum and central connections of cutaneous receptors are better known than those of receptors in other tissues. Nevertheless, it cannot be excluded that some of the receptors which are classified as nociceptors due to the fact that they seem to react to only strong and destructive stimuli have other functions which would not be detected in a routine experiment; they might be, e.g., sensors of metabolic changes. This difficulty increases with receptors in deeper tissues. Some authors have used intraarterial injections of vaso-neuroactive substances to classify these deep receptors. It has been found, for example, that bradykinin excites muscle C-fiber and Aδ-fiber afferents, but usually not muscle spindle afferents and tendon organs (15,17,22,23). Similarly, bradykinin injected intraaterially excites C-fibers with receptors in the knee joint (11). Injection of bradykinin into the splenic artery predominantly excites slow fibers in the splenic nerve (21). In contrast, afferents of the non-nociceptive Vater-Pacinian corpuscles running in visceral nerves are usually not excited. These results do not provide unequivocal proof, however, that only nociceptive enteroreceptors and proprioceptors are excited by bradykinin. It has been suggested, for example, that most bladder receptors activated by bradykinin are slowly adapting mechanoreceptors which are stimulated by contractions of the bladder wall induced by the drug (6). The crucial point is that no strict criteria are known for distinguishing between nociceptive and non-nociceptive enteroreceptors.

On the Definition of Nociceptors

In this context, a short consideration of the "nociceptor" concept might be useful. This concept was made popular by Sherrington. Originally it included two aspects: a) nociceptors are receptors excited exclusively or mainly by noxious stimuli, i.e., by stimuli which induce phlogistic reactions at least when applied over an extended period; and b) activation of nociceptors causes - due to their central connections - pain sensations in man and nocifensive reflexes in man and animals. Many researchers, especially when dealing only with peripheral nervous events, classify nerve endings as nociceptive only by the first of these two criteria. This might be misleading, since it is impossible to test the responses of a receptor to all physical and chemical stimuli possibly occurring in its physiological environment.

Direct Versus Indirect Action of Vaso-neuroactive Substances on Receptive Nerve Endings

It has been shown (Zimmermann, personal communication) that vaso-neuroactive substances such as bradykinin exert their influence only on the nerve endings. Application to the nerve fibers more proximally is without effect, even if the neurolemma is carefully removed.

Thus, the actions of bradykinin and 5-HT cannot be explained simply by a non-specific depolarization of the nerve membrane (which is effected, e.g., by K^+ injection).

Repetitive injections of bradykinin or of 5-HT often induce tachyphylaxis. It has been shown that there is no cross-tachyphylaxis between these substances. Different vaso-neuroactive substances applied to the tissue at the same time usually have a synergistic effect, which is often more than additive. Prostaglandin E, which has a very weak excitatory effect, might nevertheless potentiate the effect of bradykinin (8).

It has been concluded from these findings that different vaso-neuroactive substances react with different membrane receptors.

It has not been established, however, whether these membrane receptors are in the nerve ending itself. It must be pointed out that membrane receptors for several vaso-neuroactive substances have been demonstrated in the smooth muscle and that almost all afferents reacting to these agents are also sensitive to sustained deformations of the surrounding tissue, although their thresholds might be rather different.

An argument against an indirect effect of vaso-neuroactive substances on the nerve endings is provided by occasional simultaneous recordings of two identified afferent fibers which differ in sensitivity to different agents. An example is given in Fig. 1.

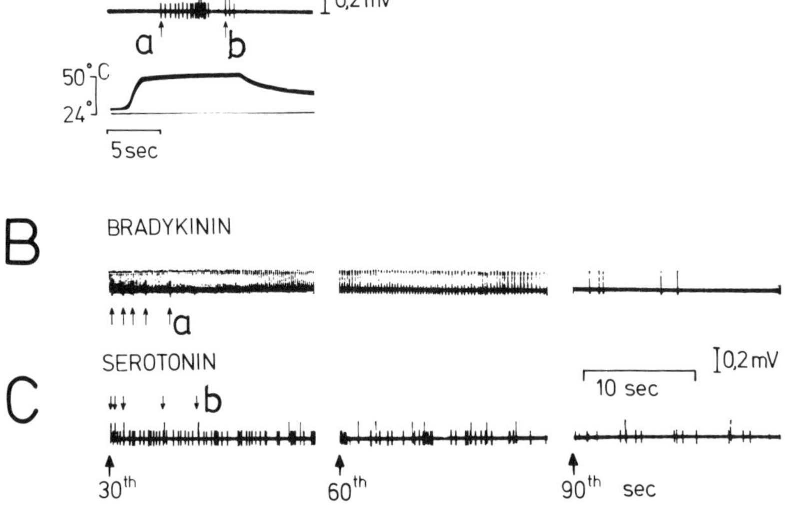

FIG. 1 - Excitation of two afferent fibers contained in one filament (A) by noxious radiant heat applied to the receptive field, (B) by close arterial injection of 5μg bradykinin, (C) by close arterial injection of 30 μg 5-HT. The smaller unit had a conduction velocity of 0.8 m/s (C-fiber), the larger one of 21 m/s (Aδ-fiber). Note the different sensitivities of the two receptors to bradykinin and 5-HT which is difficult to explain by an indirect action of these agents. Modified from (2).

Is the Excitation of Nociceptors by Physical Stimulation Produced Via Release of Vaso-neuroactive Substances?

If substances act on the membrane of the nerve endings itself (and not indirectly as conjectured above), one must ask whether they might be a causal link in the process of physical excitation of nociceptors, e.g., by heat or by strong mechanical stimulation. There are at least two arguments against this hypothesis. First, the response of cutaneous nociceptors to heat is not diminished when tachyphylaxis has rendered the fiber unresponsive to bradykinin or 5-HT. Second, aspirin-like drugs, which block the release of prostaglandins and block the action of bradykinin, do not significantly influence either the heat pain threshold in man, the threshold of a nocifensive reaction to heat in animals, or the response of nociceptors to heat. It is likely, therefore, that nociceptors are excited by heat and by vaso-neuroactive substances via different mechanisms. However, both mechanisms are unknown. The crucial point is the lack of information on membrane mechanisms of nociceptors.

Substance P: a Pain-producing Substance?

It has been known for a long time that stimulation of the C-fibers in the peripheral stump of cut dorsal roots induces vaso-dilatation in the respective dermatone (7). It has been concluded from this finding that the peripheral endings (nociceptors?) of slowly conducting afferent fibers release a vaso-active substance.

Recent histochemical studies supported the hypothesis that slowly conducting afferent nerve cells contain a peptide, substance P, which they release from their peripheral and central endings (4,10). Synthetic substance P is not very effective in exciting nociceptors (18). It has been shown, however, to excite intestinal smooth muscle and to induce vasodilatation. The latter effect might be partly indirect, since substance P appears to induce the release of histamine from mast cells (12).

A more thorough analysis of the role of substance P in peripheral nociceptive mechanisms might shed new light on this subject.

VASO-NEUROACTIVE SUBSTANCES IN CLINICAL PAIN

The neuroactive substances bradykinin, 5-HT, and histamine are released especially during the early stages of an inflammatory reaction in concentrations which might be high enough to excite nociceptive nerve endings. K^+ released from damaged cells and the low pH of inflamed tissue might have an additional effect.

It is striking, however, that many inflammations are not very painful, particularly as long as the tissue is not altered mechanically. Therefore, the vaso-neuroactive substances might be more important in potentiating rather than inducing the excitation of nociceptors. Hyperpathia and hyperalgesia of inflamed tissue presumably have their basis in the sensitization of nociceptors which has been studied in animal experiments (9).

Biochemical mechanisms involving vaso-neuroactive substances have been discussed as well in several forms of headache (headache in hypertension, cluster headache, migraine) (16). Prostaglandins, histamine, and 5-HT have been discussed as agents inducing intra- and/or extracranial vasodilatation which has been observed in some forms of migraine. The influence of the 5-HT metabolism has been studied most carefully. It has been suggested that this metabolism is altered in cranial arteries of patients suffering from migraine (1,27). Methysergide, a peripheral 5-HT antagonist, has been successfully used in the prophylaxis of this disease. Based on the phenomenology of migraine, it is very likely, however, that the pathophysiology of this disease involves central mechanisms probably including central serotonergic neurons, which might be influenced by methysergide as well (26).

CHEMICAL STIMULI AS A MEANS IN EXPERIMENTAL PAIN RESEARCH

Chemical stimuli have been used in neurophysiological and in behavioral pain research. The central organization of the nociceptive system has been studied by the use of intraarterial injection of bradykinin as a noxious test stimulus. Behavioral studies have utilized intradermal injections of vaso-neuroactive substances or of K^+ ions. Irritants which are not endogenous substances but induce a burning sensation when applied to the skin (e.g., capsaicin, naphtalene derivatives) might also be used in behavioral experiments.

For studies on central nociceptive mechanisms it is important to know (a) whether the stimulus excites only nociceptors or other receptor types as well, and (b) whether the excitation of the system by chemical agents resembles "clinical" pain.

With regard to selectivity, chemical stimulation is, as far as we know, not more selective than other types of noxious stimulation (e.g., radiant heat). Chemical stimulation might, however, be superior to physical stimulation in that it resembles the types of pain seen by the clinician more closely. Because of the slow diffusion processes, the onset of excitation of a nociceptor population is much more asynchronous in the course of chemical than of physical stimulation.

In still unpublished experiments, we have used naphtalene derivatives applied to the receptive field of nociceptive C-fibers recorded from the superficial radial nerve of conscious human subjects. The experimental subject had to match his sensation induced by the chemical stimulus with the frequency of a tone. Figure 2 shows the results from one experiment. It can be seen from this figure that the C-fiber under study started to discharge at least ten seconds before the subject felt the stimulus.

We obtained similar results from other C-fibers as well. If these C-fibers, identified as being nociceptive by their responses to physical stimuli, are indeed instrumental in pain sensation, our results demonstrate that a considerable degree of spatial and temporal summation of the impulses of a population of C-fibers is needed to induce pain sensations. The highly synchronous input induced by physical stimuli might excite the central nociceptive system in a way which is not typical of most forms of pain seen in disease.

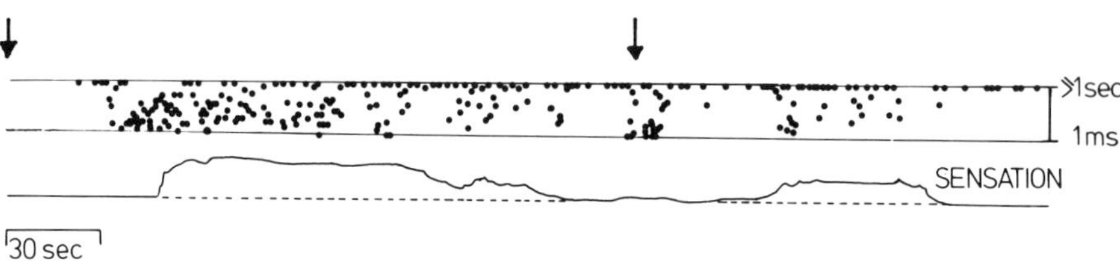

FIG. 2 - Upper trace: Interval distribution of activity of a nociceptive C-fiber (conduction velocity = 0.83 m/s) of a human subject recorded transcutaneously from the superficial radial nerve. This receptor was excited by application of naphtalene derivatives to the receptive field. Lower trace: Intensity of a burning sensation expressed by the subject by manipulating the frequency of a tone. Deflection upwards: Increase of sensation. Broken line: Base line of sensation before stimulation. First arrow: The substance was applied to the skin. Second arrow: The agent was cleansed from the skin with ether. (H. Adriaensen, J. Gybels, H.O. Handwerker, and J. Van Hees, unpublished)

Acknowledgement. The author appreciates the help of A. Müller who carefully typed this manuscript and E. Carstens who provided valuable comments.

REFERENCES

(1) Appenzeller, O. 1975. Hypothesis: Pathogenesis of vascular headache of the migrainous type: the role of impaired central inhibition. Headache 15.

(2) Beck, P.W., and Handwerker, H.O. 1974. Bradykinin and serotonin effects on various types of cutaneous nerve fibres. Pflügers Arch. 347: 209-222.

(3) Brune, K.; Glatt, M.; and Graf, P. 1976. Mechanisms of action of anti-inflammatory drugs. Gen. Pharmac. 7: 27-33.

(4) Cuello, A.C.; del Fiacco, M; and Paxinos, G. 1978. The central and peripheral ends of the substance P-containing sensory neurones in the rat trigeminal system. Brain Res. 152: 499-510.

(5) Fjällbrant, N., and Iggo, A. 1961. The effect of histamine, 5-hydroxytryptamine and acetylcholine on cutaneous afferent fibres. J. Physiol. 156: 578-590.

(6) Floyd, K.; Hick, V.E.; and Morrison, J.F.B. 1975. The responses of visceral afferent nerves to bradykinin. J. Physiol. 247: 53-54P.

(7) Folkow, B., and Neil, E. 1971. Circulation. Oxford University Press.

(8) Handwerker, H.O. 1976. Influences of algogenic substances and prostaglandins on the discharges of unmyelinated cutaneous nerve fibres identified as nociceptors. In Advances in Pain Research and Therapy, eds. J. Bonica and D. Albe-Fessard, vol. 1. New York: Raven Press.

(9) Handwerker, H.O. 1976. Pharmacological modulation of the discharge of nociceptive C-fibres. In Sensory Functions of the Skin in Primates, ed. Y. Zotterman. Oxford: Pergamon Press.

(10) Hökfelt, T.; Kellerth, J.O.; Nilsson, G.; and Pernow, B. 1975. Experimental immunohistochemical studies on the localization and distribution of substance P in cat primary sensory neurons. Brain Res. 100: 235-252.

(11) Hong, K.A.; Jänig, W.; and Schmidt, R.F. 1978. Properties of group IV fibres in the nerves to the knee joint of the cat. J. Physiol 284: 178.

(12) Johnson, A.R., and Erdös, E.G. 1973. Release of histamine from mast cells by vasoactive peptides. Proc. Soc. exp. Biol. (N.Y.) 142: 1252-1256.

(13) Juan, H., and Lembeck, F. 1974. Action of peptides and other algesic agents on paravascular pain receptors of the isolated perfused rabbit ear. Naunyn-Schmiedebergs Arch. Pharmacol. 283: 151-164.

(14) Keele, C.A., and Armstrong, D. 1964. Substances producing pain and itch. London: Edward Arnold.

(15) Kniffki, K.D.; Mense, S.; and Schmidt, R.F. 1978. Responses of group IV afferent units from sceletal muscle to stretch, contraction and chemical stimulation. Exp. Brain Res. 31: 511-522.

(16) Kudrow, L. 1974. Systemic causes of headache. Postgraduate Medicine 56: 105-111.

(17) Kumazawa, T., and Mizumura, K. 1977. Thin fibre receptors responding to mechanical, chemical, and thermal stimulation in the skeletal muscle of the dog. J. Physiol. 373: 179-194.

(18) Kumazawa, T., and Mizumura, K. 1979. Effects of synthetic substance P on unit discharges of testicular nociceptors of dogs. Brain Res. 170: 553-557.

(19) Lembeck, F.; Juan, H.; and Popper, H. 1975. Paravascular pain receptors, algesic substances and prostaglandins. Pflügers Arch. 359: R100.

(20) Lim, R.K.S., and Guzman, F. 1968. Manifestations of pain in analgesic evaluation in animals and man. In Pain, eds. A. Soulairac et al. London, New York: Academic Press

(21) Lim, R.K.S.; Guzman, F.; Rogers, D.W.; Goto, K.; Braun, C.; Dickerson, G.D.; and Engele, R.J. 1964. Site of action of narcotic and nonnarcotic analgesics determined by blocking bradykinin evoked visceral pain. Arch. int. Pharmacodyn. 152: 25-58.

(22) Mense, S. 1977. Nervous outflow from skeletal muscle following chemical noxious stimulation. J. Physiol. 267: 75-88.

(23) Mense, S., and Schmidt, R.F. 1974. Activation of group IV afferent units from muscle by algogenic agents. Brain Res. 72: 305-310.

(24) Moncada, S.; Ferreira, S.H.; and Vane, J.R. 1975. Inhibition of prostaglandin biosynthesis as the mechanism of analgesia of aspirin-like drugs in the dog knee joint. Eur. J. Pharmacol. 31: 250-260.

(25) Movat, H.Z. 1972. Chemical mediators of the vascular phenomena of the acute inflammatory reaction and of immediate hypersensitivity. Med. Clin. of North America 56: 541-555.

(26) Sicuteri, F. 1976. Headache: Disruption of pain modulation. In Advances in Pain Research and Therapy, ed. J.J. Bonica and D. Albe Fessard, vol. 1. New York: Raven Press.

(27) Ziegler, D.K. 1974. Migraine: Diagnostic and therapeutic aspects. Postgraduate Med. 56: 169-174.

(28) von Frey, M. 1914. Beobachtungen an Hautflächen mit geschädigter Innervation. Zschr. f. Biol. 63: 335-376.

Pain and Society, eds. H.W. Kosterlitz and L.Y. Terenius, pp. 339-354.
Dahlem Konferenzen 1980. Weinheim: Verlag Chemie GmbH.

The Measurement of Pain in Man

C. R. Chapman
Department of Anesthesiology RN-10, University of Washington
Seattle, WA 98195, USA

Abstract. Recent progress in the assessment of central nervous system responses to painful stimulation suggests new directions for future measurement of human pain. Amplitudes of event-related electrical brain potentials recorded during dolorimetric testing correlate with subjective pain reports and are reduced consistently by analgesic treatments. These potentials occur late, with latencies of between 50 and 500 ms. Because their origins have not yet been specified, they presently provide more information about cognitive than neurological processes. Such potentials may be a good way of assessing pain sensibility in chronic pain patients; differences in brain responsivity to painful stimulation may help in evaluating psychiatric conditions in which pain perception appears abnormal, such as hysteria. Emerging data in the literature support further exploration of evoked potentials as indicators of pain perception.

INTRODUCTION

The quantification of pain is fundamental to progress in both basic research and clinical pain control, and new trends in measurement procedures are likely to have a substantial impact on the direction of future development in these areas. Traditional methods of measuring pain threshold and tolerance have faded into the background of scientific inquiry over the last decade while newer psychological and psychometric procedures have emerged. Most recently, relationships between event-related electrical brain potentials and psychophysical scaling have seriously challenged the traditional assumption that the only approach to the measurement of human pain is through subjective report. This paper is concerned primarily with such new developments, their influence on future progress in scaling human pain, and their implications for clinical pain assessment. An overview of contemporary pain research is presented below and the development of evoked potential research in this context is described. Finally, the implications of new measurement procedures for future research and clinical evaluation are considered.

CURRENT TRENDS IN PAIN MEASUREMENT

The state of contemporary research on human pain quantification can be usefully described by analogy if we speak of pain as though it were an organism and borrow two terms from our geneticist colleagues: genotypic and phenotypic. A genotype is the fundamental hereditary constitution of an organism while a phenotype is the outward, visible expression of that constitution in a given environment. Pain is an extremely complex phenomenon which can be investigated at both genotypic and phenotypic levels since it has an underlying neurophysiology and an outwardly visible psychology that reflects both basic physiological processes and environmental influences. The analogy is appropriate clinically in chronic pain diagnosis since the same genotype (pathophysiology) may sometimes give rise to highly varied symptom constellations (phenotypes) in various patients. Conversely, two different genotypes may generate what appears to be a single phenotype in two different patients. The analogy offered here is a loose one that should not be pushed very far, but it is useful for establishing a concept that helps us gain a perspective on pain scaling.

Most published research involving the measurement of human pain has focused exclusively on the phenotypic characteristics of pain. That is, investigators have been concerned with pain behavior, pain complaint, and subjective report. Such phenomena are visible to the observer in the absence of sophisticated equipment involving invasive recording. Phenotypic approaches are the methods of choice for the quantification of clinical pain complaints since they are concerned with the emotional, attitudinal, and judgmental features of pain and not its pathophysiology. Sophisticated descriptive report systems for chronic pain based on multivariate scaling procedures are beginning to appear in the literature, for example, the McGill Pain Questionnaire (9). Moreover, psychophysicists and behaviorists have been quick to point out that subjective reports and behavior patterns can be quantified in the laboratory by a variety of methods and that the scaling procedures involved yield reliable results under controlled conditions. In recent years the proliferation of such techniques as the "Sensory Decision Theory" and magnitude estimation has helped to develop the laboratory scaling of human pain at the phenotypic level.

The genotypic study of pain in man encompasses all areas concerned with the physiologic origins of nociception, its transmission, and its modulation. Pure genotypic studies do not require conscious patients and do not involve subjective pain reports. They are biologic investigations indistinguishable from animal studies except for the ethical limitations involved. Such research permits highly refined and precise measurement of phenomena far less idiosyncratic and capricious than those observed by the investigator studying phenotypes. It incorporates recent progress in technical development as well as new advances in knowledge in biologic areas.

Between the phenotypic and genotypic poles of pain measurement methodologies lies the possible development of human pain scaling procedures that incorporate both subjective reports and physiologic measures. To be sure, in numerous studies subjective reports and physiological measures have been collected together, but this has been done in the absence of a demonstrable and reliable correlation between the two types of variables in normal perception. Investigators have simply used physiological techniques that are available and convenient with no particular insight about the relationship of the phenomena measured to behavior or subjective reports.

The search for a paradigm that incorporates both genotypic and phenotypic approaches to pain measurement calls for demonstrations of physiological correlates of human pain reports. The relationship between subjective pain judgment and measures of autonomic nervous system reactivity during noxious stimulation has been explored because such variables are related to the emotional state and because standard methods for their quantification have been developed; however, no autonomic measure has proven useful as an indicator of pain.

EVENT-RELATED BRAIN POTENTIALS AND PAIN

More recently, the search for a physiological correlate of pain has focused on central nervous system responses. By recording event-related electrical potentials from the human scalp during dolorimetric testing, one can obtain a sample of the electrical activity of the brain that occurs in response to carefully controlled painful stimulation. Broadly speaking, three classes of event-related brain potentials have been described in the literature. Far-field evoked potentials of brain stem origin, with 10-20 ms latency, are so-called because the scalp recording electrode is distant from the origin of the signals. Between 20 and 50 ms, investigators record early near-field potentials, i.e., the presumed cortical origin of the signals is relatively near the recording electrode. Between 50 and 500 ms, one obtains late near-field responses and it is with these that this paper is concerned. This late activity is, in selected cases, highly correlated with reported pain. Of course, such recordings cannot be interpreted as direct measures of pain sensation because they provide at best, physiological correlates of pain experiences that are defined on the basis of verbal reports, and such reports are imperfect indicators of perception.

The recording of brain electrical potentials (BEPs) is generally carried out by summation averaging in which multiple trials are used to provide a clear definition of the signal against the background of noise. In contrast to EEG signals, BEPs are summations of event-related brain activity that are sampled while a brief signal is delivered repeatedly to the subject. Most investigators use a "window" of time surrounding the delivery of a painful stimulus so that the EEG is averaged before and after stimulus occurrence over repeated trials.

EXAMPLES OF EVOKED POTENTIAL WAVEFORMS

Three typical late near-field evoked potentials obtained from a single subject in response to painful laboratory stimulation are provided in Figure 1. Each of these traces, collected in our laboratory, represents the averaged response recorded from 192 trials of painful electrical stimuli at a level that the subject termed strong pain. Electrical shocks were of 5 ms duration and the potentials were recorded from vertex with reference to inion, with a ground at the zygomatic arch.

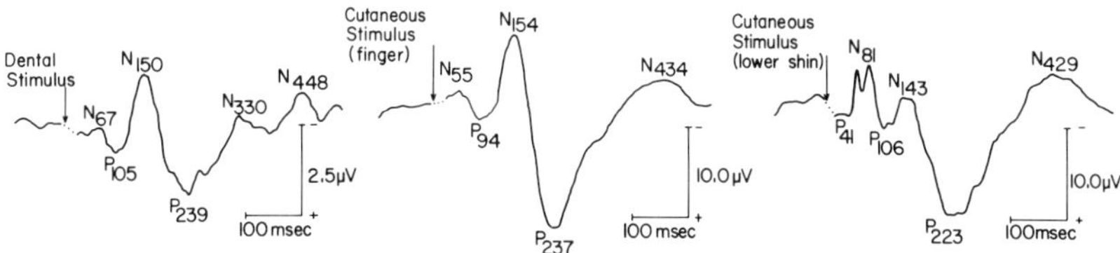

FIG. 1 - Comparison of BEPs obtained by electrically stimulating the tooth, the finger, and the shin. Somatosensory BEPs are always larger than those of dental stimuli. The latencies, in contrast, are quite similar despite the differences in conduction distances. The dental BEPs show the best morphological uniformity across subjects.

For each waveform a 600 ms interval of EEG is portrayed with a 94 ms baseline prior to stimulus onset. Beyond approximately 50 ms, four components can be defined that are consistently observed across all subjects. Peaks are identified by negative (N) and positive (P) polarity as well as by peak latency in ms, in accordance with the standard international 10-20 notation. We have found that the latencies of both the positive and negative peaks are highly stable, both within subjects and across subjects.

There are several ways to quantify the BEP waveform. We have used measures of peak-to-peak amplitude because they have been found empirically to be suited for our simple and limited recording system and because other investigators have advocated this approach to BEP scaling. Peak-to-base measures can be obtained by dividing the waveform by its pre-stimulus baseline, or one can use area measures derived from the positive and negative deflections from baseline. There is as yet no consensus in the pain literature for waveform quantification.

A BRIEF LITERATURE REVIEW

Chatrian and associates (4) first studied the dental evoked potential, stimulating the subject's tooth pulp through an implanted electrode and recording BEPs from multiple scalp sites. The most prominent BEP component was a large positive-going wave observed between 147 and 249 ms that appeared most clearly when measured at vertex with reference to inion, although it was evident with more restrictive amplitudes at other sites ipsilaterally and contralaterally. Stimulation of a devitalized tooth in a normal volunteer failed to evoke electrical scalp potentials or sensations, and a patient congenitally insensitive to all painful stimulation failed to show either evoked potentials or subjective responses to strong electrical tooth pulp shocks. Sano (10) also used a dental implantation methodology and recorded BEPs from the temporal area. Unlike Chatrian et al., Sano employed several stimulus levels. He observed a similar morphology in the BEPs from various subjects and identified the major component between 140 and 240 ms. As stimulus intensity was raised, the amplitude of the major component increased. Inhalation of 30% nitrous oxide in oxygen diminished the waveform amplitude.

Cutaneous tissue stimulation has also been used to generate BEPs. Stowell (11) delivered painful and nonpainful electrical shocks to subjects' fingers, toes, and lips. He recorded from vertex and several somatosensory areas and obtained waveforms roughly comparable to those observed by Chatrian et al. (4) and Sano (10) with the major component evident between 170 and 290 ms. Like Sano, Stowell noted that increases in component amplitudes were related to subjective reports of pain intensity. He could not determine any consistent relationship between the peak latency and subjective report. Lavine, Buchsbaum, and Poncy (8) recorded from both vertex and the somatosensory area corresponding to the hand, delivering forearm shocks at several levels ranging from barely noticeable to painful. Increased stimulus intensity was associated with increased amplitude of the waveform components and the major component occurred between 168 and 248 ms.

Carmon, Mor and Goldberg (1) stimulated forearm skin with laser energy that generated slight to severe pain and recorded from vertex and ipsilateral as well as contralateral scalp sites. Amplitudes were greatest at vertex although BEP morphology was similar at other sites, and the major component occurred between 130 and 190 ms. Again, the BEP amplitude correlated with the subject's reports as intensity varied.

Our findings have been consistent with those of other laboratories. Harkins and Chapman (6) studied the BEP to noninvasive dental electrical stimulation using stimuli giving rise to strong pain, mild pain, and very faint pain stimuli, and BEPs were recorded at vertex with reference to inion. The major BEP component occurred between 175 and 260 ms and waveform amplitudes increased as stimulus intensity was incremented. We demonstrated linear relationships between stimulus intensity and amplitudes of the various BEP components. Chen, Chapman, and Harkins (5) further explored the relationship of BEP amplitudes to stimulus intensity and subjective report. Varying order of stimulus presentation, we recorded BEPs to five dental stimulus levels ranging from very faint to strong pain. Subjects gave category judgments of the subjective painfulness of each of the stimulus levels by using visual analogue scales, and the amplitudes of the vertex waveform were measured for four different components occurring between 65 and 340 ms. We employed partial correlation methods for the statistical examination of the relationship between the measures of component amplitude and the subjective painfulness with stimulus intensity partialed out for all components. The two later waveforms, N_{175}-P_{260} and P_{260}-N_{340}, were significantly correlated with subjective painfulness. That is, as subjective painfulness increased, amplitudes of these components also increased. In contrast, amplitudes of the first component N_{65}-P_{120} showed no relationship to subjective painfulness with partial correlation analysis, and P_{120}-N_{175} was negatively correlated. Amplitudes of these components correlated positively and significantly with stimulus intensity when subjective painfulness was partialed out.

We have also investigated the effects of analgesic agents on the BEP evoked by dental stimulus. Amplitudes of major waveform components are reduced by nitrous oxide (33% in oxygen), fentanyl (0.1 mg), electrical acupuncture stimulation, and aspirin (3). The peak latencies are not altered by treatment except in the case of nitrous oxide which combines analgesic and anesthetic effects. All four BEP components are reduced in amplitude by nitrous oxide and fentanyl. Aspirin reduces only the two later components (N_{175}-P_{260}, P_{260}-N_{340}) and acupuncture reduces the two middle components (P_{120}-N_{175}, and N_{175}-P_{260}). In all cases subjective reports of reduced pain correspond to reduced BEP amplitude.

From these pioneering studies involving different modes of stimulation, variable recording sites, and several different laboratories, we can extract certain common observations: a) there are similarities in the gross general morphologies of BEPs to painful stimulation despite differences in stimulation modalities, recording procedures, and numerous other methodological details; 2) there are similarities in the latencies of the peaks of the major waveform components; c) variation of stimulus intensity results in change of BEP amplitude but the latencies of major waveform peaks are invariant; 4) different components of the waveform relate differentially to stimulus intensity and subjective painfulness; and e) analgesic treatments reduce BEP amplitudes and reports of pain intensity. The relationship between the physiological variable and the subjective pain report suggests that BEP recording may be a noteworthy step forward in the assessment of human pain. Recent findings in our laboratory indicate that the relationship between the BEP and the perceptual and judgmental aspects of pain may be indeed close.

SPECULATIONS ABOUT BEP GENESIS

While the late near-field BEPs elicited by noxious stimulation appear to be rich sources of information about pain perception, the origins of such waveforms are poorly understood and three hypotheses are generally raised. First, the specifist theorists contend that the earlier components of the waveform may reflect the arrival of information via the neospinothalamic pathways while the later two waveform components could represent paleospinothalamic transmission. This seems unlikely on several counts. First, the waveform peak latencies are so long that one would expect both neospinothalamic and paleospinothalamic transmission to be completed before the late near-field components become evident, especially for dental stimulation. In our laboratory the major negative to positive deflection obtained when the foot is painfully stimulated with electrical shock occurs at the same latency or earlier than the corresponding component seen when the central incisor is stimulated. Second, there is no evidence thus far of first and second pain in the tooth, particularly in relation to brief electrical stimuli. Third, when cutaneous electrical stimuli are used, no peak latency differences appear when BEPs to non-noxious and exquisitely noxious stimuli are compared.

One sees an amplitude difference that fails to reflect any possible distinctions between fast and slow pain transmission systems.

The second hypothesis is that the late near-field vertex BEP is a general arousal wave. Critics point out that vertex waves have long been known to be close correlates of arousal in a variety of evoked potential paradigms. Unfortunately, these critics have not considered that arousal is one aspect of pain. Indeed, the biologic function of pain is to serve as a warning system, and arousal cannot be divorced from the pain experience if we are to understand pain in a comprehensive way. In general, pain is characterized by an ability to command immediate attention in spite of other ongoing stimulation and in nature it often serves to prepare the organism for flight or fight. This criticism hardly provides a reason to dismiss BEP procedures for pain measurement since the proper study of pain seems to require measurement of arousal.

Yet another hypothesis is that the BEP indicates the activity of cortical cell populations that integrate sensory input or are involved in stimulus evaluation. There is some evidence in support of this position. Our laboratory recently examined BEP amplitudes during a stimulus discrimination task in which subjects attempted to accurately identify each of a series of potentially confusable painful and moderately painful dental stimuli delivered in random order. Our goal was to determine whether there is a relationship between measured brain function and the statistical Sensory Decision Theory model that psychophysicists use to describe the perception of discrete laboratory sensory events. This model construes the simple perception of a brief laboratory stimulus as a two-fold process involving a) the transmission of a sensory signal to higher nociceptive centers, and b) an evaluation or categorization of that signal. By recording the subject's judgments, an experimenter can specify several kinds of correct and incorrect responses. Psychophysicists use such accuracy and error rates to achieve psychophysical scaling. We summation-averaged BEPs for the various correct and incorrect judgments and compared waveform amplitudes. For brevity, only the major component amplitude, N_{175}-P_{260}, will be described here. The Sensory Decision Theory model offers a specific prediction of the rank order of the various waveform amplitudes if the N_{175}-P_{260} amplitude behaves like the hypothetical sensory signal of the psychophysical model.

Our data conformed closely (and significantly when evaluated statistically) to Sensory Decision Theory predictions. This suggests that: a) the Sensory Decision Theory and BEP measures are scaling a single perceptual process, and b) the late near-field waveforms reflect a complex perception that can be related in various ways to behavioral measures. It is tempting to hypothesize that the later components of the BEP waveform indicate the decision process component of perception. Alternatively, one might argue that the decision is made later and that the amplitude of the waveform is an indicator of the "sensation" that is delivered to the brain's decision center. Such a sensation would be the final end-product of a long process of sensory transmission and modulation. While such speculations are fascinating, the real answers to these questions will be obtained most efficiently by collecting more data that explore the relationships between earlier BEP components such as brain stem evoked potentials or early near-field recordings and the late near-field recordings now under study. Moreover, there is a need to explore alternate methods of waveform quantification and to investigate BEP changes at other scalp locations in order to approach these possibilities comprehensively.

BEP METHODOLOGY AND CHRONIC PAIN DIAGNOSIS

Recent findings suggest that the BEP approach may be useful for clinical diagnosis, particularly in patients suffering from chronic pain. The methodology appears to provide an index of pain perception, and chronic pain patients may be characterized by perceptual deficits or disorders. The successful use of BEPs obtained from auditory stimulation for the diagnosis of hearing problems provides an encouraging example, but hearing problems are essentially neurological disorders and auditory evoked potential methodologies are applied in the context of genotypic problem solving. In contrast, chronic pain problems typically involve psychological and social complications so that the issue becomes one of making a diagnosis on a phenotypic level. As we have seen, the recording of the late near-field BEP seems well suited for an approach to this problem, but it must be interpreted as cognitive rather than neurologic information. The evidence thus far available suggests that the BEP could be useful for the diagnosis of psychological problems of chronic pain which are not necessarily linked to organic pathology, for example, hysteria.

In our laboratory Yoko Colpitts is in the process of collecting evoked potentials from chronic pain patients together with controls matched on age and sex. Three levels of stimulus intensity are given to each patient, and BEP amplitudes are examined to determine whether the relationship between amplitude and stimulus intensity is the same in chronic pain patients as in normal controls. Stimulus rating procedures are employed to obtain subjective judgments. Having collected data from 11 patients, we find marked departures from normal pain modulation in most patients, but there is no single distinguishing characteristic. Several patterns of abnormal response are beginning to emerge. Some patients are hypersensitive to the dental electrical shocks while others are hyposensitive. There are some who generate abnormally low amplitude evoked potentials to all levels of stimuli (as though they were characterized by high levels of endogenous opioid peptides), while others show unusually large evoked potential amplitudes and find normally low intensity stimuli exquisitely painful (as though they were serotonin depleted). We hope to carry out a multivariate statistical analysis on a large data base of patients.

The BEP seems promising as a method for evaluating pain sensibility in patients. There is a need to extend the procedure so that both genotypic information (far-field and early near-field evoked potentials) and phenotypic information (late near-field potentials) can be obtained in a single patient evaluation session. Systematic studies of tightly restricted groups of patients will be necessary, and more basic work must be done on recording sites, methods of waveform quantification, and methods for dolorimetric stimulation.

FINAL CONSIDERATIONS

What are the implications of BEP measurements for future progress in scaling human pain? It is useful to return to the previous analogy and to reconsider the genotypic and phenotypic polarities characterizing contemporary pain research. If we take the development of BEP research as located on this bipolar continuum, it is clearly closer to the phenotypic pole than to the genotypic, since late near-field potentials are phenotypic in nature in spite of being physiological. They cannot yet be linked clearly to other activities of the central nervous system, and to the neurophysiologist they must be considered epiphenomenal. Indeed, Wall critiqued cortical evoked potential assessment in an animal experiment as follows: "If the actual cause of the potential change is unknown, it is not surprising that its functional significance is unknown beyond the fact that something is happening in the cortex. Whatever that something is, the evoked cortical potential seems a very poor indicator of a state of the entering and leaving impulse traffic from the cortex except at the threshold transition from nothing to something, when of course many measures are correlated but not causally related. A particular breakdown of the usefulness of the cortical evoked response as an index of cortical functioning occurs when its size is used. The generator of the potential change easily saturates long before the inputs and outputs reach their maximal discharge rates. Therefore, shape and size while easy to measure are either poorly correlated or not even correlated at all with the impulse traffic" ((12), p. 380).

In contrast the human BEP, apparently not a direct function of "entering and leaving impulse traffic," seems to be a step forward for phenotypic investigators since it is closely connected with perception as measured by choice behavior and subjective report.

It is clear that the actual value of the BEP paradigm depends on the perspective of the researcher judging it. While it may be of considerable use to the investigator with a phenotypic focus, its long-term worth will probably derive from its constituting an expedition into an unexplored frontier. The observations emerging from research on human BEP point to a need for basic studies that explore the links between early near-field and late near-field potentials as well as those between far-field and early near-field potentials. This can be accomplished by using correlational and regression techniques to determine what components appear to relate causally to others that occur later. If such links can be determined, a bridge will have been established between the genotypic and phenotypic camps and a comprehensive understanding of pain measurement can begin to emerge. Eventually, procedures for BEP measurement may develop as diagnostic techniques useful in the evaluation of chronic pain problems.

REFERENCES

(1) Carmon, A.; Mor, J.; and Goldberg, J. 1976. Application of laser to psychophysiological study of pain in man. In Advances in Pain Research and Therapy, eds. JJ. Bonica and D. Albe-Fessard, vol. 1, pp. 375-380. New York: Raven Press.

(2) Chapman, C.R. 1977. Sensory decision theory methods in pain research: A reply to Rollman. Pain 3: 295-305.

(3) Chapman, C.R.; Chen, A.C.N.; and Harkins, S.W. (in press) Brain evoked potentials as correlates of laboratory pain: A review and perspective. In Advances in Pain Research and Therapy, eds. J.J. Bonica, J.E. Liebeskind, and D. Albe-Fessard, vol. 3. New York: Raven Press, in press.

(4) Chatrian, G.E.; Canfield, R.C.; Knauss, T.A.; and Lettich, E. 1975. Cerebral responses to electrical tooth pulp stimulation in man. Neurology 25(8): 745-757.

(5) Chen, A.C.N.; Chapman, C.R.; and Harkins, S.W. 1979. Brain evoked potentials are functional correlates of induced pain in man. Pain 6(3): 365-374.

(6) Harkins, S.W., and Chapman, C.R. 1978. Cerebral evoked potentials to noxious dental stimulation: Relationship to subjective pain report. Psychophysiology 15(3): 248-252.

(7) Hilgard, E.R., and Hilgard, J.R. 1975. Hypnosis in the Relief of Pain. Los Altos, Calif.: William Kaufmann.

(8) Lavine, R.; Buchsbaum, M.S.; and Poncy, M. 1976. Auditory analgesia: Somatosensory evoked response and subjective pain rating. Psychophysiology 13(2): 140-148.

(9) Melzack, R. 1975. The McGill Pain Questionnaire: Major properties and scoring methods. Pain 1(3): 277-299.

(10) Sano, H. 1977. Influence of intensity-varied electrical stimulation of a tooth and 30% N_2O premixed gas inhalation on Somatosensory Evoked Potentials (SEPs). Japan. J. Dental Anesthesiology 5(1): 9-21.

(11) Stowell, H. 1977. Cerebral slow waves related to the perception of pain in man. Brain Research Bulletin 2: 23-30.

(12) Wall, P.D. 1975. The somatosensory system. In Handbook of Psychobiology, eds. M.S. Gazzaniga and C. Blakemore, pp. 373-391, New York: Academic Press.

Pain and Society, eds. H.W. Kosterlitz and L.Y. Terenius, pp. 355-364.
Dahlem Konferenzen 1980. Weinheim: Verlag Chemie GmbH.

Biochemical Assessment of Chronic Pain

L. Y. Terenius
Department of Pharmacology, Uppsala University
Box 573, 751 23 Uppsala, Sweden

Abstract. The chronic pain syndromes present considerable problems of assessment. In recent years, biochemical methods have been studied. Two lines of research are reviewed here, one aiming at the objective assessment of pain severity, the other aiming at the differential diagnosis and evaluation in mechanistic terms. The inadequacy of the present state of knowledge is emphasized. Data from analysis of cerebrospinal fluid (CSF) suggest that monoaminergic and endorphinergic systems are malfunctioning in chronic neurogenic pain. Measurements of opioid peptides in CSF seem to have a potential in evaluating the pathogenesis of a chronic pain sydrome.

INTRODUCTION

It is quite common to consider two main types of chronic pain, organic and psychogenic. As pointed by by Szasz (14), "organic pain," which is supposed to relate to a lesion in the body, is often synonymous with legitimate pain. Certainly, any chronic pain syndrome will have both somatic and psychic components. This leads to problems of definition and, more importantly, to uncertainty in relation to therapeutic approaches. It is quite surprising that despite the enormous economic significance of chronic pain syndromes, very little research has been devoted to methods of objective assessment. There is at present a high degree of empiricism in the choice of therapeutic measures and a strong tendency to use somatic approaches at the expense of psychotherapy or behavioral therapy.

Chronic pain is very unlike acute pain and should be considered a disease state, frequently with strong influence on behavior and personality. It therefore seems appropriate to analyze this disease syndrome with techniques borrowed from those used in other chronic neurologic or in psychiatric disorders. The present review will cover biochemical studies with occasional mentioning of other approaches.

GENERAL METABOLIC AND ENDOCRINE CHANGES

Several investigators have studied the general metabolic or endocrine activity in patients with chronic pain. One goal has been to establish objective measures of pain severity. Routine biochemical analysis generally shows normal values. However a certain tendency towards low $PaCO_2$ values and hyperventilation has been described which might be secondary to pain since it is relieved by analgesics (5). In a study by Keele (8), patients with strong pain from cardiac infarction, renal colic, or surgery were found to have falling levels of serum β-lipoproteins and cholesterol. There were no differences with regard to pain pathogenesis. The fall in serum lipids was therefore attributed to pain itself. Non-painful stress produced the opposite response and could be separated from pain. The procedure may therefore be used to assess acute, "hard" pain.

An extensive study by Shenkin (11) deals with the effect of pain on plasma corticoids. Unfortunately, no data were presented on the level or duration of pain in the individual patient. Cases with objective evidence for pain and cases without such evidence were separated. There were significantly higher than normal cortisol levels in cases with objective pain and also reduced diurnal variation, while cases without objective evidence for their pain showed essentially normal cortisol levels and diurnal variation. A careful study by Lascelles et al. (9) confirms several of these observations. However, both patients with pain of organic and psychologic origin tended to have higher than normal cortisol levels, and this confirms Shenkin's data, especially in the organic group. There was also less diurnal variation in the organic group.

These two studies suggest physiological differences between patients with organic and psychologic pain. Unfortunately, no information is given with respect to duration or severity of pain. Although there are significant differences in mean plasma cortisol between the groups, the difference is not enough to classify the individual patient. It will therefore have limited application in clinical work.

CHRONIC PAIN AND CNS MECHANISMS

Biochemical approaches to CNS function in man are limited by problems of access and ethical considerations. Measurements would have to be done in a body fluid, such as the cerebrospinal fluid (CSF), blood, or urine. Blood and urine have advantages in terms of access and can be sampled repeatedly but are probably less suitable than cerebrospinal fluid in terms of relevance. For instance, most monoamines which are found in the CNS also occur in peripheral tissue. Analysis of CNS serotonin activity cannot be done on blood at all since peripheral sources contribute to serotonin metabolites. It has therefore been common to use CSF analysis as an indicator of central serotonergic activity and of monoaminergic activity in general (6).

Biogenic peptides of interest in neurophysiology are distributed in the central and peripheral nervous systems and in the gastrointestinal tract. Analysis of such peptides in blood or urine will create similar questions of relevance, and probably CSF analysis is the most appropriate. A method for analysis of opioid peptides in CSF was established several years ago, based on radioreceptor analysis (16), which measures functionally active opioid peptides or endorphins. In our pilot study (16), it was observed that endorphin-like material was present in the CSF and that patients with chronic pain syndromes tended to have lower levels than patients with neurologic diseases unrelated to pain. These observations were later confirmed and amplified. We found that patients with neurogenic pain syndromes in general had lower CSF endorphin levels than healthy volunteers (Table 1).

The adequacy of the method is best illustrated by the correlations observed between the levels of endorphin-like material and various clinical and experimental variables. A positive correlation exists between endorphin levels and experimental pain thresholds and tolerance limits (19) as well as with visually evoked potentials (20). Furthermore, increases of endorphin-like material was observed on peripheral transcutaneous nerve stimulation used in the low-frequency mode (13).

Pain relief induced by this procedure is naloxone-reversible (12), which strengthens a functional relationship. Moreover, high-frequency nerve stimulation, while being clinically useful, does not produce naloxone-reversible pain relief and is not accompanied by increasing CSF endorphin levels.

TABLE 1 - Endorphin levels in lumbar cerebrospinal fluid in patients with chronic, neurogenic pain and in healthy volunteers.

Subjects	Endorphin level (pmol/ml) <0.6	0.6-1.2	>1.2
Healthy volunteers	3	12	4
Patients with chronic neurogenic pain	28	5	

As is the case with most clinical studies, this study was subject to selection. It was therefore decided to perform a study on an unselected series of patients. The series was comprised of 45 consecutive patients with chronic pain (duration over 6 months) admitted to the Neurologic Clinic at the University Hospital of Umeå. Cases with organic brain syndrome and drug or alcohol abuse were exempted. The patients were hospitalized and subjected to extensive clinical investigation, psychiatric evaluation, and tested in personality inventories. Psychophysical measures of pain thresholds, pain tolerance limits, and visual evoked potentials were performed on most patients. A spinal tap at the end of the period of investigation provided material for endorphin and monoamine metabolite measurements.

Although the investigation of these patients was so extensive, far beyond that routinely done, there were problems with regard to diagnosis. Following the classification given by others, the term "organic (somatic) pain" was reserved for those cases where there was objective evidence for such pain. Cases not meeting this criterion were called "psychogenic." These patients frequently showed neurotic behavior and abnormal scores in personality inventories. The classification, "neurogenic pain," was used when there was objective evidence for a peripheral or central nerve lesion. All these classifications were done without knowledge of the results of the biochemical measurements. In fact, the neurologic and psychiatric classifications were also done independently. However, it is realized that any chronic pain syndrome will have emotional components and there may well be organic components in the psychogenic pain syndrome. Table 2 shows the distribution of cases using the same arbitrary endorphin concentration as used in the previous study to discriminate cases with "low" or "normal" values. It is obvious that cases with neurogenic pain tend to have very low levels, confirming our previous investigation. On the other hand, patients with psychogenic pain frequently show high levels. The difference between these groups is significant at an extremely high level. There also seems to be a significant difference between organic and psychogenic pain. However, this may be true only because of the large proportion of neurogenic cases. An extended series

TABLE 2 - Endorphin levels and subdiagnosis of chronic pain (2).

Subjects	Endorphin level (pmol/ml) <0.6	>0.6	
Healthy volunteers	3	16	
Neurogenic pain	12	2	$P < 0.001$
Non-neurogenic pain	2	21	
Organic pain	14	9	$P < 0.001$
Psychogenic pain	1	16	

χ^2 analysis with Yate's correction

of patients with organic non-neurogenic pain (cancer pain, rheumatoid pain) ought to be included.

In view of the often expressed belief that depression and chronic pain may have a common pathogenesis (4,15,18), it was also investigated whether the biochemical measurements were related to psychologic and psychiatric characteristics of the patients. It was observed that endorphin levels followed depression scores, being higher in the more depressed patient (2). Furthermore, endorphin levels correlated to scores in certain personality inventories, particularly in the Zuckerman Sensation Seeking Scale. Most of the patients showed, not unexpectedly, fairly poor scores. With a low tendency to "sensation seeking" and with susceptibility to boredom, the endorphin levels were particularly high (7). It should also be noted that endorphins may be high in patients with endogenous depression, even if pain is not a major complaint (17).

Another link between depression and pain is suggested by the results of monoamine metabolite measurements in CSF. Such analyses in patients with psychiatric disorders have been carried out by several groups (6). There has been some progress particularly in depressed patients, and there is currently evidence for two subgroups with respect to levels of the serotonin metabolite, 5HIAA (3). One subgroup has very low levels, below the normal range, and this group tends to have a strong suicidal ideation and other diagnostic peculiarities. In our series of patients, a positive correlation was observed between endorphin and 5HIAA levels (1). A considerable number (about 50%) of the cases showed very low 5HIAA levels. There were significantly lower endorphin levels in the low 5HIAA subgroup than in those in the high subgroup. However, the discriminative power between the organic and the psychogenic subgroups is higher when endorphins are analyzed rather than monoamine metabolites. A compilation of the correlations observed is shown in Table 3.

It would therefore seem that the most significant observations relate to endorphin activity. What can be said about the

TABLE 3 - Fraction I endorphin values and clinical variables in patients with chronic pain (n = 44).

Positive correlation with:	Pain threshold, pain tolerance, depression scores
Negative correlation with:	Duration of pain (organic group)
Correlation with:	EEG responses to visual stimuli (V.EP), personality variables, monoamine metabolites (particularly 5HIAA)
No correlation with:	Sex, age, self-related severity of pain

functional significance? A low or a high level is not necessarily equated with a functional deficit or excess. The opioid systems are known for their capacity to develop receptor desensitation (tolerance). It is likely that the endorphins normally have a modulatory function within rather narrow constraints. Deviations in either direction may give the same phenomenological end result. Therapeutically, however, such differences may be highly significant.

CONCLUSIONS

As pointed out earlier, chronic pain is a neglected field of research. This holds for biochemical approaches as well. Essentially, two different areas have been investigated: a) methods for the objective assessment of pain and the reaction to pain and b) diagnostic and mechanistic aspects of pain. Clearly, we need much more basic work in both areas. In the former area, several possible lines can be followed. For instance, several endocrine and neuroendocrine mechanisms are very sensitive to stress and mental discomfort. As mentioned earlier, adrenal function has been investigated and found to be characteristically affected. Measurements of anterior pituitary function (prolactin, β-lipotropin/ACTH/β-endorphin) via plasma analysis could be rewarding. Techniques, such as the measurements of experimental pain thresholds with sophisticated techniques (Chapman, this volume) or patient-controlled end point titration methods with narcotics (10) could serve as correlates to the biochemical measurements. The other area of research seems to hold promise as to the definition of the underlying pathologic changes in chronic pain syndromes. The differences observed in CSF endorphin levels between patients with pain syndromes of different etiologies suggest that we are observing changes which are primary and not secondary to pain suffering. According to this view, chronic neurogenic pain would primarily derive from inadequate activation of endorphin systems.

The role of endorphin measurements in clinical practice will have to await the evaluation of the long-term response to various treatment modalities. The need for CSF sampling limits the usefulness considerably and alternative approaches should be sought.

Acknowledgement. The author is aided by the Swedish Medical Research Council.

REFERENCES

(1) Almay, B.G.L.; Johansson, F.; von Knorring, L.; Sedvall, G.; and Terenius, L. 1979. Relationships between CSF levels of endorphins and monoamine metabolites in chronic pain patients. Psychopharmacology, in press.

(2) Almay, B.G.L.; Johansson, F.; von Knorring, L.; Terenius, L.; and Åström, M. 1978. Endorphins in chronic pain. I. Differences in CSF endorphin levels between organic and psychogenic pain syndromes. Pain 5: 153-162.

(3) Åsberg, M.; Thorén, P.; Träskman, L.; Bertilsson, L.; and Ringberger, V. 1976. Serotonin depression - A biochemical subgroup within the affective disorders? Science 191: 478-480.

(4) Engel, G.L. 1959. Psychogenic pain and the pain prone patient. Amer. J. Med. 26: 899-918.

(5) Glynn, C.J., and Lloyd, J.W. 1978. Biochemical changes associated with intractable pain. Brit. Med. J. 1: 280-281.

(6) Goodwin, F.K.; Muscettola, J.; Gold, P.W.; and Wehr, F. 1978. Psychiatric Diagnosis. New York: Spectrum Publications.

(7) Johansson, F.; Almay, B.G.L.; von Knorring, L.; Terenius, L.; and Åström, M. 1979. Personality traits in chronic pain patients related to endorphin levels in CSF. Psych. Res., in press.

(8) Keele, D., and Stern, P.R.S. 1973. Serum lipid changes in relation to pain. J. Roy. Coll. Phycns. 7: 319-329.

(9) Lascelles, P.T.; Evans, P.R.; Merskey, H.; and Sabur, M.A. 1974. Plasma cortisol in psychiatric and neurological patients with pain. Brain 97: 533-538.

(10) Scott, J.S. 1970. A consideration of labor pain and a patient-controlled technique for its relief with meperidine. Amer. J. Obstet. Gynec. 106: 959-964.

(11) Shenkin, H.A. 1964. The effect of pain on the diurnal pattern of plasma corticoid levels. Neurology 14: 1112.

(12) Sjölund, B.H., and Eriksson, M.B.E. 1979. The influence of naloxone on analgesia produced by peripheral conditioning stimulation. Brain Res. 173: 295-301.

(13) Sjölund, B.H.; Terenius, L.; and Eriksson, M.B.E. 1977. Increased cerebrospinal fluid levels of endorphins after electroacupuncture. Acta Physiol. Scand. 100: 382-384.

(14) Szasz, T.S. 1975. Pain and Pleasure. New York: Basic Books.

(15) Sternbach, R.A. 1974. Pain Patients: Traits and Treatment. New York: Academic Press.

(16) Terenius, L., and Wahlström, A. 1975. Morphine-like ligand for opiate receptors in human CSF. Life Sci. 16: 1759-1764.

(17) Terenius, L.; Wahlström, A.; and Ågren, H. 1977. Naloxone treatment in depression: Clinical observations and effects on CSF endorphins and monoamine metabolites. Psychopharmacology 54: 31-33.

(18) von Knorring, L. 1975. The experience of pain in patients with depressive disorders. A clinical and experimental study. Umeå University Medical Dissertations, New Series No. 2.

(19) von Knorring, L.; Almay, B.G.L.; Johansson, F.; and Terenius, L. 1978. Pain perception and endorphin levels in cerebrospinal fluid. Pain 5: 359-365.

(20) von Knorring, L.; Almay, B.G.L.; Johansson, F.; and Terenius, L. 1979. Endorphins in CSF of chronic pain patients, in relation to augmenting-reducing response in visual averaged evoked response. Neuropsychobiology 5: 322-326.

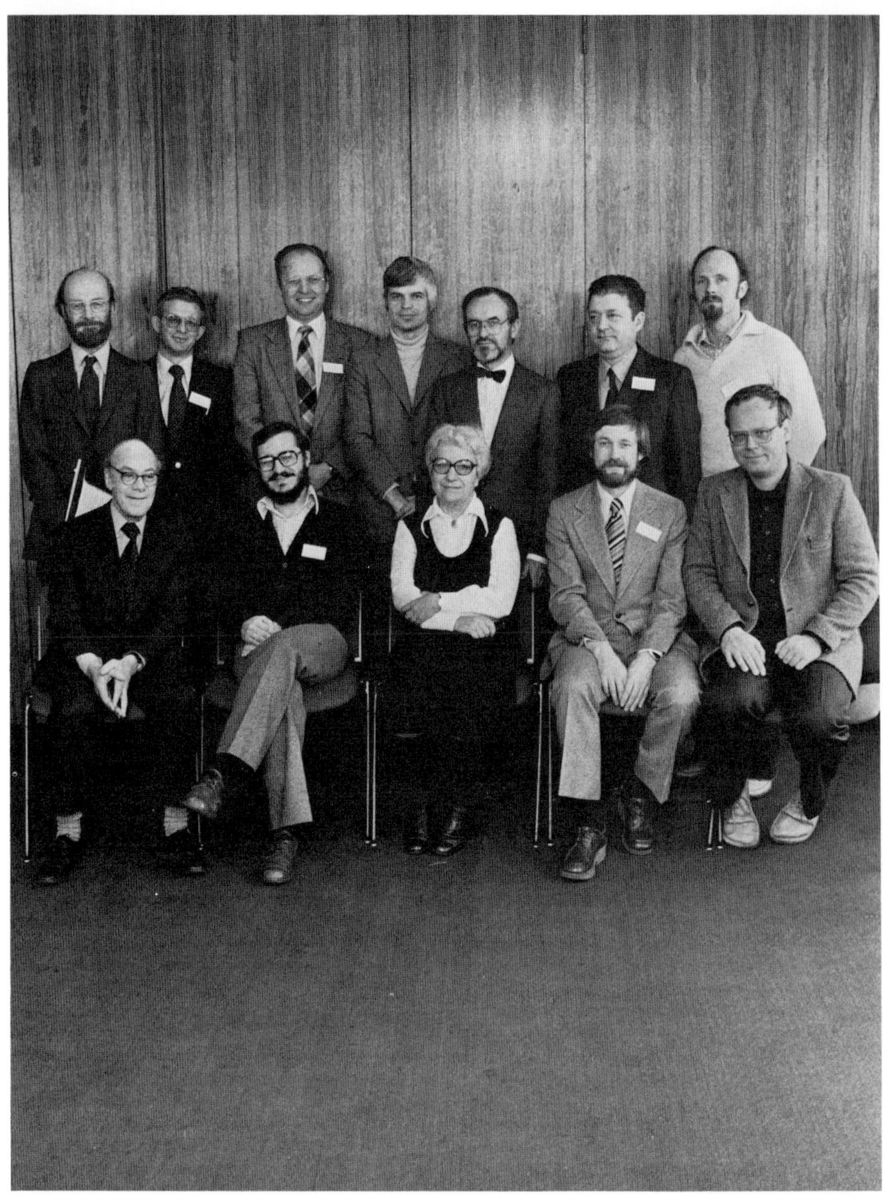

Group on <u>Recurrent Persistent Pain: Mechanisms and Models</u>:
Seated, left to right: Peter Nathan, Fernando Cervero,
Denise Albe-Fessard, Dick Chapman, Hermann Handwerker.
Standing: Pat Wall, Robert Schmidt, Klaus-Dietrich Kniffki,
Lars Terenius, Manfred Zimmermann, Paolo Procacci, Peter Reeh.

Pain and Society, eds. H.W. Kosterlitz and L.Y. Terenius, pp. 367-382.
Dahlem Konferenzen 1980. Weinheim: Verlag Chemie GmbH.

Recurrent Persistent Pain: Mechanisms and Models
Group Report

M. Zimmermann, Rapporteur
D. G. Albe-Fessard, F. Cervero, C. R. Chapman,
H. O. Handwerker, K.-D. Kniffki, P. W. Nathan,
P. Procacci, P. Reeh, R. F. Schmidt, L. Y. Terenius,
P. D. Wall

INTRODUCTION

Clinicians, neuropharmacologists, and neurophysiologists have been brought together in this group to narrow or to bridge the gap between basic science and clinical experience of pain. This was particularly necessary as the topic under discussion was chronic pain. We think that our concepts of the subject have been widened and our awareness of unsolved problems has been made clearer by our discussions. The emphasis of this report centers on the aspects of the discussion that could be shared by physiologists and clinicians. Subjects that are covered in a background paper have usually not been repeated in this report.

ACUTE AND CHRONIC PAIN

The discussion showed that no comprehensive, general definition could be formulated because of the semantic differences that existed among the participants. Physiologists and psycho-physiologists have habitually defined acute pain as a laboratory pain of short duration (e.g., radiant heat, electrical shock) that can be terminated on command. In the laboratory, the term chronic pain refers to painful stimulation that persists for hours, days or even longer, but it is still under the control of the experimenter. It may be the product of stimulation from an extraneous source (e.g., repetitive electrical pulses delivered to a nerve through an implanted electrode), or it may be the result of an experimentally induced lesion or physiological condition (e.g., neuroma produced by ligation and encapsulization of a nerve).

For the clinician and the researcher concerned with human subjects undergoing naturally produced pain experiences, acute pain may be defined as a transient pain that signals tissue injury or is commonly associated with the experience of tissue injury, and this pain diminishes in the course of the natural healing process. Recurrent pain is repeated or cyclic pain, e.g., angina pectoris, migraine headache, or tic douloureux. Chronic or persistent pain may be defined as failing to disappear as the healing process associated with injury or disease becomes complete. It can also refer to the pain associated with a progressive malignant or nonmalignant disease process that persists for a long period of time and where healing does not take place, e.g., pain associated with cancer or arthritic pain.

The aim of this group was to deal with models and mechanisms of all forms of chronic pain. Most of the basic work done in the past studied effects on the CNS produced by short experimental noxious stimuli, predominantly cutaneous stimulation. There is a lack of a suitable animal model for recurrent and chronic pain.

NOCICEPTORS AND NOCICEPTIVE AFFERENT FIBERS

A frequently recurring question in the discussion was how to define a nociceptor. Sherrington used the term to mean a receptor responding to stimuli that were likely to damage the body. In his work, these receptors triggered flexor and crossed extensor reflexes and nocifensive behavior.

At the end of this part of the discussion, we concluded that the whole concept of the existence of one group of receptors used only to signal tissue damage and of another never used for this purpose had been accepted too easily and without due criticism. Many facts do not fit into this concept. We mentioned three:

1) There are some nociceptive afferents among the Aβ fibers (4).

2) It has been shown that electrical stimulation of a nerve at a strength that evokes only an Aβ volley is not painful when single shocks are used but is painful during high frequency stimulation (28).

3) Severe pain can be triggered by slight tactile and weak thermal stimuli in various pathological states (e.g., trigerminal neuralgia, algodystrophies) (15).

An important aspect for the reevaluation of the nociceptor concept is the increasing knowledge of non-impulse events occurring in nerves - the various components of axonal transport by which information can be transferred from either end of the nerve fiber to the other. It appears that particularly long lasting - chronic - changes at a peripheral nerve might travel as signals via the axoplasma, producing chronic changes at the central terminals. It is conceivable, although speculative at present, that information travels in this manner when chronic pain is involved, in addition to nerve impulses which are sufficient to conduct the immediate effects of an acute noxious stimulus.

THE ROLE OF VENTRAL ROOT AFFERENTS IN PAIN

Stimulation of ventral roots in patients has been reported to evoke pain (12). Correspondingly, afferents which are presumably nociceptive have been found in the ventral roots (7). Labeling of ventral root afferents by horseradish peroxidase revealed that they have endings in the dorsal horn (18). However, D. Albe-Fessard reported findings in rats in which dorsal roots had been sectioned unilaterally in four to five adjacent segments. Dorsal horn neurons in the central segment of this zone did not show signs of a natural ipsilateral input. Possible explanations for this discrepancy were discussed: Species differences? Anesthesia differences? Might ventral root afferent input be supplementary, being effective only in conjunction with dorsal root input?

VISCERAL PAIN AND VISCERAL NOCICEPTORS

Compared with cutaneous nociceptors, visceral nociceptors have not been well defined to date, since they have not been sufficiently investigated. Adequate visceral noxious stimuli are difficult to define since we have no visually monitored subjective experience with such stimuli. Visceral receptors are variable in responsiveness, e.g., due to changes of tone of smooth muscle fibers with which they are arranged in series and due to chemical influences. Some visceral receptors, e.g., mechanosensitive receptors of the gall bladder, have a rather low threshold and show a steadily increasing discharge frequency when distensions are increased from a minor degree to levels that provoke signs of discomfort in animals (25). Are these nociceptors? They could be relevant to: a) pain sensations exclusively, b) to non-nocifensive control of visceral functions, or c) to both. In the first case, one might assume that a great deal of summation is needed in the CNS; in the latter case some kind of intensity coding operates in multipurpose visceral receptors so that they signal injury at a certain level of discharge frequency (16).

The density of visceral afferent innervation is lower than that of the skin. Nevertheless, pain from viscera is often more intense and aching in quality than from the skin (e.g., spasms, heart infarction). Is this because inhibitory actions on visceral input are much weaker than those on cutaneous input (24)? This suggestion conforms with the observation that visceral pain often cannot be managed by electrical nerve stimulation (Sjölund and Eriksson, this volume). Or is pain so strong despite the lower innervation density because more spatial and/or temporal summation occurs in visceral painful states?

To recognize the topology of a nonsurface pain requires a high level of experience and scrutiny of investigation. Such efforts are often of major importance for medical diagnosis of pain.

Referred pain, i.e., the referral of localization of pain originating in the inner organs to the related dermatomes of the skin, can best be explained on the basis of convergence of cutaneous and visceral afferents (see Cervero, this volume). However, as was pointed out by the clinicians during the discussion, a clear-cut referral of visceral pain to the body surface is not very common. Rather, many cases of poorly localized pain have been included in the term "referred pain," and thus caused confusion.

It has been suggested pain can be distributed according to vascular zones. In rare cases, the pain has spread to extend over a quadrant of the body (14,23), which in Germany is called the Quadrantensyndrom. Owing to this mode of spread, it has been suggested that sympathetic mechanisms are involved (10,13). Either the afferents concerned are those running along the vessels together with the sympathetic efferents, or the sympathetic efferents produce some trophic influences which in turn cause pain (see section on "the sympathetic nervous system"). An alternative proposal to explain the spreading of a painful state to contiguous regions of the body has been made by Nathan (this volume).

MUSCLE AND DEEP PAIN

The majority of afferent fibers in muscle are in the Aδ- and C-fiber ranges (>50%). Their functions, however, have been least investigated (e.g., they are dealt with in less than 2% of the text of P. Matthews' monograph on muscle afferents (20)). Thus, this is clearly a neglected field of research.

Recent work has shown that the dominant sensitivities of Aδ- and C-fibers from muscle (gastrocnemius in cat) suggest a classification into a group of nociceptors (majority of C-fibers (17)) and a group of ergoceptors (majority of Aδ-fibers (21)).

This differentiation, however, is not sharp. The researchers suggested that the functional characterization may be improved if the work could be repeated with the refined methods of investigation that emerged during the studies.

Many presumed nociceptors in muscle respond to intraarterially applied algesic substances. Of particular interest was the finding that facilitatory interactions occurred between them: e.g., prostaglandin E_2 and serotonin greatly potentiated the responses to bradykinin (21). It is conceivable that these interactions play a role in ongoing pain from muscle and in pain from joints (11).

An electron microscopic analysis (1) revealed in the Achilles tendon of sympathectomized cats at least three characteristic terminal structures of Group III or Aδ fibers and of four types of Group IV or C fibers. They end either within the perineural sheath, or in the surroundings of small arteries and veins, or in tendons or peritendinous tissue.

Only a small minority of fine caliber muscle afferents (less than 10%) responded to muscle contraction during ischemia, which causes severe pain in man (22). To explain this discrepancy between the severity of such pain and the scarcity of afferents responding, Schmidt pointed out that this scarcity might be due to a sampling bias: these fibers were found among those with the smallest action potentials and therefore their apparent incidence might have been lower than their true incidence in a muscle nerve.

It is possible that muscle contraction during ischemia may be a good model for a controlled type of chronic pain in man and animals. Therefore, it would be desirable to expand the investigation of responding afferents and their central connections. The fact that a large proportion of presumed nociceptors in muscle responds to pain-producing substances but not ischemia and contraction suggests that further work is required towards a better understanding of their functional significance.

PAIN PRODUCING SUBSTANCES

One of the modifications of nociceptors which could be relevant in chronic pain is their excitation or sensitization by pain producing or algesic substances. Although they do excite nociceptors, at low concentrations they do not excite specifically. In the cat a major proportion of slowly adapting, low threshold cutaneous mechanoreceptors (SA-receptors) are also excited at the same range of concentrations. Slowly adapting, sensitive muscle mechanoreceptors (e.g., muscle spindle), however, are not excited.

It has been postulated that such substances act via biochemical receptors located at the nociceptor. These receptors, however, have not been characterized to date. A prominent feature of nociceptor excitation by pain producing substances is the slow time course, at least when they are administered by injection into the artery supplying the area where the nociceptor is situated: signs of nociceptor excitation do not occur until about 15 s after the injection of bradykinin. This delay cannot be explained by a slow permeation and diffusion of the substance to the nociceptor. A similar delay occurs when bradykinin is applied to smooth muscle. Therefore, nociceptor excitation by algesic substances might be, at least in part, secondary to changes of smooth muscle tone in the environment of the nerve ending. Consistent with this contention is the absence of excitation by algesic substances of axons in peripheral nerves where no smooth muscles occur (Zimmermann, this volume).

It would appear to be relevant to pain mechanisms that nociceptor activity is greatly enhanced when several of the pain producing substances, e.g., prostaglandin E_2 (PGE_2) and bradykinin are simultaneously present. This is probably the situation in some painful states (e.g., inflammation), where several pain producing substances are released with different but overlapping time courses (9). PGE_2 is not a pain producing substance in the strict sense, since it does not excite nociceptors when applied alone. Hence, it has been termed a vaso-neuroactive substance.

Substance P is presumably released from both the central and the peripheral ends of small diameter afferent fibers. The peripheral effect is a powerful vasodilatation. This might contribute to hyperemia and edema following painful stimulation. The excitability of nociceptors could increase secondary to these vasoactive effects and thus produce allodynia and hyperalgesia. The question has remained unanswered whether substance P could possibly be a breakdown product of the metabolism of some neurons.

SYMPATHETIC NERVOUS SYSTEM AND PAIN

Certain aspects of pain (e.g., allodynia, hyperpathia) are related to the efferent sympathetic nervous system (see Nathan, Zimmermann, this volume). The evidence for this concept derives mainly from several clinical syndromes subsumed by the term "sympathetic algodystrophy." It has been proposed that a sympathetic reflex operated by the continuous input from nociceptors acts back onto the same nociceptors in a way that enhances their sensitivity (13). This may be interpreted as a vicious circle, a positive feedback mechanism worsening the pain - sympathetic reflex dystrophy (Fig. 4B in Zimmermann, this volume). In such cases, it has been found that repeated local anesthetic blocks of the afferent and/or the sympathetic fibers can stop the pain for weeks or months. Such therapeutic sympathetic blocks are now used for relief of pain due to heart infarction (Procacci, personal communication).

Recently experiments have been done on rats and mice to elucidate the pain that may follow amputations of limbs and traumatic lesions of the large peripheral nerves. Neuromata were induced in these animals by section of the sciatic nerves and enclosing the cut central end in plastic caps. Self-mutilation (autotomy) developed during the weeks following the nerve lesion (26). With a parallel time course, ongoing impulse activity appeared particularly in afferent Aδ fibers of the injured nerve, the impulse generators being situated at the nerve sprouts in the neuroma. Both the incidence of autotomy and of ongoing afferent impulse discharges were markedly reduced by pharmacological interference with catecholamines, for instance, by administration of guanethidine, adrenergic blockers, and 6-hydroxydopamine (27).

While these actions probably take place within the neuroma, another possibility was discussed. The spinal ganglia may have a sympathetic supply; a projection of presumed sympathetic efferents to spinal ganglion cells has been postulated (5). However, various ways of sympathetic stimulation in cats failed to produce changes in the electrical responses of dorsal root afferent fibers (6).

Future research in this neglected field should be aimed at the understanding of pathological conditions that produce such interactions of sympathetic and afferent mechanisms.

NEUROPEPTIDES AND CHRONIC PAIN

One of the possible mechanisms of chronic pain could be that persistent changes occur in neuropeptides of the central nervous system. Evidence for this comes from the measurement of the amount of endogenous opioids in the cerebrospinal fluid (CSF) (see Terenius, this volume). The rationale for this investigation was the assumption that endogenous opioids in the brain control a subject's general susceptibility to pain. In some patients with chronic pain, CSF levels of opioids were significantly reduced compared to control subjects. Acupuncture that reduced the pain produced an increase in CSF opioid levels. Consistent with this contention of brain opioids controlling pain susceptibility is a unique observation on a subject with congenital absence of pain (8). When naloxone, an opioid antagonist, was given to this patient, a marked increase occurred in spinal reflexes used as an indicator of a pain system. However, no pain sensation was reported by the patient.

However, there are arguments against this concept of a tonic control by opioids of pain perception (see Akil and Watson, this volume). For example, when naloxone is given intravenously to animals, healthy humans, and patients with chronic pain, no major changes occurred in various measures of pain sensitivity. Akil and Watson discuss the possibility that endogenous opioids may control pain in a phasic manner, e.g., when released during stimulation producing intense pain, stress, or manipulations to alleviate pain (acupuncture, stimulation of certain brain regions).

Another implication of neuropeptides relevant to pain refers to substance P, which has been proposed to be a transmitter or modulator released from nociceptive primary afferents in the spinal cord. The availability of substance P can be manipulated experimentally. Treatment with capsaicin and peripheral nerve transection produce depletion in the presynaptic terminals. Concomitant with the depletion by capsaicin, antinociceptive effects are observed in these animals. It is conceivable that manipulation of the content of substance P in the presynaptic terminals, its release by afferent nerve impulses, and its postsynaptic actions may alter transmission of noxious impulses in the spinal cord. This, however, has not been investigated systematically.

PAIN ORIGINATING IN THE CENTRAL NERVOUS SYSTEM

Pain can be produced by lesions in the peripheral and in the central nervous system. Two animal models for such pain were discussed in detail. These models used either peripheral nerve transections, as those used to perform experimental neuroma (26), or transections of dorsal roots (Albe-Fessard and Lombard, this volume). Both lesions change the properties of dorsal horn cells.

Wall reported that transections of the sciatic nerve in rat, similar to that used to induce a neuroma, produced dramatic morphological, physiological, and biochemical changes in the dorsal horn within a few days, e.g., substance P content decreased, the dorsal root potential disappeared, and new cutaneous receptive fields appeared. It is not clear whether these changes contribute to autotomy suggestive of pain behavior of the animals, since impulses originating at the peripheral site of the nerve lesion, i.e., the neuroma, are likely to determine this behavior.

Transection of dorsal roots in rats is another paradigm to induce long lasting self mutilation, e.g., production of wounds by scratching, autotomy of limbs. This preparation has been proposed as a model for deafferentation pain in man, such as anesthesia dolorosa. Deafferentation changes occur in central neurons which eventually discharge repeated trains of impulses (bursts), although they have no or a quantitatively reduced input from the periphery (Albe-Fessard and Lombard, this volume). An increase in ongoing activity has also been observed in partially deafferented dorsal horn cells of the cat. However, their responsiveness to noxious skin heating via the remaining afferents was not changed, nor was the tonic descending inhibition (3). This finding is unexpected when it is assumed that the effects of deafferentation are also related to increased pain sensation (hyperalgesia) reported by patients in the region of partial deafferentation. It might be that differences exist between species.

Various mechanisms have been proposed for the increased ongoing discharges of deafferented central neurons (see Fig. 6 of Zimmermann, this volume), all of which have been observed in various other models for plasticity of synaptic connections. However, only the unmasking of previously ineffective synapses (B in Fig. 6) has been suggested as being a possible mechanism in the dorsal horn. The contention that dorsal root transection leads to new aberrant connections (collateral sprouting) (19) has been challenged (2). An increase in the effectiveness of remaining synapses (C in Fig. 6) does not conform with the observation that the responsiveness of partially deafferented neurons to skin heating is unchanged (3). Supersensitivity of the deafferented neurons (E in Fig. 6) for a substance P analog has in fact been reported (29).

Thus, we have an animal model which might be related to an important case of human chronic pain - the central pain of anesthesia dolorosa.

MEASUREMENT OF PAIN IN MAN

At present no single, comprehensive measure of pain in man exists, but measures of some of the dimensions of the pain experience are widely used and have received some validation. The assessment of pain in man has often been compromised by oversimplification (unidimensionality), and adequate quantification involves scaling of: a) qualitative dimensions, b) quantitative dimensions, and c) physiological correlates. Qualitative measures include words of pain description, reported changes in pain over time, the social meaning of pain, and the emotional meaning of pain. The quantitative assessment of pain may involve psychophysical, psychometric, or behavioral methodologies. Evoked brain potentials, neurochemical correlates, and methods of reflex algesimetry such as psychogalvanic response, motor reflex, and pupillometry provide examples of potential physiological correlates of pain.

Experimental designs are a crucial factor in pain scaling. There is a need for further development of single subject designs in pain research, greater use of multidimensional scaling, and multivariate statistical analysis.

The issue of how laboratory research can relate to human chronic pain deserves consideration. Clearly, laboratory analogs of chronic pain are extremely difficult to achieve experimentally in the human subject. However, chronic pain patients can be tested in the laboratory and compared to normals or to one another in order to elucidate some of the perceptual and physiological abnormalities associated with, and possibly helping to maintain, pain chronicity.

Some participants expressed a need for more sophisticated descriptive studies of clinical pain and of pain occurring in nonlaboratory contexts. A continuing search for new and better strategies of measurement must be of high priority for future work in descriptive study. Moreover, cooperation in research strategy and measurement technology across laboratories will greatly foster progress in pain research and should be encouraged.

Evoked brain potentials as described in Chapman's paper (this volume) appear promising as a new advance in defining physiological correlates of pain. Such indices need to be related both to earlier evoked potentials (< 50 ms) and later evoked potentials (> 400 ms). Exploration of evoked potential work with stimuli of longer duration should be carried out. As yet there is insufficient information about such possible contaminating influences as: distraction, expectation, level of arousal, nonspecificity of painful stimulus used, and memory of previous experience.

ETHICAL PROBLEMS OF ANIMAL MODELS FOR CHRONIC PAIN

At a subsequent meeting called by K.L. Casey, scientific and ethical problems were discussed in relation to animal models for chronic pain. Such models are indispensable for clarification of the underlying mechanisms. The fact that animals might suffer, however, raises serious ethical questions. A beginning was made in the discussion to define permissible and necessary limits. It will be essential that this matter be fully debated and a policy established.

REFERENCES

(1) Andres, K.H.; von Düring, M.; Jänig, W.; and Schmidt, R.F. 1980. Ultrastructure of fine afferent terminals in the Achilles tendon of the cat. Pflügers Arch.-Eur.J.Physiol. 384, suppl.: R33.

(2) Beckermann, S.B., and Kerr, F.W.L. 1976. Electrophysiologic evidence that neither sprouting nor neuronal hyperactivity occur following long-term trigeminal or cervical primary deafferentation. Exp. Neurol. 50: 427-438.

(3) Brinkhus, H., and Zimmermann, M. 1978. Influence of partial deafferentation on spinal neurons in the cat. Pflügers Arch.-Eur. J. Physiol. 373: suppl. R90.

(4) Burgess, P.R., and Perl, E.R. 1967. Myelinated afferent fibres responding specifically to noxious stimulation of the skin. J. Physiol. (Lond.) 190: 541-562.

(5) Cajal, S. Ramon y 1909. Histologie du systême nerveux de l'homme et des vertébrés, vol. 2. Paris: Maloine.

(6) Cervero, F. 1974. Contribuciones al estudio funcional de los ganglios raquideos. Doctoral Thesis, University of Madrid.

(7) Clifton, G.L.; Coggeshall, R.E.; Waines, W.H.; and Willis, W.D. 1976. Receptive fields of unmyelinated ventral root afferent fibres in the cat. J. Physiol. (Lond.) 256: 573-600.

(8) Dehen, H.; Willer, J.C.; Prier, S.; Boureau, F.; and Cambier, J. 1978. Congenital insensivity to pain and the "morphine-like" analgesic system. Pain 5: 351-358.

(9) DiRosa, M.; Giroud, J.P.; and Willoughby, D.A. 1971. Studies of the mediators of the acute inflammatory response induced in rats in different sites by carrageenan and turpentine. J. Pathol. 104: 15-29.

(10) Davis, L., and Pollock, L.J. 1930. The peripheral pathway for painful sensations. Arch. Neurol. Psychiat. (Chicago) 24: 883-898.

(11) Enderle, T.; Meyn, H.J.; and Schmidt, R.F. 1979. Properties of afferent units subserving normal and inflammated knee joints in the cat. Pflügers Arch.-Eur. J. Physiol. 382: R50.

(12) Foerster, O. 1927. Die Leitungsbahnen des Schmerzgefühls und die chirurgische Behandlung der Schmerzzustände. Berlin, Wien: Urban und Schwarzenberg.

(13) Galletti, R., and Procacci, P. 1966. The role of the sympathetic system in the control of pain and of some associated phenomena. Acta Neuroveg. 28: 495-500.

(14) Gross, D. 1974. Pain and autonomic nervous system. In Advances in Neurology, ed. J.J. Bonica, vol. 4, pp. 93-103. New York: Raven Press.

(15) Hassler, R., and Walker, A.E., eds. 1970. Trigeminal Neuralgia. Stuttgart: Thieme.

(16) Khayutin, V.M.; Baraz, L.A.; Lukoshkova, E.V.; Sonina, R.S.; and Chernilovskaya, P.E. 1976. Chemosensitive spinal afferents: thresholds of specific and nociceptive reflexes as compared with thresholds of excitation for receptors and axons. In Progress in Brain Research 43: Somatosensory and Visceral Receptor Mechanisms, eds. A. Iggo and O.B. Ilyinski, pp. 293-306. Amsterdam: Elsevier.

(17) Kniffki, K.-D.; Mense, S.; and Schmidt, R.F. 1978. Responses of group IV afferent units from skeletal muscle to stretch, contraction and chemical stimulation. Exp. Brain Res. 31: 511-522.

(18) Light, A., and Metz, C.B. 1978. The morphology of the spinal cord efferent and afferent neurons contributing to the ventral roots of the cat. J. comp. Neurol. 179: 501-515.

(19) Liu, C.N., and Chambers, W.W. 1958. Intraspinal sprouting of dorsal root axons. Arch. Neurol. Psychiat. 79: 46-61.

(20) Matthews, P.B.C. 1972. Mammalian muscle receptors and their central actions. London: Arnold.

(21) Mense, S. 1978. Muskelreceptoren mit dünnen markhaltigen und marklosen afferenten Fasern: Receptive Eigenschaften und mögliche Funktion. (Habilitationsschrift) University of Kiel.

(22) Mense, S., and Stahnke, M. 1978. The possible role of group III and IV muscle afferents in the mediation of the pain of intermittent claudication. Pain Abstracts, vol. 1, p. 54. Second World Congress on Pain, Montreal.

(23) Pette, H. 1927. Das Problem der wechselseitigen Beziehungen zwischen Sympathicus und Sensibilität. Dtsch. Zschr. Nervenhk. 100: 143.

(24) Pomeranz, B.; Wall, P.D.; and Weber, W.V. 1968. Cord cells responding to fine myelinated afferents from viscera, muscle and skin. J. Physiol. (Lond.) 199: 511-532.

(25) Ranieri, F. 1977. Sensibilité viscerale splanchnique. Thesis, Université de Provence, Marseille.

(26) Wall, P.D.; Devor, M.; Inbal, R.; Scadding, J.W.; Schonfeld, D.; Seltzer, Z.; and Tomkiewicz, M.M. 1979. Autotomy following peripheral nerve lesions: experimental anaesthesia dolorosa. Pain 7: 103-113.

(27) Wall, P.D.; Scadding, J.W.; and Tomkiewicz, M.M. 1979. The production and prevention of experimental anaesthesia dolorosa. Pain 6: 175-182.

(28) Willer, J.C.; Boureau, F.; and Albe-Fessard, D. 1979. Role of large diameter cutaneous afferents in transmission of nociceptive messages : electrophysiological study in man. Brain Res. 152: 358-364.

(29) Wright, D.N., and Roberts, M.H.T. 1977. Supersensitivity to a substance P analogue following dorsal root section. Life Sci. 22: 19-24.

Pain and Society, eds. H.W. Kosterlitz and L.Y. Terenius, pp. 383-402.
Dahlem Konferenzen 1980. Weinheim: Verlag Chemie GmbH.

Principles of Clinical Management

R. W. Houde
Memorial Sloan-Kettering Cancer Center
New York, NY 10021, USA

Abstract. The management of patients with pain of clinical significance is a multifaceted problem and a field in which practitioners of diverse disciplines have staked out overlapping and often disputed claims of expertise and success. Although the common goal of therapy is generally stated to be the alleviation of pain, the objectives of some approaches can be more precisely stated as the relief of suffering or the development of more socially acceptable means of coping with pain. Since our knowledge of the physiological intricacies of pain is incomplete, and surely that of the bodies and minds of our patients even more so, any method which we employ will be based on debatable assumptions. The principles governing different methods of treating patients with pain are as different as the philosophies and experiences of their advocates. Pain is a universal yet very individual experience which is best managed in an individual way. There are no panaceas; eclecticism founded on a growing base of scientific knowledge should be the order of the day.

INTRODUCTION

Clinical pain is distinguishable from trivial or nonclinical pain, which virtually everyone experiences in the course of living, by the fact that it is a symptom for which the patient seeks or receives medical attention. This fact, alone, tells very little about the nature or severity of pain, but it says a great deal about the significance of pain to the patient, whether or not there are evident objective signs of bodily injury or disease. Most people will not seek medical attention for pain due to commonplace injuries, if experience has led them to believe that no matter how intense the pain at the time, it will subside and there will be no permanent damage. Paradoxically, pain of even less intensity and which is not known to be due to trauma may be viewed as an even greater threat and be more likely to compel the seeking of medical attention.

Clinical pain is characterized as being either acute or chronic. In the etymological sense, acute pain is pain of sudden and recent onset, whereas chronic pain is pain marked by long duration or repeated recurrences. Typically, acute pain is short lasting and self-limiting and, when severe, is accompanied by autonomic physical signs associated with stress. Chronic pain, even when severe, is rarely accompanied by detectable autonomic signs. Acute pain has been conceptualized as subserving the important biological function of protecting the individual from harm or of initiating behavior leading to treatment and recovery (41). Chronic pain, on the other hand, is conceived as being a malefic force which no longer serves a useful protective role and often leads to physical, emotional, and social deterioration.

Treatment of pain may be characterized as either 'definitive,' when directed at removing the cause of the pain, or 'symptomatic,' when directed at reducing perception or reaction to pain. Definitive measures may also be either those which are curative and expected to have long lasting effects, or those which are merely palliative and less likely permanent. Symptomatic measures may, in turn, be long lasting, or permanent, or short lasting. Whether they be definitive or symptomatic measures, those whose effects are prompt and short lasting are best employed earlier in the course of management of clinical pain, whereas those which have more lasting effects usually require more extensive workup, planning, and preparation.

GENERAL APPROACHES

There are three identifiable stages to the management of the patient with pain and they relate to what is done immediately, what is done in the course of diagnostic workup or while waiting for known acute pain to subside, and, finally, what is done in terms of long-range planning, should the pain persist. The relative importance of treatment in each of these stages will, quite understandably, depend upon the clinical circumstances and the nature of the pain problem. In general, treatments with prompt, but reversible and short lasting effects are are most useful in acute pain, whereas those with long lasting effects are better suited to chronic pain. Success or failure of treatment must be judged not only in terms of whether pain is relieved but also in terms of the price paid in inflicted disabilities or other forms of suffering. It is obvious that one should not produce a permanent deficit in a patient suffering from pain which is expected to be self-limiting, but there are also distinct disadvantages to the use of short acting measures which repeatedly expose chronic pain patients to the psychological impact of recurrent pain.

The large number and variety of methods employed in the management of clinical pain are indications of its complexity, of gaps in our knowledge of the nature and mechanisms of pain, and, to a large extent, to inappropriate or improper applications of knowledge that already exists (6). In treating any pain of whatever cause or type, definitive treatment should be foremost in the mind of the physician, for there is no better way of eliminating pain than by removing the cause. Definitive therapy requires not only identification of the underlying mechanism of pain, but also the availability of an effective means of altering it. If the underlying cause cannot be identified with certainty, or if it can be and there is no available effective therapy, one must then rely on measures which are purely symptomatic.

SYSTEMIC DRUGS

Pharmacological substances which affect the body generally are the most commonly employed methods of treating clinical pain. There are two major classes of these agents: the traditional analgesics and the analgesic adjuvants. The traditional analgesics include the 'simple analgesics' and the opioid, or narcotic, analgesics. In the past, the simple, or antiinflammatory-antipyretic, analgesics were designated as mild, weak, and nonaddictive drugs, whereas the opioids were equated with potent, strong, and addicting analgesics. These distinctions are no longer tenable, for there are now several simple analgesics which are strong analgesics (10,25,34) and there are opioids which are nonaddicting (23). Similarly, the distinctions between analgesics and analgesic adjuvants have become blurred, for several of the latter have also been found to have analgesic properties (3,9,12).

Simple Analgesics

Almost all of the simple analgesics are available only for oral administration and are not amenable to the immediate management of acute severe pain. However, they are the mainstay of the pharmacological treatment of mild acute pain and most chronic pains of somatic origin. In these situations, the traditional wisdom is that these drugs be given an adequate trial before resorting to the more potent opioid analgesics. There are a large number and variety of simple analgesics, and most are available without prescriptions, so that before seeking medical attention most patients have already tried one or more of these drugs.

Although the simple analgesics, with a few exceptions, produce similar adverse side effects, there are substantial differences in analgesic potency and efficacy among these drugs. Some of the newer nonsteroidal antiinflammatory drugs of this class have, in fact, been found to be quite effective in controlling severe acute and chronic pain of somatic origin (10,25,34). There are, thus, available options among drugs of this class for circumventing many of the problems of inefficacy or of adverse side effects. The administration of combinations of simple analgesics to achieve these same purposes has been controversial and not recommended (1). On the other hand, there is some evidence to support combining simple analgesics, whose major actions appear to be in the periphery, with drugs whose primary analgesic actions are exerted within the central nervous system, for, in this manner, greater efficacy can be obtained. However, the concurrent administration of simple analgesics with other classes of drugs is justifiable only on the basis of the specific indication for employing each of the drugs. There is no convincing evidence of potentiation of effects of simple analgesics by drugs which in themselves do not have analgesic properties (2).

Opioid Analgesics

The opioids are generally classified in terms of their predominant characteristics as either morphine-agonists or -antagonists. The former are comprised of the morphine surrogates and include the most potent and effective drugs for the relief of acute pain but, because of their identification with drug addiction, their use in chronic pain has been controversial. On the other hand, the narcotic antagonist analgesics are considered to have relatively low addiction potentials and have been looked upon as promising potent analgesics for patients with severe chronic pain (23). In low doses, the narcotic antagonist analgesics have many morphine-like properties in patients not already receiving narcotics, but quite different effects when given in high doses to patients who have become physically dependent on narcotics (17).

The classical narcotics include the naturally occurring opium alkaloids, their semisynthetic congeners, and an increasing variety of purely synthetic compounds. The range of analgesic potencies of these drugs is of several orders of magnitude. However, when employed in maximal tolerated doses the differences in efficacy between the weak and potent drugs are considerably less striking (16). Nevertheless, individual patients do differ appreciably one from another in their responses to narcotics, presumably because of inherent or acquired differences in their capacity to absorb, metabolize, or eliminate these drugs (37). The choice of drug and dose must be individualized with due attention paid to the patient's physical state and past history of exposure to narcotics.

In the immediate treatment stage of severe acute pain, the morphine surrogates are without peers. They can be administered by any of several parenteral routes; their effects are prompt, predictable, and reversible. There are only minor differences in the actions and side effects of these drugs, if used in equianalgesic doses (14). This is not true for the narcotic antagonists for, when high doses are needed for severe pain, there is, paradoxically, a greater risk of limiting adverse effects than encountered with the morphine agonists (15).

In contrast to the situation in acute pain, the oral route is generally the most convenient and preferred way of administering drugs to patients with chronic pain. When simple analgesics are judged to be no longer adequate in controlling pain, the customary recommendation is to add one of the weak, orally administered opioids to the regimen, for reasons which have been stated above. Codeine and propoxyphene are commonly employed for this purpose, usually in combination with simple analgesics, and in such small fixed doses that there would be little likelihood of significant tolerance or physical dependence developing. This is also the most advantageous time for employing the narcotic antagonist analgesics since they do not produce dependence of the morphine-type. Unfortunately, few of the narcotic antagonists with desirable analgesic attributes are presently available in the oral form, and the practical advantages of the oral route of administration of mixtures of weak narcotics with simple analgesics far outweigh those of resorting to the parenteral administration of narcotic antagonist analgesics.

Patients with chronic pain due to advanced malignant disease should not be denied narcotic analgesics if that is what is necessary to control their pains or suffering. However, even in these patients, it is usually preferable to administer the narcotic by the oral route, and in combination with a simple analgesic, for as long as possible. Oral administration permits great flexibility in dosage, an important consideration when employing drugs to which tolerance can develop to their repeated administration. In patients with terminal illnesses, there are several advantages to administering drugs of this type on a regular time schedule and in doses adequate to prevent pain from recurring. Indeed, it has been found that the daily amount of narcotics taken in this manner is less than on conventional on-demand schedules (39). The advantages of this approach must, however, be weighed against the risks of masking pain heralding a serious complication which, if not promptly treated definitively, could result in irreversible injury and additional suffering (16).

The use of parenterally administered narcotics in patients with chronic pain is generally reserved for those situations in which oral medication is contraindicated or in which there is an urgent need to control severe pain. The major problems arise in those types of chronic pain which are characterized by recurrent bouts of severe pain interspersed with periods of relatively little or no pain. When the condition is remediable by some form of definitive therapy, or can be prevented by a long lasting or permanent regional block, it is usually recommended that the use of narcotics be restricted to as short a period as possible. If for some reason, these procedures are not feasible, one may employ a potent analgesic adjuvant or narcotic antagonist analgesic if there is concern that the patient is likely to develop drug seeking illness behavior. However, care must be taken if the patient has already been receiving regular doses of narcotics, for none of the analgesic adjuvants will fully suppress the narcotic abstinence syndrome in abruptly withdrawn patients, and even weak narcotic antagonists can precipitate acute withdrawal signs in some narcotic dependent patients (15).

Analgesic Adjuvants

There are a number of drugs which are not customarily classified as analgesics even though they are often successfully employed, either alone or in conjunction with classical analgesics, in the management of patients with pain. A few of these, such as colchicine, carbamazepine, phenytoin, and the corticosteroids have selective analgesic actions for specific painful states, and drugs such as these should be used as one would use indicated definitive therapy. There remain, however, several drugs of diverse chemical nature which appear to be effective as analgesics or analgesic adjuvants in a wide range of painful states (12,18,29). All of these drugs have appreciable central nervous system actions; they include the major and minor tranquilizers, sedative-hypnotics, antihistamines, sympathomimetics, and antidepressants. A few have been found to be truly effective analgesics, but all are primarily used for other therapeutic indications (12,33). The demonstration of the analgesic effectiveness of a drug does not imply that other members of the class will share that attribute. This has been a matter of some controversy in the case of the phenothiazines (11,14). The major tranquilizers have given little reason for concern about problems of addiction, but this has not been so for some of the other analgesic adjuvants of the minor tranquilizer, sedative-hypnotic, and sympathomimetic classes (12). Although many of the pharmacological actions of these drugs are similar to those of the opioids, all have other properties which, in particular clinical states, make them useful alternatives or supplements to the standard analgesics (14).

Stress and anxiety are frequent companions of acute pain, and the analgesic adjuvants which have been most useful in these situations are those with tranquilizing, anxiolytic, or sedative properties. However, the narcotic analgesics also possess these qualities and are more firmly established as effective analgesics, so that there is usually little need to add an analgesic adjuvant in the immediate stage of treating acute severe pain. In the later stages, they may be considered desirable substitutes or supplements for standard analgesics because of their other special properties, such as their antiemetic actions. In general, though, the analgesic adjuvants have lower potential than narcotics for controlling very severe pain without producing undesirable side effects and, when given together with narcotics, they are likely to produce more sedation and mental confusion than analgesia (14).

Depression is more commonly associated with chronic pain, and there are a number of reports in the literature attesting to the value of antidepressants given either alone or concurrently with a major tranquilizer, anticonvulsant, or simple analgesic in the management of chronic pain patients (9,12,18,29, 33). Combinations of phenothiazines and tricyclics have been reported to be particularly effective in relieving some types of neuralgias and other painful conditions which have proven to be refractory to standard analgesics (13,38). Whether the effects of these drugs are primarily due to the relief of depression or to specific actions on neural structures subserving pain perception, or both, remains an unresolved issue. Experience with minor tranquilizers with predominant anxiolytic or sedative properties have revealed that these analgesic adjuvants are less apt to be helpful in patients with chronic pain and may, in fact, often precipitate overt depression (12,33).

LOCAL ANESTHETIC AND NEUROLYTIC AGENTS

Pharmacological substances capable of blocking the transmission of impulses along nociceptive pathways are of inestimable value in the diagnostic and/or therapeutic management of clinical pain. As diagnostic tools, local anesthetic blocks can provide insights as to the probable mechanism of pain and the more likely effective means of treating it. When pain is confined to a localized region of the body, local anesthetic and neurolytic agent blocks of peripheral nerve pathways can provide complete and long lasting pain relief. These methods are applicable to the management of both acute and chronic pain, and the outcomes are, in large measure, dependent upon the skill and diligence of the physician performing the blocks. In addition to highly trained physicians, special facilities are needed for the monitoring and performace of some of these procedures. Serious complications are rare, but some can be formidable and irreversible (26).

Therapeutic nerve blocks are often employed in conjunction with other modalities of treating pain. They are particularly useful in the management of chronic, localized, severe 'incident pain' - pains that come on suddenly with certain movements, activities, or other precipitating events (26). Even when the latter can be anticipated, it is often virtually impossible to control sudden pain of this sort with systemic analgesics without producing undesirable side effects. Methods capable of producing long lasting effects have the potential advantage of reducing both the physical and psychological impact of recurring or persistent pain, as well as the complications of drug therapy or other temporary means. A discussion of the indications, limitations, and complications of the various local anesthetic or neurolytic agent blocks is beyond the scope of this paper, but several excellent reference sources are available (4,5,19,36).

NEUROSURGICAL PROCEDURES

The neurosurgical procedures represent a stage beyond that of the nerve block techniques in their complexity, need for special facilities and trained personnel, and in their sites of attack on the neural apparatus subserving the perception and reaction to pain. There are basically three different neurosurgical approaches for relieving clinical pain: the interruption of known ascending pathways for pain (19); the stimulation of nerves capable of inhibiting synaptic or impulse transmission along the antinociceptive pathways (32); and the production of hormonal deficits which are capable of relieving pain in selected patients (31). The last of these appears to be specific to particular painful illnesses and will not be discussed further.

The neurosurgical approaches for interrupting ascending pain pathways differ from the nerve block techniques primarily in that they may not only be directed at peripheral sites but also at pathways within the central nervous system itself. These are obviously more formidable procedures than nerve blocks and more likely to produce lasting irreversible results, whether desired or undesired. These procedures are used to best advantage in patients with severe persistent or recurrent regional disease which cannot be effectively controlled by nerve blocks or by noninvasive methods. In general, procedures involving the interruption of ascending pathways identified with the perception of pain have greater applicability and have been less controversial than procedures directed at altering the affective component of pain. The latter methods are considered to be last resort measures and reserved for patients suffering from intractable pain which cannot be effectively controlled by any other means (30).

By the use of implanted electrodes, neurosurgeons are now able to activate pain inhibitory mechanisms in the central nervous system. These techniques generally do not produce any irreversible neural deficits and have the advantage of being free of the adverse side effects of some of the pharmacologic approaches, even though it appears that tolerance does develop to repeated stimulation of the dorsal columns and periaqueductal and periventricular areas of the brain. Stimulation techniques would seem to provide promising alternatives to the destructive neurosurgical methods of relieving pain and suffering, but most of these procedures must still be considered experimental at this time (21).

OTHER PHYSICAL METHODS

There is a bewildering array of other physical methods which have been designed to relieve pain by mechanical, electrical, and thermal means. Most of these involve stimulation of the skin or superficial structures by the application of heat or cold, rubbing or massage, or the use of counterirritants. These methods are often effective in relieving pain which is localized and not too severe and they are worth considering as adjunctive therapy in certain types of acute and chronic pain. Transcutaneous electrical stimulation, which is believed to relieve pain by the same mechanism, may be an even more effective way of achieving the same results (27,40). More controversial, however, has been the use of acupuncture which presumably produces pain relief by stimulating the release of opioid peptides (24), or, at least, by acting through some mechanism similar to that of needling trigger points (19,20,28). Its place in the management of patients with acute or chronic pain, however, is still uncertain and there is a need for additional controlled studies of its potential therapeutic role (6,22).

PSYCHOLOGICAL METHODS

Pain is one of the most frequently encountered presenting symptoms in medical practice, and it is often an important diagnostic clue to the nature of an underlying disease or injury. However, language tends to be imprecise when describing pain and there are no reliable physical signs of the presence or severity of pain, even those observed in patients with acute pain may be merely manifestations of anxiety or of stress relating to suspected or actual bodily injury. Pain is an important molder of behavior, so that past experiences with pain and its treatment will, in large measure, determine how a patient perceives and reacts to pain. Conditioned stimuli and responses have been so identified with the development of characteristic pain behavior that chronic pain is considered by many to be a separate nosological entity and not to be treated in the same manner as acute pain (7,35). Exception is usually made for patients with chronic pain due to malignant or terminal disease, even though there is little reason to believe that the pain behavior of these patients should be different from those with chronic benign pain of somatic origin (7).

It has long been known that both perception and reaction to pain can be modified by psychological means. Various forms of suggestion and distraction are commonly employed in the management of both acute and chronic pain, often in conjunction with or as an integral part of other methods or strategies. More highly structured methods requiring training, counseling, or guidance include hypnosis, operant conditioning, biofeedback, and various forms of individual or group psychotherapy. These formal approaches usually require substantial investments in time and effort, well motivated patients, and access to therapists with special interests and training in the field of pain management.

The major thrust of the psychological approach is to modify 'pain behavior' often with techniques designed to get the patient to ignore pain or to cope with it. One of the risks entailed is the denial or deferral of indicated definitive medical therapy because of a misdiagnosis of psychogenic pain. The term 'psychogenic pain' is commonly used when an organic cause cannot be identified or if it is felt that the patient should not be having as much pain as he reports. However, anxiety, neuroticism, and depression are just as likely to occur in patients with chronic pain due to organic disease as they are in patients whose origins of pain are in the mind (35). The behavioral approach to the treatment of patients with chronic pain has a sound scientific basis, but it is one probably best practiced in a setting of ready access to medical expertise.

CONCLUSIONS

Pain is a common symptom encountered in medical practice either as a presenting chief complaint or merely as one of a number of symptoms implying bodily injury or disorder, and signifying an appeal for its relief. The physician's responsibilities are not only to determine and treat the cause for pain but also to treat the pain itself. Pain should not be treated without at least a presumptive diagnosis of its etiology, and first consideration should always be given to definitive treatment, whether the underlying disorder is curable or can be merely temporarily alleviated. However, if prompt relief cannot be provided by definitive means, one should not withhold purely symptomatic measures. Effective definitive symptomatic treatment requires an understanding not only of the pain and underlying disease but also of the patient, his circumstances, and his perception of the significance of his pain.

In the broader sense of the term, 'purely symptomatic measures' are employed in every patient with pain, for they include everything from the effects of the laying on of hands to invasive neurosurgical procedures. Each in its own way may have both desired and undesired effects which are, in large measure, determined by the setting in which it is employed.

In the management of acute pain, the objective should be to provide relief of pain and suffering by the simplest means which will provide prompt and adequate relief. Systemic analgesics are most commonly relied upon in these circumstances. The choice of drug and dose should be based on the provisional diagnosis, the patient's prior drug experience, and the physician's familiarity with the drug. There is no predetermined optimal dose for any type of pain; there are merely recommended starting doses from which the optimal dose is determined by titration and the maximal dose limited only by adverse effects. Severe acute pain is often attended by anxiety; a calm, confident, reassuring, and attentive attitude on the part of the physician should, along with the effective use of analgesics, provide the best means of its alleviation. Tranquilizers and anxiolytic drugs can be useful adjuvants, but should not be relied upon merely to provide or potentiate analgesia.

Chronic pain is a far more complex problem and a variety of methods have been developed for the treatment of chronic pain patients. The simplest means of providing early and effective relief of pain should be employed in the hope of preventing the central imprinting of pain and its consequent refractoriness to peripherally directed measures. Procedures which have little risk of producing a permanent neural deficit or disability should always be given first consideration. However, nondestructive measures with long lasting effects are to be preferred to those whose effects are so short lasting as to require their repeated administration. When localized, incident pain is best managed by blocking or interrupting the afferent nociceptive pathways, preferrably by the least destructive means directed at the peripheral nervous system. Psychological factors play an important role in chronic pain and due account of this should be taken in the management of every patient. Most chronic pain patients show signs of depression and/or psychoneurosis for which appropriate antidepressant medication and counseling are indicated. Invasive neurosurgical procedures and measures that will produce permanent neural defects should not be undertaken without prior psychiatric evaluation and an adequate trial of less destructive methods.

The most effective use of any single method of treating patients with chronic pain will, in large measure, depend upon the training, skills, and experience of the therapist, and the assessment of results will frequently reflect discipline bias. Of the pharmacological approaches, the simple analgesics and analgesic adjuvants - in particular, the tricyclic antidepressants - and local anesthetic and neurolytic blocks should be tried first. Various combinations of analgesics, analgesic adjuvants, and nerve blocks are often complementary and their concurrent use should be explored when feasible. Narcotic analgesics should be used with discrimination but should not be withheld, especially in patients with chronic pain due to malignant or terminal disease, if there are no effective acceptable alternatives. When employing a narcotic, it is usually advisable to give it together with a simple analgesic, for their analgesic effects are additive and the rate of tolerance development will be slowed. Of the physical methods, cutaneous stimulation by any of the variety of thermal, mechanical, or electrical techniques are worthy of a trial where indicated, and their effects may be complemented by simple analgesics and/or analgesic adjuvants. Neurosurgically implanted percutaneous and dorsal column stimulators are worthy of consideration in patients with chronic benign pain refractory to the aforementioned procedures. Neurosurgical methods of brain stimulation, pituitary ablation, and of interruption of nociceptive pathways within the central nervous system are generally reserved for patients with chronic pain due to malignant disease, but are employed to best advantage before the patient reaches the terminal stages of disease. Individual or group psychotherapy is indicated in patients with pain due primarily to emotional disorders, and behavioral techniques when psychological assessment reveals that pain is primarily serving the patient as a means of drawing attention to himself or avoiding unpleasant activities. Biofeedback and hypnosis are very effective methods of controlling pain but only in a very small selected group of patients. No physician or therapist can claim expertise in all methods of management of the patient with chronic pain, and patients who present particularly difficult problems are best referred to centers equipped to provide care in a multidisciplinary clinic setting.

Acknowledgement. Supported in part by the National Institute on Drug Abuse Grant DA 01707 and the National Cancer Institute Core Grant CA 08748.

REFERENCES

(1) AMA Department of Drugs. 1977. Mild analgesics, In Drug Evaluations, 3rd Ed., Ch. 21, pp. 340-363. Littleton, Mass.: Publishing Sciences Group, Inc.

(2) Beaver, W.T. 1965-6. Mild analgesics: A review of their clinical pharmacology. Am. J. Med. Sci. 250: 577-604; 251: 576-599.

(3) Beaver, W.T., and Feise, G. 1976. Comparison of the analgesic effects of morphine, hydroxyzine, and their combination in patients with postoperative pain. In Pain Research and Therapy, eds. J.J. Bonica and D. Albe-Fessard, vol. 1, pp. 553-557. New York: Raven Press.

(4) Bonica, J.J. 1953. The Management of Pain. Philadelphia: Lea and Febiger.

(5) Bonica, J.J. 1959. Clinical Applications of Diagnostic and Therapeutic Blocks. Springfield, IL: Charles C. Thomas.

(6) Bonica, J.J. 1979. Current status of pain therapy. In The Interagency Committee on New Therapies for Pain and Discomfort. Report to the White House, pp. 110-114. U.S. Dept. Health, Education and Welfare.

(7) Bonica, J.J. 1979. Importance of the problem. In Advances in Pain Research and Therapy, eds. J.J. Bonica and V. Ventafridda, vol. 2, pp. 1-12. New York: Raven Press.

(8) Bonica, J.J. 1979. Important clinical aspects of acute and chronic pain. In Mechanisms of Pain and Analgesic Compounds, Eleventh Miles International Symposium, eds. R.F. Beers, Jr. and E.G. Bassett, pp. 15-29. New York: Raven Press.

(9) Budd, K. 1978. Psychotropic drugs in the management of chronic pain. Anesthesiology 33: 531-534.

(10) Cooper, S.A., and Sullivan, D. 1978. Relative efficacy of zomepirac sodium compared with an APC/codeine combination. Clin. Pharmacol. Ther. 23: 111-112.

(11) Dundee, J.W.; Love, W.J.; and Moore, J. 1963. Alterations in response to somatic pain associated with analgesia and further studies with phenothiazine derivatives and similar drugs. Br. J. Anaesth. 35: 597-609.

(12) Halpern, L.M. 1979. Psychotropics, ataractics, and related drugs. In Advances in Pain Research and Therapy, eds. J.J. Bonica and V. Ventafridda, vol. 2 pp. 275-283. New York: Raven Press.

(13) Hatangdi, V.S.; Boas, R.A.; and Richards, E.G. 1976. Postoperative neuralgia: Management with antiepileptic and tricyclic drugs. In Advances in Pain Research and Therapy, eds. J.J. Bonica and D. Albe-Fessard, pp. 583-587. New York: Raven Press.

(14) Houde, R.W. 1974. Medical treatment of oncological pain. In Recent Advances on Pain, eds. J.J. Bonica, P. Procacci, and C.A. Pagni, pp. 168-188. Springfield, IL: Charles C. Thomas.

(15) Houde, R.W. 1979. Analgesic effectiveness of the narcotic agonist-antagonists. Br. J. clin. Pharmac. 7: 297S-308S.

(16) Houde, R.W. 1979. Systemic analgesics and related drugs: Narcotic analgesics. In Pain Research and Therapy, eds. J.J. Bonica and V. Ventafridda, vol. 2, pp. 263-273. New York: Raven Press.

(17) Jasinski, D.R. 1979. Human pharmacology of narcotic antagonists. Br. J. clin. Pharmac. 7: 287S-290S.

(18) Kocher, R. 1976. Use of psychotropic drugs for the treatment of chronic severe pain. In Advances in Pain Research and Therapy, eds. J.J. Bonica and D. Albe-Fessard, pp. 579-582. New York: Raven Press.

(19) Levine, J.D.; Gormley, J.; and Fields, H.L. 1976. Observations on the analgesic effects of needle puncture (acupuncture). Pain 2: 149-159.

(20) Lewit, K. 1979. The needle effect in the relief of myofascial pain. Pain 6: 83-90.

(21) Loeser, J. 1979. Panel: Future needs, goals and directions. In Advances in Pain Research and Therapy, eds. J. J. Bonica and V. Ventafridda, vol. 2, p. 676. New York: Raven Press.

(22) Lynn, B., and Perl, E.R. 1977. Failure of acupuncture to produce localized analgesia. Pain 3: 339-351.

(23) Martin, W.R. 1979. History and development of mixed opioid agonists, partial agonists and antagonists. Br. J. clin. Pharmac. 7: 273S-279S.

(24) Mayer, D.J.; Price, D.D.; Rafii, A; and Barber, J. 1976. Acupuncture hypalgesia: Evidence for activation of a central control system as a mechanism of action. In Advances in Pain Research and Therapy, eds. J.J. Bonica and D. Albe-Fessard, vol. 1, pp. 751-754. New York: Raven Press.

(25) Martino, G.; Ventafridda, V.; Parini, J.; and Emanuelli, A. 1976. A controlled study on the analgesic activity of indoprofen in patients with cancer pain. In Advances in Pain Research and Therapy, eds. J.J. Bonica and D. Albe-Fessard, vol. 1, pp. 573-578. New York: Raven Press.

(26) Mehta, M. 1973. Intractable Pain. London: W.B. Saunders Co. Ltd.

(27) Melzack, R. 1975. Prolonged relief of pain by brief, intense transcutaneous somatic stimulation. Pain 1: 357-373.

(28) Melzack, R.; Stillwell, D.M.; and Fox, E.J. 1977. Trigger points and acupuncture points for pain: Correlations and implications. Pain 3: 3-23.

(29) Mersky, H., and Hester, R.N. 1972. The treatment of chronic pain with psychotropic drugs. Postgrad. Med. J. 48: 594-598.

(30) Pagni, C.A. 1979. General comments on ablative neurosurgical procedures. In Advances in Pain Research and Therapy, eds. J.J. Bonica and V. Ventafridda, vol. 2. New York: Raven Press.

(31) Pearson, O.H.; Ray, B.S.; Harrold, C.C.; West, D.C.; Li, M.C.; McLean, J.P.; and Lipsett, M.B. 1956. Hypophysectomy in treatment of advanced cancer. JAMA 161: 17-21.

(32) Richardson, D.E., and Akil, H. 1977. Pain reduction by electrical brain stimulation in man. Part I: Acute administration in periaqueductal and periventricular sites; Part II: Chronic self-administration in periventricular gray matter. J. Neurosurg. 47: 178-183; 184-194.

(33) Shimm, D.S.; Logue, G.L.; Maltbie, A.A.; and Dugan, S. 1979. Medical management of chronic cancer pain. JAMA 241: 2408-2412.

(34) Stambaugh, J.E., and Sarajian, C. 1978. Relative analgesic efficacy of zomepirac sodium as compared to oxycodone/APC combination in the treatment of cancer pain. Clin. Research 26 (3): 594A.

(35) Sternbach, R.A. 1974. Pain Patients: Traits and Treatment. New York: Academic Press.

(36) Swerdlow, M. 1978. Relief of Intractable Pain. 2nd Ed. Amsterdam: Excerpta Medica.

(37) Szeto, H.H.; Inturrisi, C.E.; Houde, R.W.; Saal, S.; Cheigh, J.; and Reidenberg, M.M. 1977. Accumulation of normeperidine, an active metabolite of meperidine in patients with renal failure or cancer. Ann. Int. Med. 86: 738-741.

(38) Taub, A., and Collins, W.F., Jr. 1974. Observation on the treatment of denervation dysesthesia with psychotropic agents. Postherpetic neuralgia, anesthesia dolorosa, peripheral neuropathy. In Advances in Neurology, ed. J.J Bonica, vol. 4, pp. 309-315. New York: Raven Press.

(39) Twycross, R.G. 1979. Overview of analgesia. In Advances in Pain Research and Therapy, eds. J.J. Bonica and V. Ventafridda, vol. 2, pp. 617-633. New York: Raven Press.

(40) Ventafridda, V.; Sganzerla, E.P.; Foci, C.; Pozzi, G.; and Cordini, G. 1979. Transcutaneous nerve stimulation in cancer pain. In Advances in Pain Research and Therapy, eds. J.J. Bonica and V. Ventafridda, vol. 2, pp. 509-515. New York: Raven Press.

(41) Wall, P. 1979. On the relation of injury to pain. Pain 6: 253-264.

Pain and Society, eds. H.W. Kosterlitz and L.Y. Terenius, pp. 403-414.
Dahlem Konferenzen 1980. Weinheim: Verlag Chemie GmbH.

Pain Clinics

H. U. Gerbershagen
Institute of Anesthesia, Johannes Gutenberg-Universität
6500 Mainz, F. R. Germany

Abstract. Acute and chronic intractable pain states should be evaluated and treated in specialized units. The classification of pain centers in major comprehensive, comprehensive, syndrome oriented, and modality oriented pain centers of the American Society of Anesthesiologists is presented The effectiveness of each type of facility will depend on the selection of its mono- or multidisciplinary staff, its pain evaluative procedures, and its therapeutic modalities. A German pain center is quoted in regard to staff selection, organized evaluative processes for screening of pain patients, organized standardized patient work-up schemes in all disciplines, and in planning of treatment. It is emphasized that pain centers, even if well staffed and organized, are no panacea, achieving only limited satisfactory long-term results.

INTRODUCTION

The sociologic, psychologic, economic, and medical importance and impact of chronic pain have been intensely studied by many research teams worldwide and were reemphasized during this conference. Until recently these research results were rarely considered in pain patient care. Bonica (3-6) and Alexander (1) were the first proponents for the establishment of interdisciplinary pain clinics to serve the patient suffering from chronic pain. Today, some twenty years after the original proposition of these specialized pain units, mono-, multi-, and interdisciplinary pain units (pain relief center or clinic, pain treatment center, pain control center, pain management center or unit, chronic pain service or rehabilitation center, pain evaluation and treatment center) have been established. These specialized units will help in preventing pain states from growing into a "pain illness," will reduce human suffering, will diminish medical expenditure, will contribute to a better cooperation between basic scientists and clinicians, will help to disseminate new information on pain mechanisms and diagnostic and treatment modalities, and will lead to a better understanding of the complex problem of chronic pain.

The scope of these pain units will depend on their size, staff, and local conditions. We expect a pain unit to
1) evaluate, treat, guide, and rehabilitate patients suffering from chronic pain,
2) evaluate and treat those acute and subacute pain states (e.g., wide-spread herpes zoster, cancer pain, pancreatic pain, idiopathic neuralgias), which do not respond to therapeutic modalities applied by other physicians,
3) counsel colleagues by telephone or writing,
4) train physicians and other health-professionals of the pain unit,
5) teach physicians in training, pain therapists, and private physicians,
6) bear expert witness for chronic pain patients,
7) organize and carry out postgraduate meetings on pain for all health professional groups,
8) perform interdisciplinary pain studies, and
9) carry out basic research.

CLASSIFICATION OF PAIN CENTERS

Pain units around the world are presently being classified, and a new pain center directory is being prepared by the Committee on Pain Therapy, American Society of Anesthesiologists (7).

The questionnaire distributed worldwide distinguishes the following four different types of pain units:
1) Major Comprehensive Pain Center
2) Comprehensive Pain Center
3) Syndrome Oriented Pain Center, and
4) Modality Oriented Pain Center.
This classification - as deficient as it may be - will help

physicians and pain patients around the world to recognize some of the characteristics of the individual pain service offered.

A Comprehensive Pain Center will have its own space, own beds, full-time professional and supportive staff, will insist on a patient's record review prior to admission, will emphasize a preadmission patient screening, will routinely carry out a psychological assessment, will involve consultants of several specialties, will organize teaching, training and research programs, will provide a large variety of therapeutic modalities, and will follow-up patients.

Syndrome Oriented Pain Centers provide thorough evaluation and treatment of particular pain syndromes, such as low back pain, orofacial pain, headache. They are mono- and multidisciplinary inpatient or outpatient facilities, such as arthritis centers, causalgia and reflex sympathetic dystrophy centers, and cancer pain centers.

Modality Oriented Pain Centers may utilize mono- or multidisciplinary patient work-up schemes and will apply certain limited treatment modalities, such as nerve blocks, psychotherapy, transcutaneous stimulation, and neurosurgery. A typical example is the diagnostic and therapeutic nerve block clinic directed by anesthesiologists. Modality oriented pain centers may or may not provide extensive evaluative procedures (3,8,9,11).

ORGANIZATION OF THE MAINZ COMPREHENSIVE PAIN CENTER

We have studied the pain clinic problem carefully, established the first German pain clinic in 1971, and have run a fairly successful service since. We feel that proper care of patients with complex chronic pain requires the team work of specialists of all medical disciplines, clinical psychology, and medical sociology. Due to our conviction and experience that monodisciplinary modality oriented pain centers will only achieve up to 40% satisfactory long-term results (follow-up one year) and multidisciplinary groups up to 65% satisfactory long-term results, we established a comprehensive pain center (8).

Our inital core group of some twenty-five physicians represented eighteen disciplines (anesthesiology, dental and general surgery, gastroenterology, gynecology, medical statistics and documentation, nephrology, neurology, neurosurgery, ophthalmology, oral surgery, orthopedic surgery, otorhinolaryngology, psychiatry, psychology, psychotherapy, radiology, and rheumatology and rehabilitation medicine. It has been our experience that a pain group member will effectively work on a part-time basis for about three years only, due to the typical staff fluctuation within a university setting.

Members of our pain clinic group are characterized by: (a) special interest in pain as a "pain illness" and chronic pain behavior, (b) extensive knowledge of pain syndromes, (c) extensive knowledge of diagnostic and therapeutic possibilities of psychology, sociology, and the various medical fields, (d) specialized skills, e.g., the anesthesiologist or neurosurgeon offers methods of electrical stimulation, the psychiatrist operant conditioning programs and biofeedback methods, the orthopedic surgeon diagnostic and therapeutic procedures of osteopathic medicine, (e) special knowledge of clinical and research literature on pain in his special field, (f) interest in standardized methods for recording medical and pain histories, work-up and examination schemes, and (g) interest in teaching and education programs. Some twenty physicians are loosely associated with the group in addition to the regular consultants within various departments, who are infrequently involved in the activities at our pain clinic (Fig. 1).

Our pain clinic is organized, coordinated, and headed by the anesthesia department. Generally, it is of little importance which department leads a pain clinic group. The head must have sufficient time for organization, coordination, and

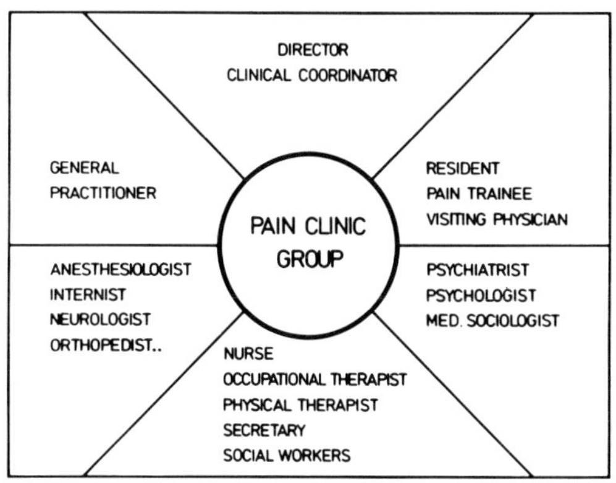

FIG. 1 - Selection of staff in the Mainz pain unit.

public relations work, be accepted by all group members, and of course, fulfill the criteria for a member of the clinic.

FUNCTIONAL ORGANIZATION OF THE MAINZ COMPREHENSIVE PAIN CENTER

Pain units have to be well organized and managed. Thus, from the beginning we felt that pain diagnostic procedures should be started well ahead of the patient's first visit to a pain unit (Fig. 2).

For the past nine years we have practiced and evaluated a screening procedure, which is terminated several weeks prior to the patient's first interview. In order to obtain a useful summary of the patient's pain problem and his pain behavior, we ask the patient to: (a) fill in a detailed pain questionnaire, (b) complete several psychometric tests, (c) daily record his physical activities for at least 8 days and note down all medications taken, and (d) compile reports of all previous medical examinations and hospitalizations (or record addresses of physicians and hospitals involved in his care in order to allow us to contact them).

As soon as the pain clinic secretary has completed the record of a patient, an experienced physician reviews the screening results, makes a preliminary diagnosis, arranges

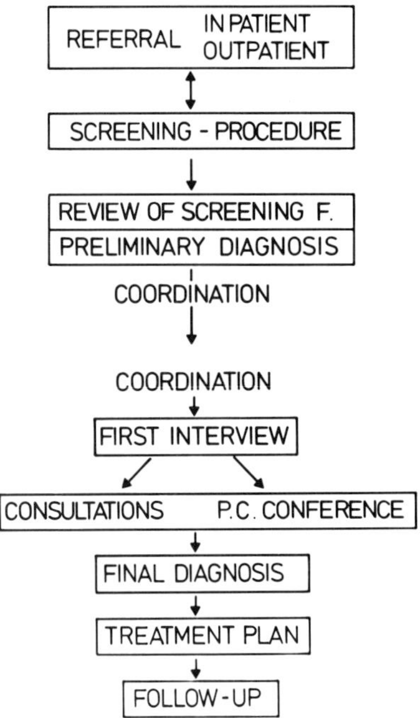

FIG. 2 - Functional organization of the Mainz pain unit

interviews and examinations in the appropriate departments, and orders special laboratory (e.g., EEG, EMG, SCANS) and additional X-ray studies several weeks in advance. This screening physician will be the patient's personal physician later on, responsible for the patient from the start of the screening procedure to the discharge letter and for the follow-up of the patient.

We estimate that the average screening procedure prior to the first appointment requires 1,5 hours of a secretary's time and 1,0 hour of a physician's time.

The screening procedure and planning in advance allow for a detailed work-up of the chronic pain patient within a two to three day period. We do feel, and our results seem to justify our opinion, that the work-up of pain patients should not be spread over several weeks as is done in some pain units. It is more acceptable to the patient to experience two to three tiring and stressful days than to live through eight to twelve frustrating and costly weeks. Furthermore, the physicians involved will be more familiar with the compiled patient's data and the patient in a two day work-up period.

At the first interview, when a detailed medical and pain history is taken and a thorough physical examination is done, it is decided whether the appointments made with the various specialists have to be kept, can be cancelled, or whether (rarely) others have to be arranged for.

Our team is convinced that a standardized patient work-up scheme in each speciality, discussed and set up with all members, is essential for the work of a pain clinic, because otherwise team members cannot rely on what has been checked, tested, evaluated, and considered. Such a procedure is time- and money-saving, and avoids repetition of laboratory and radiological studies. Three to four specialists, including radiologists specially interested in pain problems, are usually consulted in our pain unit. Our studies on the neccessity of diagnostic procedures and consultations clearly demonstrated that more consultations did not add to the final diagnosis and are not to the patient's advantage.

After evaluation of all diagnostic information, and in close consultation with the specialists involved, a final diagnosis is made and a treatment plan, directed towards the total care of the patient, is arranged. In most cases with chronic pain a polymodal, multidimensional plan of therapy is chosen.

Some patients with very complex pain problems (about 7% at our pain clinic) will have to be presented to as many group members as possible. This is best achieved at a regularly held pain conference. Our weekly two hour meeting seems to be optimal. At this conference two to three patients can be interviewed and briefly examined, especially by members who have not been involved in this patient's care. The discussions most often lead to significant diagnostic and/or therapeutic proposals and aid towards the correct diagnosis. The conferences are also utilized to present short papers on special pain subjects in order to promote further training of members, guests, trainees, medical and psychology students, nurses and physiotherapists, and to stimulate interest in pain problems. About 40% of these pain patients are presented by their own physicians practicing outside the university hospital. Private physicians and staff from other hospitals eagerly seize the opportunity to become actively engaged with problem patients. This joint meeting serves as an excellent form of exchange of information on pain problems, diagnostic and therapeutic ideas of the various specialists, indications, limitations, and complications of various treatment modalities, ongoing clinical and basic research, and finally it helps group members to become a team.

We also feel that in a comprehensive pain center - in contrast to some syndrome oriented (e.g., headache) or modality oriented pain centers (e.g., operant conditioning) - some 80% of the chronic pain patients can and should be diagnosed and treated on a money-saving outpatient basis. Today in our pain unit, which is part of a university hospital (1900 beds), 55% of the patients evaluated are referred by university hospital facilities, 20% are sent by other hospitals and institutions, and 30% are referred by general practitioners and other specialists. No patient is accepted for evaluation and/or treatment unless referred by a physician.

We do accept all pain patients, in spite of our extensive screening procedure, because frequently the abnormal illness behavior is obvious, but quite obviously previous "diagnostic labels" are incorrect. Thus, we have to evaluate some patients in whom satisfactory treatment cannot be expected, such as unsettled compensation claims, chronic post herpetic neuralgia, pain states involving the whole body, and patients who have undergone, multiple surgical procedures for their pain.

Due to our way of thinking, due to limited space and personnel, we can only evaluate 550 problem patients suffering from chronic pain per year. Patients with acute pain referred to us with the label "intractable pain" have not yet been a therapeutic problem and are considered to be patients of the anesthesia department and not of the pain unit. It is characteristic for pain centers to record the number of previous outpatient appointments a patient has had for evaluation and treatment. Some 75% of our patients have had at least six visits, some 20% at least eleven appointments, and some 2.5% sixteen visits or more (e.g., cancer pain patients on a drug rotation schedule). We firmly believe that the total number of visits - and this is especially true for modality oriented pain centers - is directly related to the correct diagnosis. The time spent on the review and evaluation of the screening records and coordination procedure does save many diagnostic and treatment sessions later on.

PLANS FOR A MAJOR COMPREHENSIVE PAIN CENTER

In most established hospital settings the number of pain patients evaluated and treated is relatively limited by space, medical and supportive staff, and time. In order to provide the best treatment for patients with pain, the problem has to be tackled on a wide scale. Therefore, we now plan to take over a 100 bed hospital as a major comprehensive pain center. Physicians (anesthesiologists, general practitioners, neurosurgeons, orthopedic surgeons, psychiatrists, rheumatologists, and physiatrists) and psychologists who have been working in pain units for several years, will form the core group. A well-selected supportive staff of nurses, physical and occupational therapists, secretaries, and technicians will guarantee a well-organized center. This center will have wards for psychiatric-psychological evaluation and treatment, drug detoxification, orthopedic and neurological pain surgery, physical medicine and rehabilitation, and general pain and cancer pain diagnosis and treatment. A large outpatient facility is planned. Physicians, interested and already well-trained in the management of pain, of the university hospital and in private practice will be consultants. This pain center will provide all traditional and modern non-invasive and most invasive therapeutic modalities. In particular, the necessity for the rehabilitation of the pain patient will be emphasized. Clinical and basic research programs are presently being set-up. Our experience has shown that a pain center will work at its best when interdisciplinary studies are undertaken.

REFERENCES

(1) Alexander, F.A.D. 1954. The control of pain. In Anesthesiology, ed. D. Hale, pp. 579-610. Philadelphia: F.A. Davis.

(2) Baar, H.A., and Gerbershagen, H.U. 1974. Schmerz, Schmerzkrankheit, Schmerzklinik, pp. 49-78. Berlin-New York: Springer.

(3) Bonica, J.J. 1953. The Management of Pain. Philadelphia: Lea and Febiger.

(4) Bonica, J.J. 1974. Current status of pain clinics. In Interdisziplinäre Schmerzbehandlung, eds. R. Frey, J.J., Bonica, H.U. Gerbershagen, and D. Gross, pp. 83-95. Berlin-New York: Springer.

(5) Bonica, J.J. 1979. Important clinical aspects of acute and chronic pain. In Mechanisms of Pain and Analgesic Compounds, eds. R.F. Beers, Jr. and E.G. Bassett, pp. 15-29. New York: Raven Press.

(6) Bonica, J.J., and Black, R.G. 1974. The management of pain clinic. In Relief of Intractable Pain, ed. M. Swerdlow, pp. 116-129. Amsterdam-New York: Excerpta Medica.

(7) Committee on Pain Therapy, American Society of Anesthesiologists, 515 Busse Highway, Park Ridge, Il. 60068, USA.

(8) Gerbershagen, H.U.; Frey, R.; Magin, F.; Scholl, W.; and Müller-Suur, N. 1975. The pain clinic: an interdisciplinary team approach to the problem of pain. Brit. J. Anaesth. 47: 526-529.

(9) Gerbershagen, H.U.; Magin, F.; and Scholl, W. 1975. Die Schmerzklinik als neuer Aufgabenbereich für den Anästhesisten. Anästh. Inform. 16: 41-44.

(10) Howland, D.E., and Howland, L.A. 1987. An outpatient pain service. In Outpatient Anesthesia, ed. B.R. Brown, Jr., pp. 55-70. Philadelphia: F.A. Davis.

(11) Swerdlow, M. 1967. 4 years pain clinic experience. Anaesthesia 22: 568-574.

Pain and Society, eds. H.W. Kosterlitz and L.Y. Terenius, pp. 415-430.
Dahlem Konferenzen 1980. Weinheim: Verlag Chemie GmbH.

Stimulation Techniques in the Management of Pain

B. H. Sjölund and M. B. E. Eriksson
Department of Neurosurgery (Clinical Neurophysiology and Physiology), University of Lund
221 85 Lund, Sweden

Abstract. Dating back in history, stimulation techniques for pain relief have recently gained revived interest. Essential to the increasing use of such treatment have been the recent experimental findings of pain control mechanisms in animals and in man as well as the technological advances enabling the design of pocked-sized but still adequate stimulation equipment. Two main lines of approach have emerged: electrical (or mechanical) stimulation of peripheral tissues and direct stimulation of nervous structures belonging to pain control systems in the CNS. Still, however, long-term therapeutic success is more rare than failure, reflecting our insufficient knowledge of the control mechanisms and how to address them and also of the multi-dimensional problems of the pain patient.

INTRODUCTION

"For any type of gout, a live black torpedo should, when pain begins, be placed under the feet. The patient must stand on a moist shore by the sea, and he should stay like this until his whole foot and leg, up to the knee, is numbed. This takes away present pain and prevents pain for coming on if it has not already arisen" (Scribonius Largus, C.E. 46, (see (22)). Sensory stimulation for pain relief, even if performed with electrical fishes, is indeed an ancient technique (21). It is in the Far East, however, that we find the earliest notions of this kind. In the classical textbook of Oriental medicine Nei Ching from about B.C. 2600, there is already a description of acupunctural techniques, where different pathological conditions are claimed to be healed (=becoming painless?) by inserting and manipulating sharp, thin objects (bamboo sticks, fish bones) into certain points of the body tissues. Later on the art of acupuncture was usually performed with thin metal (bronze) needles inserted into very well defined points along a number of lines (meridians) on the body surface. An alternative was to heat the tissue by the burning of certain weeds (moxa) on the skin. In fact, similar methods of physically manipulating the tissues by suction or heat ("cupping") has been known from Western folk medicine since medieval times.

In France, at the beginning of the nineteenth century, needles were used as electrodes for discharging Leyden bottle condensors into the tissues to achieve pain relief. With the development of devices generating and storing electricity in the eighteenth and nineteenth centuries, "electroanalgesia" became widely used in Western countries to alleviate low-back pain, arthritis, toothache, and other chronic pain conditions, as well as the acute pain from tooth extraction and other surgical procedures. However, with the appearance of effective volatile anesthetic agents and of oral analgesics, the stimulation methods were gradually forgotten, probably because they gave a varying and unpredictable therapeutic response. Moreover, the equipment used was non-portable and often insufficient.

It is everyday knowledge that non-painful sensory stimulation of several kinds can divert our attention from nociceptive stimuli. To rub a painful part of the skin or to massage an aching muscle group are pain relieving measures probably as old as man. As regards the distracting or pain alleviating effect of a painful stimulus in itself, several reports have appeared on the use of counter-irritation for analgesia (29) as well as on "pain free" states in man (6), and in animals (footshock analgesia) (7) elicited by weak painful stimuli. Sensory inflow via other modalities also influences the perception of painful stimuli under certain circumstances, e.g., the pleasant earphone music or white noise as used in dentistry ("audio analgesia," see (32)). Furthermore, the individual obviously selects internally what attention should be paid to one or the other kind of sensory, even noxious stimuli received. With increasing knowledge of the control mechanisms behind the above-mentioned phenomena it will be, and is in fact already, possible to address some of them in an artificial manner.

From a general point of view, mechanisms that interrupt or modulate the transmission of a nociceptive input may act at any level in the paths from the nociceptors to the cerebral cortex. In addition, the perception of, and the reaction to, the pain stimulus message may be influenced by mechanisms acting at cortical and hypothalamic limbic levels. Indeed, the knowledge of such control mechanisms is still fragmentary, even if data accumulating during the last decade have dramatically increased our understanding (see (5,28) and this symposium). This rapid development was initiated by a series of circumstances, notably the postulates of the now classical gate control theory (31), the findings of Reynolds (38) on analgesia from brain stem stimulation, and the revival of acupunctural techniques during the Chinese cultural revolution with its impact on Western observers (20). The interest in this field was further promoted by the identification of the endogenous opioids ((17) and see (50)), which may well participate in pain controlling mechanisms. Basic and clinical research has already resulted in a number of therapeutically useful stimulation techniques for pain alleviation, i.e., for activation of endogenous control mechanisms mainly by electrical stimulation of peripheral or central nervous structures.

STIMULATION OF PERIPHERAL STRUCTURES

Conventional Transcutaneous Nerve Stimulation (TNS)

After the proposal of a spinal gating mechanism that would inhibit the transmission from thin pain afferents to relay cells with increasing input via course tactile afferents, it was a logical step to electrically stimulate large diameter afferents in chronic pain patients to achieve analgesia. Large diameter afferents have a low activation threshold on electrical stimulation as compared to small diameter afferents (18) since the inner longitudinal resistance varies inversely with the fiber diameter. Hence, it is possible to selectively activate large diameter afferents by low intensity electrical pulses delivered via electrodes placed over nerve branches (on the skin). The first attempt to perform such stimulation was partly successful (54), but the technique was soon abandoned in favor of implantation techniques (see below). However, further trials proved the transcutaneous nerve stimulation (TNS) method clinically useful (33,42), and very soon equipment for such stimulation became commercially available.

The first stimulators usually produced pulses of constant voltage, i.e., the stimulus charge was dependent on the impedance presented by the electrode-patient-electrode circuit. A number of mono- and biphasic waveforms were tried, with, however, no convincing proof that any was superior to a simple monophasic rectangular pulse as regards pain relief, tolerable stimulation paresthesia, or minimum energy optimization (37). A problem related to that of impedance load is the design of electrodes for TNS. After initial trials with metal discs, most manufacturers turned to conductive elastomers coated with highly conductive gel. This design has the advantage of conforming well to the skin surface and of providing some longitudinal resistance in the electrode proper, preventing sudden high current densities when the skin-electrode contact is altered with movements, etc. Unfortunately, however, there are significant capacitive impedance components of the electrode-skin interface and of the skin, resulting in no less than 1000-2500 ohms total load at the effective frequencies of commonly used waveforms (1-10 kHz) ((37) and own unpublished observations). This load must thus be taken into consideration when designing the stimulator output, as must the minimum effective pulse width and charge per pulse for stimulation of large fiber afferents. Linzer and Long (24) found the minimum effective width to be about 50-150 µs and the charge per pulse to be 1-7 µA.s in twenty-three carefully studied patients with good to excellent pain relief from TNS. Taken together, these data indicate that an "ideal" TNS-stimulator should provide monophasic rectangular pulses of preferably 150 µs duration, each containing up to 7 µA.s into 2500 ohms, which would demand a maximum output current of 50 mA into 2500 ohms. To allow conditions with a stable charge per pulse and calibration of the amplitude control, the output circuit should be of constant current design (42). Stimulators with specifications of this kind have only recently come into general use which may explain some of the early therapeutic failures encountered (see below).

During the last five years a number of follow-up studies have been published on the use of TNS for pain alleviation in chronic pain conditions. The results of TNS treatment appear to vary markedly (Table 1), undoubtedly mainly due to selection of patients, criteria of success, and lack of characterization of stimulus parameters.

TABLE 1. - Long-term success rate with conventional TNS in chronic pain.

Authors	No. of patients	Continuing treatment after < 1 month	2-6 months	12 months
Cauthen & Renner, 1975 (9)	113		32%	
Ebersold et al., 1975 (10)	230	60%	35%	
Loeser et al., 1975 (25)	198	68%		12.5%
Long & Hagfors, 1975 (27)	~3000		25-30%	
Long, 1976 (26)	197?			38%

It is interesting to observe that the most effective pain relief seems to be produced when the patient feels stimulation paresthesia in the painful area proper, either by placing the electrodes over a nerve branch from that area/dermatome or on either side of it (13), indicating that the control mechanism has a "local sign." Such paresthesia cannot readily be produced in visceral structures, and visceral pain is, as a rule, not susceptible to TNS treatment. It is also necessary to fulfill the charge per pulse conditions (above) to ensure that a sufficient number of large diameter fibers be activated. Empirically this means a still not painful stimulus current of 2-3 times that at perception threshold (13).

The stimulation frequency selected by the patients is most commonly 10-100 Hz (14,37), which is well within the physiological range for these afferents. However, such signal frequencies probably occur only for very short periods of time under normal conditions, whereas the patients may use stimulation from 10 minutes a day up to almost continuous stimulation. This variation of the length of the stimulation periods reflects the duration of the "poststimulation analgesia" (12,27). In fact, the mere existence of this phenomenon necessitates additional postulates to the gate control theory (such as reverberation mechanisms or slow temporary changes in synaptic efficiency) or may indicate other mechanisms of action of TNS. Thus, it has been suggested that TNS might produce pain relief by activating nociceptive fibers, inducing fatigue and conduction failure (49). In fact, spontaneous activity in Aδ fibers from experimental neuromas (53) can be silenced by high frequency electrical stimulation. However, the fact that patients do not experience pain from TNS argues against the view that a significant number of nociceptive afferents are stimulated. Moreover, conditions other than neuromata are alleviated by this treatment. For example, several acute pain conditions, such as postoperative and childbirth pain, have been shown to respond significantly to TNS treatment (4,52). Most reports, however, have dealt with chronic "benign" pain such as neuralgia, rhizalgia, dorsalgia, and pain after lesions in the CNS. Common to these reports (Table 1) is the fact that even if 2/3 of the patients report satisfactory pain relief at the start of treatment, this figure drops rapidly to 1/3 or less within 6-12 months. This may be due to the fact that some patients cannot at first distinguish a mere distracting effect of stimulation from true pain relief. In addition, there may be an initial placebo effect of TNS as with any other pain treatment. In a prospective study of the pain relief from TNS versus that from placebo, however, the pain relief from stimulation was significantly greater (51). Unfortunately, no prospective randomized studies have been performed to date, where the pain relief from stimulation treatment has been compared to that from pharmacological or surgical pain treatment.

Obviously then, TNS in its present form is not an ideal method for pain relief. Vital to further development of this treatment is of course to clarify its mechanism of action in man. In a double blind study on patients with chronic pain, we found no inhibition of the pain relief induced by conventional TNS by administration of the opioid antagonist naloxone (45), indicating that endogenous opioid peptides do not participate in pain relief from conditioning stimulation of cutaneous large diameter afferents. Few experimental investigations have been made on the effect of TNS on sensory perception thresholds or on changes in experimental pain tolerance. To date, no or only a weak (transient) increase of the pain threshold has been reported, whereas hyperesthesia seems to be reduced (3,8,22,40). Simultaneously, tactile thresholds appear to be markedly increased. To clarify this point further, we are currently studying the influence of TNS on the thermal sense in man, assuming that spinothalamic cells mediating temperature are subject to control mechanisms similar to those mediating pain. In preliminary experiments we found bilateral, often long-standing decreases in thermal sensitivity after TNS (11). Still, however, few hard data bridge the gap between the clinically produced pain relief and the characterization of the underlying mechanisms.

Acupuncture, Electroacupuncture, and Acupuncture-like TNS

In acupuncture treatment, needles are inserted through very well-defined points on the body surface into the subcutaneous tissue (20). These points show a remarkable correlation to so-called trigger points which can be mechanically manipulated to precipitate or relieve pain in various regions (organs) (30), but the morphological substrate for these effects is highly uncertain. The needles inserted are either manipulated manually or used as electrodes for stimulation of the tissue with a current usually of low frequency (1-4 Hz). Local muscle contractions are often seen around the needles and it has been claimed that an afferent input from deep structures (muscle?) is necessary for the effect (see ((20)). After 15-20 minutes, a feeling (te-ch'i) of soreness is produced and pain relief is sometimes experienced. Several well-controlled studies have shown an increase in the experimental pain threshold after acupuncture (2,28,48), even if a marked inter-individual variation seems to exist. Andersson and co-workers (2,3) found that to achieve an increase in pain threshold with electroacupuncture, it is unnecessary to insert needles; rather large surface electrodes can be used provided that the current applied is sufficient to evoke muscle contractions in related segments (myotomes). Unfortunately, when tried in chronic pain patients, the high intensity low frequency stimulation (Fig. 1 B) was usually not tolerated, and hence the analgesia produced was not sufficient. To overcome this problem we have introduced a new kind of peripheral conditioning stimulation (12,14) where nerves to myotomes segmentally related to the painful area are stimulated with brief tetani, still at a low repetition rate (Fig. 1 C). It is then possible to achieve forceful muscle contraction at a tolerable stimulation intensity using standard TNS surface electrodes. By using this method (acupuncture-like TNS) when the conventional TNS does not give sufficient pain relief, it has been possible to improve the overall long-term results of TNS by 40% (14). However, about 50% of the patients with chronic pain from somatic origin still fail to get satisfactory pain relief for long-term use.

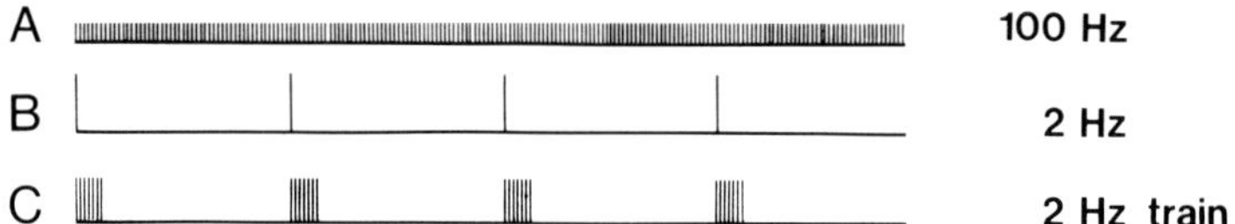

Fig. 1 - Different kinds of peripheral conditioning stimulation for pain relief. Note differences in amplitude (see text).

Following the demonstration by Mayer et al. (see (28)) that the increase in experimental pain threshold after needle acupuncture was reversed by the opioid antagonist naloxone indicating that endogenous opioid peptides participate in the underlying mechanisms, we found in double blind experiments that the pain relief caused by acupuncture-like TNS in chronic pain patients is likewise counteracted by low doses of naloxone, whereas that from conventional TNS is not (43,45). From measurements of the CSF content of opioid peptides before and after stimulation, it would appear that these values seem to increase locally at the level of the segment of stimulation (44,47). This notion of a spinal, opioid-mediated action of acupunctural or acupuncture-like stimulation has recently been confirmed in animal experiments, where a suppression of the transmission from C-fibers to motoneurons in spinal cats was observed for several hours after a period of conditioning low frequency stimulation of group III muscle afferents (46).

Other Forms of Peripheral Stimulation

As mentioned previously, pain relief can also be produced by painless and painful physical manipulations. As regards non-painful stimulation, it should be considered a distinct possibility that physical therapy and massage may activate central control mechanisms similar to those activated by electrical stimulation and acupuncture.

With painful stimuli, as in various forms of counter-irritation (15,29), many reports exist of pain relief long outlasting the period of stimulation. Here, we may deal either with a very powerful activation of the same mechanisms as are underlying TNS and acupuncture or with specialized negative feedback loops for pain inhibition (5) which may come into play in dangerous stress situations. Such loops would have a high "survival value" and may well persist in man.

CENTRAL STIMULATION

A technology for implanting stimulators in tissues is well developed due to the widespread use of pacemakers. Special problems pertaining to the CNS exist with respect to electrolysis, scar formation (gliosis), and initiation of epileptic fits (kindling) (36), as well as the risks of infection, hemorrhage, and dislocation of electrodes.

Dorsal Column Stimulation (DCS)

After the initial observations of Wall and Sweet (54), methods were devised to implant electrodes near the dorsal funiculi in man, the purpose being to activate many branches of large diameter cutaneous afferents simultaneously in the antidromic direction. This would create an intense barrage at the segmental level and effectively "close the gate." From an initial enthusiasm with many implants (35), the use of this method has gradually become more restricted with a careful selection of patients including psychiatric evaluation and a period of test stimulation with non-permanent electrodes (41). In fact, properly applied TNS should replace DCS in most instances (14).

For practical purposes, the patients considered should be those in whom a sufficient number of afferents cannot be stimulated due to the cause or the location of the pain (cf. (34)). As with conventional TNS, a condition for pain relief seems to be that paresthesia is felt in the painful area. Also in other respects, the properties of this treatment resemble those of conventional TNS (cf. above).

On the other hand, it cannot be excluded that fibers other than those ascending in the dorsal funiculi are stimulated with DCS. Should this be the case, pain relief may be caused by stimulation of descending control systems (5). However, the available clinical evidence does not support this notion.

Intracranial Stimulation

Chronic stimulation of deep brain structures for pain relief was first reported by Hosobuchi et al. (see (1)), using the sensory thalamus as target, and by Richardson and Akil (39), using the periventricular gray matter for the same purpose. The former method was based on clinical observations during stereotactic thalamotomy for pain relief, where the stimulation used for the localization procedure was sometimes found to create longlasting pain relief. Initially, five patients with severe anesthesia dolorosa of the face had electrodes implanted in the ventroposteromedial nucleus of the thalamus and four of these reported satisfactory pain relief from intermittent stimulation. With increasing experience, this treatment has been used for different kinds of chronic pain and particularly that due to presumed lesions of sensory paths in the nervous system. Such pain ("deafferentation pain") often responds poorly to opioids (Hosobuchi, personal communication) or to non-opioid analgesics and is a major clinical problem. However, about half of these patients respond well to stimulation, whereas those with pain after thalamic infarction ("thalamic syndrome") often do not experience sufficient relief even if the electrodes are placed in the posterior limb of the internal capsule (1). The mechanism of pain relief, when present, is completely unknown.

A different approach, emanating from results of animal experimentation on descending control systems from the brain stem periaqueductal area (5), was made by Richardson and Akil (39). They stimulated the corresponding structures in man, creating pain relief but also untoward effects such as vertigo and nausea. By moving the electrode more rostrally, into the vicinity of the gray matter surrounding the posterior part of the third ventricle, pain relief without side effects could be produced in 6 out of 8 of their first patients, usually concomitant with a decreased sensitivity to experimental pain (39). There is preliminary evidence that this form of stimulation-evoked analgesia is brought about by release of opioid peptides, as evidenced by naloxone tests and direct measurements of the CSF content of opioid peptides (1,39,50). Furthermore, the patients responding best seem to be those with satisfactory relief from exogenous opioids (Hosobuchi, personal communication). Interestingly, tolerance to the stimulation frequently appears, but this can be counteracted by temporarily interrupting the treatment or by administration of the serotonin precursor l-tryptophan (19), indicating that serotonergic fibers participate in this effect. The pain relief usually outlasts the stimulation which is not associated with sensory paresthesia aside from an occasional feeling of warmth (1). However, the clinical use of this treatment has recently been questioned by Gybels (16), who has not been able to reproduce the abovementioned results in spite of seemingly identical electrode localizations.

CONCLUDING REMARKS

To summarize, it is evident that our use of stimulation techniques for alleviation of pain is still inadequate in many respects. First of all, our knowledge of the underlying mechanisms is fragmentary or even nonexisting. Second, we probably do not know the most appropriate methods to address these mechanisms. Third, the design and biocompatibility of the stimulation equipment is not optimal. Fourth and perhaps most important, the criteria for proper selection of patients for the use of stimulation treatment in clinical practice have yet to be defined.

Acknowledgements. Supported by the Swedish Medical Research Council (proj. no. 05658 to B.S.) and by Greta and Johan Kocks Foundations.

REFERENCES

(1) Adams, J.E.; Hosobuchi, Y.; and Linchitz, R. 1977. The present status of implantable intracranial stimulators for pain. Clin Neurosurg. 24: 347-361.

(2) Andersson, S.A.; Ericson, T.; Holmgren, E.; and Lindqvist G. 1973. Electro-acupuncture. Effect on pain threshold measured with electrical stimulation of teeth. Brain Res. 63: 393-396.

(3) Andersson, S.A., and Holmgren, E. 1976. Pain threshold effects of peripheral conditioning stimulation. In Advances in Pain Research and Therapy, eds. J.J. Bonica and D. Albe-Fessard, vol. 1, pp. 761-768. New York: Raven Press.

(4) Augustinsson, L.-E.; Bohlin, P.; Bundsen, P.; Carlsson, C.-A.; Forssman, L.; Sjöberg, P.; and Tyreman, N.O. 1977. Pain relief during delivery by transcutaneous electrical nerve stimulation. Pain 4: 59-65.

(5) Basbaum, A.I., and Fields, H.L. 1978. Endogenous pain control mechanisms: Review and hypothesis. Annals Neurol. 4: 451-462.

(6) Beecher, H.K. 1959. Measurement of subjective responses. Oxford University Press.

(7) Buckett, W.R. 1979. Peripheral stimulation in mice induces short duration analgesia preventable by naloxone. Eur. J. Pharmacol. 58: 169-178.

(8) Callaghan, M.; Sternbach, R.A.; Nyqvist, J.K.; and Timmermans, G. 1978. Changes in somatic sensitivity during transcutaneous electrical analgesia. Pain 5: 115-127.

(9) Cauthen, J.C., and Renner, E.J. 1975. Transcutaneous and peripheral nerve stimulation for chronic pain states. Surg. Neurol. 4: 102-104.

(10) Ebersold, M.J.; Laws, E.R.; Stonnington, H.H.; and Stilwell, G.K. 1975. Transcutaneous electrical stimulation for treatment of chronic pain. A preliminary report. Surg. Neurol. 4: 96-99.

(11) Eriksson, M.B.E; Rosén, I.; and Sjölund, B.H. 1980. Thermal sensitivity is decreased by a central mechanism after transcutaneous nerve stimulation. Submitted.

(12) Eriksson, M.B.E., and Sjölund, B.H. 1976. Acupuncturelike electroanalgesia in TNS-resistant chronic pain. In Sensory Functions of the Skin, ed. Y. Zotterman, pp. 575-581. Oxford and New York: Pergamon Press.

(13) Eriksson, M.B.E., and Sjölund, B.H. 1979. Transkutane Nervenstimulierung für Schmerzlinderung, pp. 1-111. Heidelberg: Edwald Fischer Verlag für Medizin.

(14) Eriksson, M.B.E.; Sjölund, B.H.; and Nielzén, S. 1979. Long term results of peripheral conditioning stimulation as an analgesic measure in chronic pain. Pain 6: 335-347.

(15) Gammon, G.D., and Starr, I. 1941. Studies on the relief of pain by counterirritation. J clin. Invest. 20: 13-20.

(16) Gybels, J. 1979. Electrical stimulation of the central gray for pain relief in humans: A critical review. In Advances in Pain Research and Therapy, ed. J.J. Bonica, vol. 3, pp. 499-509. New York: Raven Press.

(17) Hughes, J.; Smith, T.W.; Kosterlitz, H.W.; Fothergill, L. A.; Morgan, B.A.; and Morris, H.R. 1975. Identification of two related pentapeptides from the brain with potent opiate agonist activity. Nature 258: 577-579.

(18) Hill, A.V. 1936. Strength-duration relation for electric exitation of medullated nerve. Proc. Roy. Soc. 119: 440-453.

(19) Hosobuchi, Y. 1978. Tryptophan reversal of tolerance to analgesia induced by central grey stimulation. The Lancet II:47

(20) Kaada, B.; Hoel, E.; Leseth, K.; Nygaard-Östby, B.; Setekleiv, J.; and Stovner, J. 1974. Acupuncture analgesia in the People's Republic of China. T. Norsk Laegeforen. 94: 417-442.

(21) Kane, K., and Taub, A. 1975. A history of local electrical analgesia. Pain 1: 125-138.

(22) Kellaway, P. 1946. The part played by electric fish in the early history of bioelectricity and electrotherapy. Bull. Hist. Med. 20: 112-137.

(23) Lindblom, U., and Meyerson, B.A. 1975. Influence on touch, vibration and cutaneous pain of dorsal column stimulation in man. Pain 1: 257-270.

(24) Linzer, M., and Long, D.M. 1976. Transcutaneous neural stimulation for relief of pain. IEEE Trans. Biomed. Eng. BME-23: 341-345.

(25) Loeser, J.D.; Black, R.G.; and Christman, A. 1975. Relief of pain by transcutaneous stimulation. J. Neurosurg. 42: 308-314.

(26) Long, D.M. 1976. Cutaneous afferent stimulation for the relief of pain. Progr. Neurol. Surg. 7: 35-51.

(27) Long, D.M., and Hagfors, N. 1975. Electrical stimulation in the nervous system: the current status of electrical stimulation of the nervous system for relief of pain. Pain 1: 109-123.

(28) Mayer, D.J., and Price, D.D. 1976. Central nervous system mechanisms of analgesia. Pain 2: 379-404.

(29) Melzack, R. 1975. Prolonged relief of pain by brief, intense transcutaneous somatic stimulation. Pain 1: 357-373.

(30) Melzack, R.; Stilwell, D.M.; and Fow, E.J. 1977. Trigger points and acupuncture points for pain: correlations and implications. Pain 3: 3-23.

(31) Melzack, R., and Wall, P.D. 1965. Pain mechanisms: a new theory. Science, 150: 971-979.

(32) Melzack, R.; Weisz, A.Z.; and Sprague, L.T. 1963. Stratagems for controlling pain: contributions of auditory stimulation and suggestion. Exp. Neurol. 8: 239-247.

(33) Meyer, G.A., and Fields, H.L. 1972. Causalgia treated by selective large fibre stimulation of peripheral nerve. Brain 95: 163-168.

(34) Miles, J., and Lipton, S. 1978. Phantom limb pain treated by electrical stimulation. Pain 5: 373-382.

(35) Nielson, K.D.; Adams, J.E.; and Hosobuchi, Y. 1975. Experience with dorsal column stimulation for relief of chronic intractable pain. Surg. Neurol. 4: 148-152.

(36) Pudenz, R.H.; Bullara, L.A.; Jacques, S.; and Hambrecht, F.T. 1975. Electrical stimulation of the brain. III. The neural damage model. Surg. Neurol. 4: 389-400.

(37) Ray, C.D., and Maurer, D.D. 1975. Electrical neurological stimulation systems: A review of contemporary methodology. Surg. Neurol. 4: 82-90.

(38) Reynolds, D.V. 1969. Surgery in the rat during electrical analgesia induced by focal brain stimulation. Science 164: 444.

(39) Richardson, D.E., and Akil, H. 1977. Pain reduction by electrical brain stimulation in man. Part 2. Chronic self-administration in the periventricular gray matter. J. Neurosurg. 47: 184-194.

(40) Satran, R., and Goldstein, M.N. 1973. Pain perception: Modification of threshold of intolerance and cortical potentials by cutaneous stimulation. Science 180: 1201-1202.

(41) Shealy, C.N. 1975. Dorsal column stimulation: Optimization of application. Surg. Neurol. 4: 142-145.

(42) Shealy, C.N., and Maurer, D. 1974. Transcutaneous nerve stimulation for control of pain. A preliminary technical note. Surg. Neurol. 2: 45-47.

(43) Sjölund, B.H., and Eriksson, M.B.E. 1976. Electro-acupuncture and endogenous morphines. The Lancet II: 1085.

(44) Sjölund, B.H., and Eriksson, M.B.E. 1979. Endorphins and analgesia produced by peripheral conditioning stimulation. In Advances in Pain Research and Therapy, ed. J.J. Bonica, vol. 3, pp. 587-592. New York: Raven Press.

(45) Sjölund, B.H., and Eriksson, M.B.E. 1979. The influence of naloxone on analgesia produced by peripheral conditioning stimulation. Brain Res. 173: 295-301.

(46) Sjölund, B.H., and Eriksson, M.B.E. 1979. Naloxone-reversible depression of C-fiber evoked flexion reflex in low spinal cats after conditioning electrical stimulation of primary afferents. Neurosci. Lett. suppl. 3: 264.

(47) Sjölund, B.H.; Terenius, L.; and Eriksson, M.B.E. 1977. Increased cerebrospinal fluid levels of endorphins after electro-acupuncture. Acta Physiol. Scand. 100: 382-384.

(48) Stewart, D.; Thomson, J.; and Oswald, I. 1977. Acupuncture analgesia: an experimental investigation. Brit. Med. J. 1: 67-70.

(49) Taub, A., and Campbell, J.N. 1974. Percutaneous local electrical analgesia: peripheral mechanisms. In Advances of Neurology, ed. J.J. Bonica, vol. 4, pp. 727-735. New York: Raven Press.

(50) Terenius, L., and Wahlström, A. 1978. Physiological and clinical relevance of endorphins. In Centrally Acting Peptides, ed. J. Hughes, pp. 161-178. London: The Macmillan Press Ltd.

(51) Thorsteinsson, G.; Stonnington, H.H.; Stilwell, G.K.; and Elveback, L.R. 1978. The placebo effect of transcutaneous electrical stimulation. Pain 5: 31-41.

(52) Van der Ark, G.D., and McGrath, K.A. 1975. Transcutaneous electrical stimulation in treatment of postoperative pain. Am. J. Surg. 130: 338-340.

(53) Wall, P.D., and Gutnick, M. 1974. Properties of afferent nerve impulses originating from a neuroma. Nature 248: 740-743.

(54) Wall, P.D., and Sweet, W.H. 1967. Temporary abolition of pain in man. Science 155: 108-109.

Pain and Society, eds. H.W. Kosterlitz and L.Y. Terenius, pp. 431-444.
Dahlem Konferenzen 1980. Weinheim: Verlag Chemie GmbH.

Psychological Techniques in the Management of Pain

R. A. Sternbach
Pain Treatment Center, Scripps Clinic and Research Foundation
La Jolla, CA 92037, USA

Abstract. Current psychological techniques in the management of pain share certain concepts with the new trends in behavioral medicine. Behavioral analyses and behavior modification techniques are applied to diagnosis, treatment, rehabilitation, and prevention of disease. Pain treatment programs typically share in each of these processes, and include modification of chronic pain behaviors, drug withdrawal or detoxification programs, physical rehabilitation, and operant conditioning of physiological processes related to the pain syndrome. More traditional techniques include hypnosis, group therapy, and the use of psychotropic medications, but even these are somewhat modified for specific applications to pain problems. There are special difficulties associated with understanding hypnotic mechanisms, recidivism, abnormal illness behavior, and coping with socioeconomic forces which promote perpetual pain disability.

INTRODUCTION

The application of psychological techniques in treating or helping to control pain is but one instance of a larger movement of the use of behavioral methods in medicine. In order to set the proper context for the particular instance, we should first make some remarks about the general behavioral movement.

THE NEW BEHAVIORAL MEDICINE

Behavioral medicine refers to the application of behavioral sciences to medical problems. It derives from the successful use of conditioning principles in understanding and treating problems of learning and the application of these to other areas, such as the modification of maladaptive (psychiatric) behaviors. Both Pavlovian (respondent) and Skinnerian (operant) conditioning principles are applied in the analyses of behaviors. Behavioral analyses and behavior modification techniques can be and are increasingly used in the diagnosis, prevention, treatment, and rehabilitation of diseases.

Behavioral medicine is wide-ranging. It has been used in crises to stop infantile projectile vomiting, adolescent anorexia nervosa, and senile inappropriate behavior. It has been used in rehabilitation programs to correct foot drop and teach sphincter control in stroke and spinal cord injury patients. It has been used to foster patient compliance in chronic management programs of diabetes, coronary disease, and renal dialysis. programs. It has been used in weight control, aerobic, and anti-smoking preventive health programs, and it has been used as well in the treatment of muscle contraction and vascular headaches, Raynaud's disease, colitis and functional bowel disorders, spasmodic torticollis, and various chronic pain states.

The essence of the behavioral approach is that illness (or pain) behavior is, like any behavior, governed by its consequences. That is, it can be enhanced, maintained, or extinguished by the appropriate delivery of (or witholding of) positive, negative, or aversive reinforcers. The behavioral analyst determines what the reinforcers and contingencies are and proposes a conditioning or learning or desensitization schedule that is most appropriate under the circumstances.

There is a clear distinction if not actual opposition between behavioral medicine and psychosomatic medicine. Psychosomatic medicine derived from the psychoanalytic tradition and attempted to emphasize the whole person with a disease, in opposition to the narrow specialization in medicine in the 1930s and 1940s which studied diseases at the expense of the whole person. Psychosomatic medicine was "holistic" several generations ago. However, the movement has always been psychodynamically oriented and emphasized the psychogenic factors in all illness: the personality types susceptible to ulcers, hives, asthma, etc., or the psychodynamic conflicts and mechanisms that resulted in such illness. The assumption was that with such analyses, psychodynamic therapy would cure or ameliorate the underlying unconscious pathology, and then the external symptoms would resolve.

Behavioral medicine, on the other hand, is more empirical and relatively a-theoretical. Inner mechanisms are not postulated. Rather than changing the inner person (underlying pathology) to relieve symptoms, the symptoms themselves are modified directly, and any generalization of improvement is assumed to benefit the inner person, although this is a secondary or incidental effect. Thus, whereas the psychosomatic approach might diagnose a case of migraine as reflecting repressed rage against mother and attempt long-term psychodynamic therapy to resolve the symptom, the behavioral approach would treat the migraine with short-term biofeedback training and, with evidence that symptom-substitution is quite uncommon, assume that the patient's relationships with mother might have improved.

The increasing popularity of behavioral medicine is in large part due to its efficiency. Psychosomatic medicine has long been known not only for its interesting psychodynamic formulations, but also for its ineffectiveness in producing meaningful changes in symptoms. Behavioral medicine, on the other hand, produces quite boring analyses and treatment paradigms, but large numbers of successful results with relatively brief treatments.

With these generalizations about behavioral medicine to set the context, we can now describe specific application of these principles to the problems of patients with pain.

BEHAVIORAL DIAGNOSTIC TECHNIQUES IN PAIN

For many years, psychiatrists and psychologists have struggled with ways to answer the question, "Is this pain in this patient organic or functional in origin?" Aside from the difficulties inherent in assuming such a dualism, it has proved very difficult to apportion weights to psychogenic and to organic factors. Partly this is because one can always find, in retrospect, potential psychodynamic rationales for psychogenic pain in almost any patient; and partly, because the effects of organic pain on the psyche are quite similar in manifestation to that which one finds in pain-prone (psychogenic) patients.

The behavioral approach is much simpler. The questions to be answered are, What are the pain behaviors (signs of pain)? What maintains these? Which are respondent (reflex-like) behaviors which appear elicited by an organic pain generator, and which are operant pain behaviors which are maintained by environmental contingent reinforcers (e.g., bedrest, social attention, narcotics, disability income, etc.).

Although early behaviorists may have denied the role of innate drives or motives in behavior, recent studies by ethologists, personality theorists, and others have shown that such modern equivalents of the "instincts" must be considered in any comprehensive view of the person. For example, Craig (2) has shown that social modeling has a significant effect not merely on pain tolerance, but on autonomic responses to noxious stimuli. Presumably, this involves perceptual and cognitive processes which go beyond simple conditioning.

But the modern behaviorist, more pragmatic and empirical, is not concerned with such theoretical considerations and would merely incorporate such findings in his behavioral analysis. Assuming that most of a particular patient's pain behavior is maintained by such social reinforcers as described, the behaviorist would plan to control such reinforcers so as to make their delivery contingent upon healthy, pain-incompatible behavior. A pain-tolerant role model might be introduced to help elicit such behavior from the patient in order to permit a more rapid learning process. In other words, there is no denial of intrapsychic, cognitive, affective, or motivational factors, but because of the relative ineffectiveness of psychosomatic (psychodynamic) formulations and therapy and the success of behavior therapy, these factors are considered simply less relevant than formerly.

BEHAVIORAL TREATMENT TECHNIQUES FOR CHRONIC PAIN

Fordyce (5) has made the most systematic presentation of the application of behavioral principles to pain rehabilitation and management, and these are now used in many if not most of the inpatient pain treatment programs in the United States.

Operant Conditioning of Pain Behavior

Pain behaviors are usually expressions of suffering which normally elicit expressions of sympathy and support from others, for example, grimaces, gasps or moaning, staggering gait, requests for pain relief, withdrawal from social interactions, remaining bedfast, etc. Experience has shown that these behaviors extinguish when they are ignored, as they are usually maintained by attention from others. When social attention is given instead to the patient in response only to healthy, pain-incompatible behaviors (e.g., normal conversations, exercises, participating in work projects, etc.), the latter occur more frequently, and pain behaviors occur with decreasing frequency (4).

Narcotic overuse occurs because, in part, tolerance to narcotics develops, and in part because narcotics are taken in response to pain increases, and as positive reinforcers, thus make more likely subsequent increases in pain. Therefore, drug withdrawal is started by giving the analgesics on a clock schedule rather than on demand. This breaks the association between pain increases and narcotic intake. Then, with amount or dosage of analgesic kept from the patient's knowledge (in a capsule or liquid masking vehicle), the strength is so gradually reduced that the patient is unaware of any withdrawal symptoms and experiences no anxiety as well. Almost always, patients experience some reduction in pain levels with withdrawal.

Many patients with chronic pain become relatively inactive and thus deconditioned, showing both loss of muscle tone and obesity. Physical therapy would not be effective if it were regularly followed by an increase in pain. Thus the behavioral approach to exercise (or any pain-limited activity) is not to work to tolerance, that is to a point which causes pain to become more severe, but to establish a time or exercise quota which is below tolerance, so that the patient can stop before a pain increase occurs. Thus accomplishment is rewarded by rest, not punished by pain. Quotas can be increased very gradually to an optimal level, always staying within tolerance limits.

Weight loss can be similarly treated. It is not enough merely to prescribe a diet. Eating behavior must be shaped, so that snacking is extinguished, special places and times and ways of eating are reinforced, and changes are made sufficiently gradually that neither hunger nor anxiety are increased.

As pain behavior is gradually extinguished and physical conditioning and socialization are improved, the patient is shedding the role of chronic invalid. This can be done more effectively if there are explicit career-like goals of the patient's own choosing toward which the rehabilitation effort is directed. It is not enough to give up invalidism; some other rewarding role must replace it, and this must be specified in advance and worked at during treatment.

Biofeedback

The specific application of operant procedures to physiological processes is termed biofeedback. Any function which can be detected, transduced, amplified, and displayed instantaneously and continuously to the patient can be brought under voluntary control. In practice, striped muscle, smooth muscle, and cardiovascular variables are the more frequently used, especially as part of pain treatment programs. Electromyographic biofeedback of frontalis or cervical paraspinal muscles is routinely used in many centers as the treatment of choice for muscle contraction headaches and/or the sustained muscle contractions due to "whiplash" injuries or torticollis. Similar treatment is used for muscle spasms and cramping elsewhere, as in lumbosacral strain, and for general relaxation training. Gastrointestinal biofeedback has been used for painful cramping associated with colitis and functional bowel disease. And digital plethysmography or temperature feedback has been shown successful in treating both vascular headaches and Raynaud's disease (13).

There is a long history of animal research showing that such physiological functions, even including single motor units and single cortical cells, can be brought under "voluntary" control, that is, their activity can be emitted by the organism in connection with response-contingent reinforcement. In the human patient, the reinforcement apparently consists in the satisfaction of making a response in the desired direction of decreased or increased activity, knowing that such will result in pain relief. Reinforcers are usually more effective if they immediately follow a response. Thus biofeedback training can be relatively efficient because feedback of responses is instantaneous and continuous.

A similar system, but one perhaps not quite as efficient, is the well-known autogenic training. In this method, which is rather like hypnotic auto-suggestion, patients repeat phrases such as "My hands are heavy and warm," and vividly imagine holding their hands in front of a fire, or in a tub of hot water. This technique has been shown effective for conditions similar to those treated by biofeedback, and in many centers the two methods have been combined for greater efficiency. The use of autogenic phrases and imagery helps patients make the initial desired responses sooner; the feedback from the instrumentation reinforces these responses quickly and speeds the rate of learning.

Hypnosis

As we have mentioned hypnosis, it is appropriate to consider it here. Hypnosis of course has long been used in the control of pain, both chronic and acute, and there is an enormous anecdotal clinical literature. Only recently has there been any attempt at systematic investigation of hypnotic analgesia. A recent review of clinical and experimental studies (9) confirms that it is a genuine phenomenon whose effectiveness is in part dependent upon the patient's hypnotic responsiveness, which is approximately normally distributed in the population. Thus approximately 20% will get little or no analgesic effect, and 20% will get an excellent result, with the others showing mixed or inconsistent or incomplete results. The upper end of the distribution may be bimodal, with about 5% being "hypnotic virtuosos" capable of remarkable feats and experiences. Hypnotic responsiveness may be a trait relatively unsusceptible to modification, but this is still a debated issue. The findings in normal subjects may not be entirely applicable to patients whose motivation (or "desperation") to achieve hypnotic analgesia may be strong and for whom instructions in self-hypnosis may be quite effective.

The mechanisms of hypnotic analgesia are not known, although of course there have been speculations, and it is assumed that the process must share in the mechanisms of hypnotic phenomena in general. Psychoanalytic theories have described the relaxation of ego boundaries and incorporation of the hypnotist. More recently Hilgard (8) has described a neo-dissociation theory with a splitting off of various personality functions - perceptual, motor, cognitive, etc. - and Frankel suggests that this may be merely an extreme case of a process which occurs in daily life, with varying frequencies and varying degrees of success in different persons, without formal trance induction (6).

It is also possible, of course, to describe the phenomena of hypnosis in simple conditioning terms in a quite parsimonious way. Images are elicited in the patient by verbal instructions, and these images have in the past been associated with physiological changes, and so re-create them. It is a simple Pavlovian paradigm, the verbally-mediated images being the conditioned stimuli which elicit the desired physiological responses. The result is quite effective with autonomically-innervated variables, as Finer has shown (3). The chief function of trance is to reduce competing stimuli and thus competing responses. Barber has shown that comparable results can be achieved with waking imagination, but others have demonstrated that trance-induced analgesia is more effective than that from waking imagination, and both are more effective than relaxation alone (8,13).

Group Therapy

Although individual psychotherapy has been of little benefit with chronic pain patients, group therapy has its advocates. Short-term, didactic therapy is said to provide patients with a different orientation than their habitual chronic invalidism, so that different role concepts develop. In the groups, there is little emphasis either on individual unconscious motives or on group process. Rather, the emphasis is on rehabilitation goals, ways of achieving these, and "games" or other habits the patients may unwittingly use to sabotage their progress.

Whatever rationale the advocates of this approach may propose, it is probable that social learning is an important element in the process. From Craig's (2) studies it appears that modeling has a highly significant effect both on subjective pain and respondent physiological events. Thus the content of the group's discussion may well be important in maintaining the interest and attention of the patients, but the effect of the therapy may be due more to the learning of adaptive responses by modeling than by the acquisition of cognitive strategies.

Psychotropic Medication

Many have reported that psychotropic medications are helpful in managing pain patients (10). These seem not merely to modulate affective responses to pain, but to have a direct analgesic effect as well. Benzodiazepines, and quite modest doses of the phenothiazines, are particularly helpful in reducing the anxiety associated with acute pain. They also increase pain threshold and tolerance, and this seems to be a sensory effect rather than only a change in response bias or criterion for reporting. Similarly, tricyclic antidepressants are not only helpful in treating the depression associated with chronic pain, but also seem to increase pain tolerance, particularly those which increase the level or activity of brain serotonin. Some general outlines for the reasons underlying such observations are beginning to emerge with reports on the neurochemistry of the descending inhibitory systems in the brain stem and spinal cord. These aspects are dealt with in other chapters of this volume.

Apart from these neurochemical processes, mood states have long been known to affect pain. Not only does acute pain cause anxiety, but anxiety can cause, or exacerbate, pain.

This is a daily observation in the emergency room and the dentist's office. Similarly, chronic pain is known to result in depression in most patients, but it is less well known that about 50% of patients with depression develop pain as one of their symptoms - which clears when the depression is treated. Thus when depression results from chronic pain, it is not surprising that it makes the pain worse. It is for this reason that psychotropic medications are an essential part of most pain treatment programs.

PROBLEM AREAS

In the management of patients with chronic pain, three major problems seem to plague those who administer rehabilitation programs.

Recidivism does occur, although it is not systematically reported. Informal reports suggest the figure may be 10%-20%, and since many of those patients who are recidivists (i.e., return to medical care for additional relief) may not return to the same treatment program but may go elsewhere, the rate of recidivism may be as high as 20%-40% of those who "successfully" complete a pain treatment program. This area clearly needs more systematic study, both with respect to the actual percentages of treatment failures and to the identification of the characteristics of such patients. Only with such basic information can we know the extent and nature of the problem and plan strategies for coping with it.

One of the possible characteristics of recidivists, and the second major problem in this area, is that unique combination of chronic invalidism and hypochondriasis which Pilowsky (11) has termed "abnormal illness behavior." It apparently consists of the wholesale adoption of the sick role, and a fascinated absorption in the symptom of pain as evidence of deterioration. It is remarkably resistant to change except when secondary to a treatable affective disturbance. We need to develop a more effective system for treating such patients.

A third major problem area involves forces much larger than the clinic. In many of our societies there are socioeconomic forces that predispose the laboring class, especially, to develop and maintain pain behaviors. There are social status and financial reinforcers which make it virtually impossible to return a disabled worker to his or her former occupation, and in many cases, even vocational rehabilitation is discouraged. Health insurance programs, employers' liability insurance, government disability programs, trade union rules, etc., all conspire against the rehabilitation program's efforts to salvage the worker from the refuse pile of permanent disability. Some possibility should be built into our systems for a no-risk trial of vocational rehabilitation to replace the present punitive attitude toward such programs.

AN INTRIGUING PROBLEM FOR RESEARCH

One additional area which needs investigation has to do with the neurophysiology and neurochemistry of hypnotic analgesia. Hypnotic analgesia has been shown not to be reversed by naloxone (1,7), except in a single case report (12). This suggests a different mechanism than the presumed conditioned enkephalin response in placebo analgesia. Furthermore, hypnotic analgesia can be very rapid and last much longer than, for example, stimulation-produced analgesia. This all suggests a different pathway and different processes than are currently known. Can the preliminary reports of the microinjection in brain of the dibutyryl derivative of cyclic GMP be relevant? With respect to cortical evoked potentials, there is marked inconsistency in the handful of reports, perhaps due to methodological differences. Hysterical analgesia and hypnotic analgesia are reported to either enhance or reduce the late components of evoked responses to noxious stimuli, and this area clearly needs resolution. In summary, hypnotic analysis gesia is an apparently real phenomenon for a certain percentage of the population. If its underlying mechanisms could be known, it might be possible to extend its benefits to others who are not now capable of using it.

REFERENCES

(1) Barber, J., and Mayer, D. 1977. Evaluation of the efficacy and neural mechanism of a hypnotic analgesia procedure in experimental and clinical dental pain. Pain 4: 41-48.

(2) Craig, K.D. 1978. Social modeling influences on pain. In The Psychology of Pain, ed. R. A. Sternbach, pp. 73-109. New York: Raven Press.

(3) Finer, B. 1974. Clinical use of hypnosis in pain management. In Advances in Neurology, ed. J.J. Bonica, vol. 4, pp. 573-579. New York: Raven Press.

(4) Fordyce, W.E. 1976. Behavioral Methods for Chronic Pain and Illness, pp. 1-236. St. Louis: C. V. Mosby Co.

(5) Fordyce, W.E. 1978. Learning processes in pain. In The Psychology of Pain, ed. R. A. Sternbach, pp. 49-72. New York: Raven Press.

(6) Frankel, F.H. 1976. Hypnosis: Trance as a Coping Mechanism, pp. 1-185. New York: Plenum Publishing Company.

(7) Goldstein, A., and Hilgard, E.R. 1975. Lack of influence of the morphine antagonist naloxone on hypnotic analgesia. Proc. Nat. Acad. Sci. 72: 2041-2043.

(8) Hilgard, E.R. 1978. Hypnosis and pain. In The Psychology of Pain, ed. R. A. Sternbach, pp. 219-240. New York: Raven Press.

(9) Hilgard, E.R., and Hilgard, J.R. 1975. Hypnosis in the Relief of Pain, pp. 1-262. Los Altos, CA: W. Kaufmann, Inc.

(10) Merskey, H., and Hester, R.N. 1972. The treatment of chronic pain with psychotropic drugs. Postgraduate Medical Journal 48: 594-598.

(11) Pilowsky, I. 1978. Psychodynamic aspects of the pain experience. In the Psychology of Pain, ed. R. A. Sternbach, pp. 203-217. New York: Raven Press.

(12) Stephenson, J.B.P. 1978. Reversal of hypnosis-induced analgesia by naloxone. Lancet 2: 991-992.

(13) Sternbach, R. A. 1978. Clinical aspects of pain. In The Psychology of Pain, ed. R. A. Sternbach, pp. 241-264. New York: Raven Press.

Pain and Society, eds. H.W. Kosterlitz and L.Y. Terenius, pp. 445-460.
Dahlem Konferenzen 1980. Weinheim: Verlag Chemie GmbH.

Abnormal Illness Behavior and Sociocultural Aspects of Pain

I. Pilowsky
Department of Psychiatry, University of Adelaide
Adelaide, S.A. 5001, Australia

Abstract. Abnormal illness behavior presenting as chronic intractable pain is a particularly challenging problem for the clinician and society at large.

In this paper the concept of sick role, illness behavior and illness, and abnormal illness behavior are defined. Relevant forms of abnormal illness behavior are described. The literature dealing with sociocultural influence on the sick role and illness behavior is reviewed, and the relevance of these phenomena to the pain experience is discussed. The need to distinguish between sociocultural and intrapersonal influences on pain and illness behavior is emphasized.

INTRODUCTION

The experience of pain is virtually inseparable from the phenomenon of illness behavior (27). Indeed, Wall (35) has proposed that "just as hunger is associated with the search for food and eating....pain is associated with the search for treatment and optimal conditions for recovery."

It would probably be true to say that to a considerable extent, recent interest in pain has been a consequence of the need to manage patients whose pain does not conform to well recognized disease patterns and, perhaps more importantly, does not respond to treatment as might be expected. Patients with atypical and intractable pain may be variously diagnosed, but existing categories are not always adequate and are easily misapplied. Thus patients with chronic pain may be regarded as suffering from conditions such as "hysteria," "hypochondriasis," and even "malingering" without any clear understanding of the criteria for such diagnoses.

The concept of "abnormal illness behavior" (AIB) was introduced in the hope that it might help to bring some order to this difficult area of diagnosis and treatment (23, 24, 25, 26). It is a concept which stands on the borderland between sociology and psychiatry since, on the one hand, it is based on the concepts of the sick role and illness behavior while, on the other hand, it refers to states which are predominantly determined by intrapersonal and interpersonal processes. In order to clarify the concept of abnormal illness behavior it is therefore necessary to consider the "sick role," "illness behavior," and the notion of "illness."

Parsons introduced the concept of the sick role in 1951 (20). He maintained that in Western societies the sick role is characterized by two rights and two duties. The two rights associated with sick role status consist of an exemption from responsibility for the condition and relief from normal social role responsibilities. The duties require the individual to recognize and acknowledge the undesirability of the illness to try to get well, and to seek help from someone who is socially recognized as competent and appropriate to treat the condition.

Parsons' conception of the sick role (21) has often been criticized as constituting an ideal role-type rather than an empirically derived one. Furthermore, it has been considered to apply essentially to acute short-term illnesses and not to states such as chronic illness, alcoholism, psychiatric illness, and pregnancy. Nonetheless, Arluke et al. (3) have presented evidence based on a study of 490 patients which suggests that Parsons was not that far off the mark in his description of the sick role.

ILLNESS BEHAVIOR

Related to and complementing the concept of the sick role is that of "illness behavior" introduced by Mechanic and Volkart (17, 18) which refers to the ways in which symptoms are perceived, evaluated, and acted (or not acted) upon by individuals. This concept has proved to be an exceedingly useful one since it facilitates the empirical study of behaviors which are of considerable importance to clinicians and other health-care providers. Of course, these behaviors are also exceedingly important to the individual's family and society at large, but for the moment it seems useful to take an iatrocentric view of this process since the doctor occupies such a pivotal social role in its development and resolution. Although useful as it stands, further consideration suggests that illness behavior as defined by Mechanic (16) is perhaps too restrictive, for since it refers to "symptoms" as the focus of the behavior, it deemphasizes actions directed toward the avoidance of illness. In other words, since it is clearly quite possible for individuals to manifest illness behavior without having "symptoms," it may be more useful to define illness behavior as "the ways in which individuals experience and respond to those aspects of themselves which they are predisposed to evaluate in terms of an illness-health frame of reference."

As can be seen this definition emphasizes the conceptual categories utilized by the individual in evaluating himself rather than his "objective" state, since even the use of the term "symptom" implies "illness," and it is obvious that a person might show illness behavior in the absence of what he himself would consider a symptom, when he seeks medical care and attention in order to avoid becoming ill in whatever way. In some cases, this might be considered appropriate and adaptive (e.g., in seeking regular medical checks) and in other cases, not. It is also interesting to consider whether illness behavior should include reactions to the health status of significant others. Certainly, this would seem to be a legitimate extension of the concept in the case of parent-children interaction.

ABNORMAL ILLNESS BEHAVIOR

Having thus defined illness behavior, we may turn to the question of abnormal illness behavior. Before doing so, however, it is necessary to consider the definition of "illness." This is not an easy matter and certainly the word is used in a variety of ways. Usually a distinction is drawn between "disease" and "illness" - the latter referring to the entire experience of "being ill" and the former to the "objective" pathological processes associated with illness. What seems to be required is a definition of illness which would allow the identification and classification of certain states on a reasonably operational basis and in a manner which would facilitate comparisons between and within cultures both synchronically and diachronically. The definition suggested is as follows: "an illness is an organismic state which fulfills the requirements of a relevant reference group for admission to the sick role" (25).

It will be appreciated that a particular organismic state may fulfill requirements for a sick role at one time and not at another. For example, alcohol dependence as such, was not recognized as an illness for many years and in some places is still not so regarded.

It is for this reason, of course, that the concept of "illness" must be separated from that of "disease," which often refers to organismic states which are the same as those considered illnesses, but which may not coincide with them in all cultures or at all times. In some ways, a "disease" may best be conceived as an organismic state which doctors believe ought to be regarded as an illness (but which it may take them some time to persuade society to accept as such). If we separate "disease" and "illness" in this way, we can see that in each transaction with a patient, a doctor has at least two important decisions to make. The first is to ascertain whether the patient shows evidence of "disease," and the second is to establish whether he has an "illness." (It should of course be borne in mind that the patient can manifest a complex organismic state, part of which may fulfill the requirements for admission to a sick role, part for relegation to criminal status and part, indeed, for admission to sainthood - depending on the reference group one has in mind.)

Another important reason for distinguishing clearly between illness and the sick role (while linking them closely), is that under certain conditions the presence of illness may be acknowledged but, for various reasons, the granting of a sick role may not be possible, e.g., in a military triage context. The position of a doctor examining a patient can, to some extent, be compared to that of a currency exchange agent at an airport in relation to a traveller who wishes to obtain local currency. Thus the traveller presents the agent with what he has and the latter is required to indicate first, which currencies he is prepared to accept, and second, what they are worth. In some situations, therefore, he may indicate that certain notes and coins do indeed constitute legal currency in the countries where they were issued, but that he does not wish to accept them. In other words, they are being presented to the wrong reference group. Similarly, the patient presents to the doctor with what he has and asks whether it is an illness and, if so, how many "sick role units," i.e., rights, it may be worth. In the majority of cases, of course, the patient does not distinguish between "disease" and "illness" although there are situations where this can happen - for example, in the case of a chronic neurological condition which the patient might agree was a "disease" but where there might be disagreement as to whether the stage it had reached constituted an "illness." Certainly, the presence of a genetic predisposition to certain illness (such as Huntington's chorea) might be designated a disease but may not be considered an actual illness at all stages.

Thus the doctor not only decides whether the individual is entitled to the rights conferred by a sick role, but to what degree and for how long. The fact that the doctor has this function is particularly clear when he is required to provide the patient with a certificate testifying to his need for a sick role. By so doing, he not only gives permission for the conferring of certain rights, but also indicates that the individual has fulfilled the duties associated with sick role status.

The issue of "abnormal illness behavior" arises most sharply in the context of a disagreement between a doctor and a patient. Indeed, strictly speaking, a precisely defined form of such a disagreement is required for the diagnosis to be made definitively. This can be made difficult by the fact that the patient may often not disagree overtly, but may simply not cooperate, on the basis of a private view of his health status at variance with that held by his doctor.

Abnormal illness behavior is defined as: the persistence of an inappropriate or maladaptive mode of perceiving, evaluating, and acting in relation to one's own state of health, despite the fact that a doctor (or other appropriate social agent) has offered a reasonably lucid explanation of the nature of the illness and the appropriate course of management to be followed, based on a thorough examination and assessment of all parameters of functioning (including the use of special investigations where necessary) and taking into account the individual's age, educational, and sociocultural background (25). Forms of abnormal illness behavior (AIB) may be classified into those where the focus of disagreement is on organic pathology, and those in which the focus is on emotional illness. Both categories may be further subdivided on the basis of whether the patient affirms or denies illness and, in each case, whether the motivation is predominantly conscious or predominantly unconscious.

In the case of pain, our main interest is in those forms of abnormal illness behavior characterized by illness affirmation, i.e., those conditions in which the doctor believes and conveys that the illness behavior manifested by the patient is inappropriate and excessive in relation to the degree of objective somatic pathology.

Clearly, since it is the patient's response to the doctor's explanation and advice that is important in deciding the diagnosis, a heavy responsibility devolves upon the doctor to ensure that his behavior is appropriate for the demands of the situation. This is particularly so if he decides that the patient is "malingering," i.e., consciously affirming and enacting illness while not being unwell at all. As is well known, society has a particular horror of the malingerer which often spills over onto other patients whose illnesses are suggestive of malingering.

It will be appreciated that abnormal illness behavior is a rather unique diagnosis in medicine to the extent that it depends so largely on the interpretation of a doctor-patient disagreement. For this reason, it is a diagnosis which should not be made lightly. And yet, it too often is made following a disagreement with a patient as a result of communication difficulties or time constraints (9).

Forms of Abnormal Illness Behavior

The two main neurotic forms of abnormal illness behavior associated with an excessive preoccupation with illness or a disability out of proportion to the objective pathology are hypochondriacal and conversion reactions, and both syndromes are very commonly associated with pain. Hypochondriacal reactions are characterized by three main features: somatic preoccupation, disease phobias, and disease conviction with resistance to reassurance (22). Two subtypes may be identified: the first characterized by a fear of illness (nosophobia), and the second by a worried concern about pathology which is believed to be actually present. In both instances, the patient is constantly preoccupied with issues relating to his own state of health. In conversion reactions, the picture is different. The patient generally denies a preoccupation or even particular concern with the disability or pain, although he may express considerable dissatisfaction with the perceived consequences. In the classical case, the pain is presented with a type of serenity known as "la belle indifference." According to Ziegler and Imboden (38), the patient with a conversion symptom may be usefully considered as "someone enacting the role of a person with 'organic illness'." Quite often, however, it is difficult to distinguish between conversion and hypochondriacal patterns so that what seems to be present is relatively undifferentiated abnormal illness behavior.

It is also not always easy to draw a clear distinction between neurotic and psychotic forms of abnormal illness behavior. In general terms, however, the latter are diagnosed on the basis of a fixed false belief concerning one's own state of health, quite inaccessible to reasoned argument, and associated with other features of a depressive or schizophrenic psychosis.

SOCIOCULTURAL STUDIES

The frame of reference provided by the concepts discussed thus far offer a useful universe of discourse within which to consider social and cultural aspects of pain. When one considers that pain is regarded as the most important initial warning sign of illness (33), it is clear that the sick role, illness behavior, and abnormal illness behavior, serve as helpful conceptual bridges in attempts to delineate the individual and societal forces which influence and shape the experience of pain. For these reasons, it may be anticipated that sociological studies of the sick role and illness behavior will complement and prove congruent with studies of pain and illness behavior in the clinical context.

Studies concerned with sociocultural influences on experimental pain have been well reviewed by Wolff and Langley (36), who indicate that no firm conclusions can be drawn from the available evidence. The typical finding that emerges from U.S. studies (31) is that "Yankees" have the highest pain tolerance followed by Jews, Irish, and Italians. In addition, it appears that attitudes to pain vary, e.g., Jews express concern about the meaning of the pain while Italians focus on the immediacy of the pain and the need for relief. Having reviewed the field, Wolff and Langley (36) suggest that it is an area which calls for close cooperation between anthropologists and medical scientists if further progress is to be made.

Away from the laboratory, the effect of ethnic influences on sick role expectations and illness behavior have been studied in various ways, and while illuminating, do suffer from difficulties in operationalizing the concepts being examined. What is important, nonetheless, is that most studies have undermined stereotypes, or at least revealed some of the complex motivations and meanings underlying the illness behaviors encountered by physicians in patients of other cultures (28, 32, 34, 37, 39, 40). Suchman's (32) study of almost 2000 New York subjects is particularly interesting. Contrasting "parochialism" and "cosmopolitanism," he found that "membership in closely-knit, ethnocentric, traditionalistic community, friendship and family groups, appears to symbolize a parochial way of life which finds expression in the health area as (an orientation)....characterized by low factual knowledge about disease, suspicion of outside professional medical care and reliance upon members of one's own group for help and support during illness." However, women (who were more "parochial") showed a lower commitment to non-scientific medicine! This may reflect their greater responsibility for family health. Similarly, Pilowsky and Spence (28) found that age, sex, and degree of ethnicity all made significant contributions to illness behavior in general practice populations.

Socioeconomic status (SES) has been shown to influence sick role expectations in a number of ways. Arluke et al. (3) found that patients with a lower socioeconomic status were more likely to agree that one has a right not to be held responsible for one's illness. Kassebaum and Baumann (10), in a study of 201 chronically ill patients, found that blue collar workers were more likely to score high on scales measuring dependency, concern with role performance, and denial of affect with emphasis on autonomy. Gordon (7) similarly found that subjects of low socioeconomic status were more likely to accept dependency as an appropriate response to illness. On the other hand, Apple (2) found no relationship between social class and the definition of "illness."

Important associations have emerged between social class and various aspects of illness behavior. Thus individuals of low socioeconomic status show in a psychiatric setting "a tendency to see their presenting problem as physical rather than emotional" (4, 8). However, more recently (6) it would appear that these effects of low socioeconomic status are becoming less apparent in the U.S. and that is is more important to take educational levels into account. For example, Kulka et al. (11) found education influenced whether a problem was defined in mental health terms and that income determined whether professional help was sought - the wealthier being more likely to do so. Others (13) have found that low income, and not type of symptom, exerts the strongest influence against seeking medical care. Furthermore, McBroom (14) found no evidence that individuals of low socioeconomic status "overreact to, or overreport their symptomatology."

It is not easy, of course, to separate the effects of low socioeconomic status and restricted education. Thus a comparison of depressed patients with low back pain patients (15) has shown the latter to be mainly blue collar workers, with less education and from large families. Interestingly, Fabrega et al. (5) have shown that "problem patients" of low socioeconomic status are more likely to volunteer social concerns among their difficulties, than similarly placed controls.

Apart from their characteristic view of the sick role and their illness behavior, individuals of low socioeconomic status have also been found to differ in their attitudes to doctors; they tend to be impressed by a doctor's social status as reflected by his address and office (29), while a high socioeconomic status is associated with a more "rational approach to choosing a physician." As might be anticipated, a low socioeconomic status is frequently associated with problems of language and language level which interfere with the doctor-patient transaction (12, 30).

Finally it may be said that, in general, clinical studies of chronic pain associated with conversion and hypochondriacal states suggest that these syndromes are also associated with a low socioeconomic status and therefore support the validity of sociological analysis (4, 8, 19).

Despite these conclusions, it is equally clear that these syndromes can occur at all social levels and that early developmental factors are probably of particular importance in the more severe forms of abnormal illness behavior.

It is important, therefore, to draw a distinction between sociocultural factors, which influence patients' style and language when they communicate their pain experience, and more personal factors which determine the tendency to use pain and abnormal illness behavior as a maladaptive mode of coping with stress. Since childhood experiences are likely to be extremely significant determinants of later abnormal illness behavior (1), it is of importance to identify such problems as early as possible. It is equally necessary, however, that doctors treating adults acquire a) the skills of communicating with patients from other sociocultural backgrounds so that abnormal illness behavior is not incorrectly diagnosed and b) the ability to detect abnormal illness behavior very early in a clinical encounter so that unnecessary investigations and treatments may be avoided. The need to respond to abnormal illness behavior is a task which particularly challenges a society's capacity to modulate its altruistic respons appropriately. For this reason, medical science needs to make greater efforts to delineate and understand abnormal illness behavior syndromes.

This view of abnormal illness behavior places emphasis on the doctor's central and extremely vulnerable role in the process of allocating the sick role status and deciding on its precise nature. In the case of chronic pain, the consequences of his role require him to be well informed on a number of psychobiological and sociocultural issues and, therefore, carries important implications for medical education.

REFERENCES

(1) Apley, J., and MacKeith, R. 1968. The Child and His Symptoms. Oxford: Blackwell.

(2) Apple, D. 1960. How laymen define illness. J. Hlth. Hum. Behav. 1: 219-225.

(3) Arluke, A.; Kennedy, L.; and Kessler, R.C. 1979. Reexamining the sick-role concept: An empirical assessment. J. Hlth. Soc. Beh. 20: 30-36.

(4) Brill, N.Q., and Sorrow, H.A. 1960. Social class and psychiatric treatment. Arch. Gen. Psychiat. 3: 340-344.

(5) Fabrega, H.; Moore, R.J.; and Strawn, J.R. 1969. Low income medical problem patients: Some medical and behavioral features. J. Hlth. Soc. Beh. 10: 334-343.

(6) Frank, A.; Eisenthal, S.; and Lazare, A. 1978. Are there social class differences in patients' treatment conceptions? Arch. Gen. Psychiat. 36: 61-69.

(7) Gordon, G. 1966. Role Theory and Illness: A Sociological Perspective. New Haven: College and University Press.

(8) Hollingshead, A.B., and Redlich, F.C. 1958. Social Class and Mental Illness. New York: John Wiley and Sons.

(9) Hornung, C.A., and Massagli, M. 1979. Primary care physicians affective orientation toward their patients. J. Hlth. Hum. Beh. 20: 61-76.

(10) Kassebaum, G.G., and Baumann, B.O. 1965. Dimensions of the sick role in chronic illness. J. Hlth. Hum. Beh. 6: 16-27.

(11) Kulka, R.A.; Veroff, J; and Douvan, E. 1979. Social class and the use of professional help for personal problems. 1957 and 1976. J. Hlth. Soc. Beh. 20: 2-17.

(12) Koos, E. 1954. The Health of Regionville. New York: Columbia University Press.

(13) Ludwig, E.G., and Gibson, G. 1969. Self perception of sickness and the seeking of medical care. J. Hlth. Soc. Beh. 10: 125-133.

(14) McBroom, W.H. 1970. Illness behavior and socioeconomic status. J. Hlth. Soc. Beh. 11: 319-326.

(15) Maruta, T.; Swanson, D.W.; and Swenson, W.M. 1976. Pain as a psychiatric symptom: Comparison between low back pain and depression. Psychosom. 17: 123-127.

(16) Mechanic, D. 1968. Medical Sociology. New York: Free Press.

(17) Mechanic, D., and Volkart, E.H. 1960. Illness behavior and medical diagnosis. J. Hlth. Hum. Beh. 1: 86-96.

(18) Mechanic, D., and Volkart, E.H. 1961. Stress, illness behavior and the sick role. Am. Sociol. Rev. 26: 51-58.

(19) Merskey, H., and Spear, F.G. 1967. Pain: Psychological and Psychiatric Aspects. London: Bailliere, Tindall and Cassell.

(20) Parsons, T. 1951. The Social System. New York: Free Press.

(21) Parsons, T. 1964. Social Structure and Personality. London: Collier-MacMillan.

(22) Pilowsky, I. 1967. Dimensions of hypochondriasis. Br. J. Psychiat. 113: 89-93.

(23) Pilowsky, I. 1969. Abnormal illness behavior. Br. J. Med. Psychol. 42: 347-351.

(24) Pilowsky, I. 1971. The diagnosis of abnormal illness behavior. Aust. N.Z. J. Psychiat. 5: 136-138.

(25) Pilowsky, I. 1978. A general classification of abnormal illness behaviors. Br. J. Med. Psychol. 51: 131-137.

(26) Pilowsky, I. 1978. Pain as abnormal illness behavior. J. Hum. Stress 4: 22-27.

(27) Pilowsky, I. 1978. Psychodynamic aspects of the pain experience. In The Psychology of Pain, ed. R.A. Sternbach. New York: Raven Press.

(28) Pilowsky, I., and Spence, N.D. 1977. Ethnicity and illness behavior. Psychol. Med. 7: 447-452.

(29) Rosenblatt, D., and Suchman, E. 1966. Awareness of physicians' social status within an urban community. J. Hlth. Hum. Beh. 7: 146-153.

(30) Samora, J.; Saunders, L.; and Larson, R.F. 1961. Medical vocabulary knowledge among hospital patients. J. Hlth. Hum. Beh. 2: 83-92.

(31) Sternbach, R.A., and Turskey, B. 1965. Ethnic differences among housewives in psychophysical and skin potential responses to electric shock. Psychophys. 1: 241-246.

(32) Suchman, E.A. 1965. Social patterns of illness and medical care. J. Hlth. Hum. Beh. 6: 2-16.

(33) Suchman, E.A. 1965. Stages of illness and medical care. J. Hlth. Hum. Beh. 6: 114-128.

(34) Twaddle, A.C. 1969. Health decisions and sick role variations: An exploration. J. Hlth. Soc. Beh. 10: 105-115.

(35) Wall, P.D. 1979. On the relation of injury to pain. The John J. Bonica lecture. Pain 6: 253-264.

(36) Wolff, B.B., and Langley, S. 1968. Cultural factors and the response to pain. Am. Anthrop. 70: 494-501.

(37) Zborowski, M. 1952. Cultural components in responses to pain. J. Soc. Issues 8: 16-30.

(38) Ziegler, F.J.; Imboden, J.B.; and Meyer, E. 1960. Contemporary conversion reactions: A clinical study. Amer. J. Psychiat. 116: 901-909.

(39) Zola, I.K. 1963. Problems of communication, diagnosis and patient care. J. Med. Educ. 38: 829-838.

(40) Zola, I.K. 1966. Culture and symptoms-analysis of patients presenting complaints. Amer. Sociol. Rev. 31: 615-630.

Pain and Society, eds. H.W. Kosterlitz and L.Y. Terenius, pp. 461-480.
Dahlem Konferenzen 1980. Weinheim: Verlag Chemie GmbH.

Ethical Issues in Pain Management

H. T. Engelhardt, Jr.
Kennedy Institute of Ethics, Georgetown University
Washington, D.C., 20057, USA

Abstract. The ethical issues that arise in pain management reflect tensions concerning who will decide on the character of particular approaches to pain management and which approaches are best. Insofar as one sees ethics as a means of negotiating disputes in a way that is not grounded in force, the central problems will be those of procedure (e.g., free and informed consent) and of tolerance of diverse choices (i.e., the decisions as to what are the best modes of pain management will be as much creations as discoveries of what is important in life, and therefore in suffering). In concrete instances, the forms these conflicts will take will depend upon how the therapist (pain management consultant)/patient (client) relationship is perceived.

INTRODUCTION

In this paper I will advance a few philosophical reflections raised by attempts to control pain. By philosophical reflections I mean endeavors to become clearer about the role and function of the ideas involved in, or presupposed by, attempts to manage pain. I will not simply forward a set of answers, but rather offer a set of questions in the sense of suggesting where puzzles do or could arise. A philosophical approach to ethics is after all not a program for imposing a particular cultural view, a religious faith, or a professional etiquette for conduct. It is instead an endeavor to forge a means of negotiating moral intuitions, of framing a logic of a pluralism, of fashioning ways by appealing to reasons, of choosing better answers to moral questions, given interests in certain goods and values. That is, philosophical ethics is a reflective analysis towards the goals of discerning the grounds for general rational agreement about moral issues and of outlining as far as possible the character of such possible agreement. Though it is not likely to provide final or best answers, philosophical ethics as a disciplined mode of puzzling can show us which answers are worse and which are better, given our particular initial commitments. It is a means of making our moral ideals and sentiments clearer. Insofar as this view of ethics is correct, the hard core of ethics will be respecting freedom and the nexus of obligations it creates. This dimension of ethics will be procedural; it will involve negotiation among free agents. There will also be a core of values that many individuals will take to be important, but this importance will be perceived in different ways. This might be termed the soft core of ethics, which is given a firm structure through the agreement of the individuals concerned. In terms of pain management, these issues will display themselves in discussions about who chooses which way to manage pain (i.e., the pain manager, the person in pain, the care-giving institution, society) and what values are involved in different modes of managing pain.

In beginning a consideration of the ethical issues raised by pain management, one must recognize the ambiguity of the term 'pain' itself. One might at first blush think that pain is a univocally negative quality, the character of which is disclosed fully in the experience itself. However, the experience in general and medicine in particular show this not to be the case. Rather, pain appears to have, given certain qualifications, a neutral quality that, when set in its most frequent contexts, is usually judged negatively and indeed becomes a central element of suffering. Thus the masochist may observe, 'It hurts so good,' and the person with disconnected or damaged frontal lobes may remark with la belle indifference, 'Oh, yes, it hurts terribly,' and then smile. The relation of a pain to anxiety, or to a negative minding of the sensation, appears to be necessary for the pain 'causing' suffering. This can as well be captured in a distinction between pain as a sensation taken in isolation and pain as an indication of a threat to one's existence, as anxiety evoking (2). An analysis of this sort is forwarded, for example, in Melzack and Casey's distinction between a sensory and an affective (motivational-affective) dimension of pain, between that element of pain that distinguishes it as a sensation of a certain sort and one's minding it, disliking it (3,20). As George Pitcher has argued, it is best to speak of the sensory element as pain and of the second element as the context that provides the evaluation of pain (27). Then, one can understand in a nonoxymoronic fashion the report of individuals with frontal lobotomies or of those who have taken morphine, that they feel a pain, but that it does not really bother them.

This distinction is important for the ethics of pain management in that it directs us to the fact that though pain may in all circumstances in a very primitive sense be unpleasant, it becomes suffering only in an affective context that makes it something to be disliked. It is a distinction that directs us to where the disvalues exist which invite pain management. The goal of pain management will often be to make pain less evocative of suffering even when the pain itself may remain. Moreover, the suffering evoked by pain may be magnified by other suffering unassociated with physical pain, but due to mental anguish arising out of such circumstances as loss of physical capacities, isolation, or anxiety about impending death. Managing pain is likely, then, to be a complex endeavor involving more than simply controlling pain and as a result will engender a range of ethical issues as well as other value questions. However, despite the importance of the aforementioned distinctions, I will continue to speak simply of pain and pain management and trust the reader to import these distinctions as required.

Severe and chronic pain have a disruptively intrusive character. The intrusiveness of pain into the lives of humans and the consequent importance of its management in the practice of medicine is reflected in the fact that the symptom pain is often treated as a disease entity in its own right. It appears in and of itself as the focus of medical concern. However, given our modern view of diseases as based on pathophysiological or pathoanatomical derangements, there is an understandable ambivalence on the part of many physicians with regard to addressing pain as a disease entity. There is often also a prejudice against symptomatic as opposed to etiological treatment. However, major elements of the history of clinical medicine reflect a recognition that pain as such is a proper focus for medical management. The clinical phenomenological nosologies of Francois Boissier de Sauvages (1707-1764) and Carl von Linnaeus (1704-1778) listed among their clinical classes of diseases (e.g., fevers, spasms, weaknesses, fluxes) the category pain (Sauvages: dolores; Linnaeus: dolorosi) (19,28). Sauvages' class dolores embraced five orders: unlocalized, of the head, of the chest, of the internal abdomen, and pains that are external and of the limbs. Moreover, pains could exist like essential fevers, standing in their own right unreduced to more basic processes. One might think here of Sauvages' category dolores vagi qui nomen a sede fixa non habent - unlocalized pains that do not have name from a fixed site ((28), p.94). In short, pain was a cardinal basic category in organizing the world of medical diagnosis, and in directing treatment.

However, this very natural recognition of pain as a medical problem in its own right has led to two sets of conflicts. On the one hand, recognizing pain as a medical problem has tended to suggest perhaps too strongly that its control is properly under the aegis of medical experts. On the other hand, it has suggested that patients complaining of chronic pains that lack a clear somatic basis have less of a claim upon care than those with a demonstrable basis. One might, employing Ivan Illich's metaphor, characterize the first as the medicalizing of pain (15). The second one could term the need for somatic vindication of pain - a view that is likely a side effect of the largely successful pathophysiological reduction of clinical phenomenological categories during the nineteenth century. That is, the true significance of the clinical findings was held to be their underlying patho-anatomical lesions and physiological processes (12). Both of these phenomena suggest the extent to which the appreciation of pain and suffering is a function of the conceptual framework within which they are understood. This is a general point. A pain which is understood to be associated with heart disease will be appreciated differently than one understood as due simply to swellings of the costal cartilages. Or one might think, for example, of the difference between the way a pain is likely to be experienced when it is thought to be functional, versus when it is held to be due to a carcinoma. So also, whether a pain leads to financial compensation or not will change its significance. Pains do not simply exist by themselves, but are understood a) through the pathophysiological explanatory models that account for their appearance and b) through the social roles they authorize for their bearers, which roles provide excuses from certain duties and claims to attention and compensation. These issues have been explored, for example, in analyses of the social significance of the sick role (22-26,30) and of the explanatory and evaluative functions of concepts of diseases (7).

Because of the multiple functions of classification of pain, one should not view them simply as true or false, but as rather more or less useful towards the goals of pain management. Henrik Wulff has argued this point with regard to nosologies. In clinical sciences, so he holds, one should choose one classification over another because of the advantages it affords for therapy and for prognosis (34). This is true as well in the case of pain management for, as indicated above, the significance of a pain is embedded in a particular pathophysiological explanatory account, and the diagnosis provides a social role which, among other things, can allocate welfare benefits. Thus classifications of pains are not only descriptive and evaluative, they are performative. They create social roles. They indicate, in addition, which pains are worse, more severe. In the process they allocate concomitant rights, duties, and expectations (e.g., special roles of dependency with rights to financial compensation and support).

One should note as well that a great deal of the difficulties surrounding the descriptions of pains is due to the difficulties attendant to describing the mind-brain relationship. In order to avoid Cartesian interactionist dualism (i.e., that the mind and body are two things, two substances interacting), some investigators assert that a pain _is_ a physiological process of a particular character and location. However, a pain sensation _as_ an experienced phenomenon is not identical with a pain _as_ a physiological process. What is often meant is that a certain pain is the property of certain physiological processes. Which is to say, a materialist can employ a dualism of properties, holding that certain very complex material objects can be fully described only by identifying both physicalist properties (e.g., the character of neural structures or physiological processes) and mentalistic properties (e.g., the qualities of a pain of a certain kind - "crushing"), while rejecting a dualism of substances (i.e., that there is a mind-thing, a res cogitans, and a brain-thing, a res extensa). In fact, such a parallelism of properties was suggested by the British neurologist John Hughlings Jackson (1835-1911) in his proposal that neurologists act as if mental events and physiological processes occurred concomitantly without interaction. He suggested that one make this assumption in order a) to remove physiological language from neurological explanation so as b) to facilitate the exploration of the extent to which one could succeed in giving physiological and anatomical explanations in neurology without the _deus ex machina_ of asserting that the mind had done this or felt that. In this fashion Jackson proposed an instrumentalist or pragmatic solution of the mind-brain problem: one should explore the possibilities of a physio-anatomical account of brain functions, while eschewing all psychological terms and models, though correlating such physiological findings with psychological occurrences where appropriate. The result was a methodological parallelism that avoided metaphysics and instead addressed the issue of scientific method in neurology (6,8,16,17). Similarly, one can correlate pain as an experience with certain physiological processes without holding that the pain as an experience is those processes, or for that matter that it is the behaviors associated with such experiences.

In summary, when one moves to manage pain, one will not be addressing a theory or value-neutral sense of pain. Rather, pain and our classifications of pain, will reflect theoretical, clinical, and general societal interests. In that those classifications will therefore reflect various explanatory, therapeutic, and societal goals, these classifications will as a consequence incorporate value judgments, many of which will have ethical force. Again, for example, when an individual is having severe chronic pain, one will likely offer a sick role which imposes obligations and gives excuses which have moral force. As a result, it would be morally wrong, ceteris paribus, to blame someone for not working if he is unable to, due to such a state of chronic pain. Value judgments, including ethical judgments, will thus often pass unnoticed in what may be taken to be merely descriptions of states of affairs. In addition, the language of pain descriptions will reflect views about the nature of the mind-brain relation and of the sciences and arts of pain study and management. The world of pain terms and classifications is therefore the result of a complex interplay of facts, theories, social institutions, social goals, and conceptual views of reality and science. It is within this complex context, which can only be indicated here, that ethical issues of pain management must be analyzed.

ETHICAL IMPLICATIONS OF VARIOUS MODELS OF PAIN MANAGEMENT

The professionalization of pain care and the scientific approach to accounting for pains have had the partial successes and failures that characterize human endeavors and engender ethical conflicts. Since pain is often the central constituent element of severe suffering, and since there are dangers involved in many forms of pain management, there are inter- and intra-professional disputes concerning modes of, and prerogatives in, pain management. These concerns include problems of sympathetic suffering on the part of pain managers. There are therefore conflicting views as to the proper weightings of possible risks and benefits and as to the proper division of rights and duties in the development and execution of plans for pain management. It is here that the core areas of possible value divergence exist: control of pain management. If one invokes the image of an economy of pleasures and pains, one can speak of problems in characterizing and controlling exchanges in that economy.

Ethical issues in pain management can as well be analyzed using the contrast between medical and non-medical models of care and cure. Such a contrast is, however, helpful only if one means by the dyad "medical model of pain management" versus "non-medical model of pain management," the dyad "patient-therapist model of pain management" versus "client-service provider model of pain management." This dyad signals various differences in the amount of active participation in the management of pain by the person in pain ranging from the patient who accepts the management provided by the therapist to the client who decides upon the form and circumstances of pain management to be provided. This spectrum from self to other determination of pain management is to be distinguished from the universe of discourse, which includes somatic, psychological, behavioral, and social models of pain therapy - models for theoretically accounting for pain states and their therapy. Medical versus non-medical models in the first stipulated senses thus involve different degrees of a) providing information concerning the nature of the pain management to be employed, including its benefits, drawbacks, and possible adverse effects, b) providing information concerning the nature, advantages, and disadvantages of possible alternate models of pain management, and c) allowing the person in pain to adjust his or her own pain management plan. The considerations influencing where a given model of pain management falls on this spectrum are a) the extent to which the therapist is seen to be in possession of specialized information about pain management that cannot be accurately communicated to the person in pain due to differences in education and experience, or due to the debilities incident to the condition of the person in pain; b) the extent to which the therapist is seen to be in possession of specialized knowledge concerning the significance of particular choices of pain management because the therapist is an objective observer who has witnessed the consequences of many such choices; c) the extent to which the person in pain is seen to have the right to determine his or her own plan of pain management, even if such a choice is made with far from ideal comprehension of technical information or with insufficient knowledge of the consequences of a choice for his or her future life; and d) the extent to which the choices of the person in pain at the time (t_o), though wholeheartedly embraced, must be respected even if they are likely to be repudiated by that person in the future (t+n) - one might think here of severely burned but salvageable patients refusing life-saving treatment because of the pain involved, but who after treatment is completed do not object to being alive. These considerations define the extent to which pain management will be paternalistic or libertarian, fashioned in the best interests of the afflicted person as the experts define those interests, or fashioned by the free choice of the person in pain.

Depending on how one interprets this spectrum, different ethical issues are made salient. If the spectrum is seen as one moving from an ethic of best interests to an ethic of respect of freedom, as a condition for morality, one will move from a teleological ethics focused on achieving certain goods and values (health, avoidance of addiction, optimally diminishing suffering) to a deontological ethics focused on an obligation to respect freedom not as one good among others, but as the condition for morality in the sense of a community based not on force but on mutual respect of reason-giving. Of course, freedom can also be viewed as one good among others in a hierarchy of values, and this would be a second interpretation of the spectrum. If the spectrum is interpreted in the first way, which itself turns on accepting one fundamental view of ethics, there will be irresolvable disputes between interests in achieving certain goods and values in pain management and the need to respect the free, even if bizarre, choices that persons make. There will in many cases be a conflict between what experienced clinicians know to be the best choices and what individuals freely choose. If the spectrum is interpreted in the second way, one will confront the difficulty of all hypothetical choice theories. One will have the problem of establishing that one's view of the proper ordering of goods to be achieved corresponds with the objective ordering, or in fact that there is an objective ordering, an ordering that would be given by a perfectly informed, disinterested observer or group of observers. Such a view presupposes that, ceteris paribus, one can univocally rank the goods of pain control, risk of addiction, risk of untoward side effects, etc. The first view can function even if concrete hierarchies of values are created or invented, not objectively discovered, because its central presupposition is respect of individual freedom. Concrete ethical obligations can then be derived contractually. But to complicate matters, one is likely to achieve different sorts of contracts depending on the value one gives to free choice beyond one's acknowledging respect for free choice. That is, though one may endorse the negative right of individuals not to be interfered with in their attempts to achieve whatever therapeutic contracts they can with regard to self determination in pain management, still many, if not most, major institutions may be unwilling to contract for much latitude in the patient/ client control over pain management by those suffering from pain.

There can in short be profound value conflicts with respect to pain management because of the quite different ways in which one can view the place of patient/client participation in pain management. Such conflicts will as well reflect the divergent ways in which the secondary values of pain are perceived. Pain can be appreciated as that which should be borne silently and patiently, that which justifies tears and anger, that which can save one's soul, that which can be an occasion for personal growth, or simply that which reflects the blind, senseless forces of the cosmos. These and other views express how pain comes to play a role in a general economy of pleasure and suffering. One might think here, for example, of a Christian account of suffering as redemption in which the man-God is portrayed as accepting great suffering in order to buy back man from sin and perdition. Christians are then, within this view, enjoined to bear pain and suffering because of the positive effect of such endurance in the economy of salvation. Suffering, not simply pain, thus receives positive value and the suffering borne gains meaning and purpose.

Such economies of suffering are geographies of values. They signal the acceptable ways of controlling pain - for example, a) bearing pain stoically, b) using only that minimum of surgical, pharmacological and other interventions that will return one to a "productive life," c) employing liberal self-medication, d) resorting to suicide when, as Seneca states, further life is not worthwhile (29). Choice of a particular means of pain management involves a choice of lifestyle, as Robert Veatch has argued with regard to the control of behavior through drugs (33). In choosing a particular way of managing pain, one is usually making a choice among interventions which are in varying degrees disruptive of one's lifeplan. One is as well, in providing or tolerating particular forms of pain management, giving more or less weight to particular social institutions and practices, including styles of professional practice, symbols of practice and symbols of status such as the right to prescribe controlled drugs.

The ethical problems raised by pain management therefore cluster around disputes concerning a) the proper ranking of the goods and values affected by such management, and b) the proper mediation of the freedom of those with pain and the freedom of those who are the professional pain managers. Insofar as pain management presupposes a) understanding how particular pains are part of specific contexts of suffering, as well as b) appreciating the role of suffering in any person's economy of pains and pleasures, one will then be pressed into analyzing ethical as well as non-ethical values concerning the quality of life under particular life circumstances and the secondary significance of pain as a part of suffering seen to be meaningless, redemptive, etc. This point is made in discussions of the nature of transactions made among those in pain, those who treat pain, and surrounding social groups. Such points, though, are usually advanced in psychological terms (31), and often placed within a transactional paradigm or developed with regard to not reinforcing manipulative behavior on the part of those in pain (10,11). Such psychological accounts are surely in part useful. However, in addition, choices of modes of pain management involve value judgments about issues such as the seriousness of risks associated with more invasive, less reversible modalities of pain management (e.g., chordotomies, rhizotomies, thalamotomies, lobotomies), the risks of addiction, the risks of other side effects, the risks of premature tolerance to analgesic agents, and the thresholds at which suffering makes the quality of life intolerable. Such gradings of states of affairs, such rankings of risks and benefits are value judgments. Some involve issues of a moral nature, others various ideals of a pleasing lifestyle. The central and in part intractable ethical core of controversy here, however, concerns whose judgment in these matters should prevail in areas of disagreement - those of the therapists, of the persons in pain, of the social institutions developed to manage pain, or of society generally.

The issue of who decides, signals tensions between paternalistic interests and respect for freedom. Such tensions are, however, not necessarily irresolvable in all cases. Insofar as the object of the paternalism consents as in a fiduciary trust, there is no conflict with a principle of regard for the self-determination of persons. There have been attempts to expand this notion of consented-to paternalism to cover those paternalistic interventions that function as social insurance policies. It is under that rubric, it has been argued, that one should place practices of ignoring the choices of individuals who are seriously misinformed about life endangering risks, who are under overbearing psychological or social pressure, or who have not sufficiently understood or appreciated the dangers involved in their choices (4). Such arguments if successful would support an experienced therapist's setting limits for choices with regard to pain management, where one could reasonably show that such 'insurance policies' had been agreed to. It would also support physicians, under such circumstances, regarding the act of agreeing to be a patient as a case of agreeing to a special fiduciary relationship in which the physician is expected to be directive in virtue of greater knowledge, experience, and objectivity. Others would defend an even greater scope and stronger foundation for paternalism by appealing to policies that will achieve a convincing balance of value over disvalue (for a recent discussion of paternalism in medicine, see (5,14)). And of course there are strong utilitarian arguments for setting patterns for pain management on the basis of maximizing institutional and team efficiency in delivering care.

However, if one takes seriously the notion of the ethical community as one based not on the use of force, but on respect for freedom in the adjudication of disputes, one will be pressed closer to full-fledged libertarian policies, such as the decriminalization of the sale and possession of controlled substances (letting clear warnings of their dangers suffice), which would allow increased self-medication for pain. One will be pressed as well to the decriminalization of attempted suicide and the abetting of the suicide of competent individuals. In any event, the patients' rights movement (1) and recent debates concerning free and informed consent have strongly forwarded the right of autonomy in medical decision making (21). The right to autonomy or liberty in medical care is, as Charles Fried has put it, "the right to dispose of one's self, that is of one's person, one's body, mind and capacities according to a plan and a conception fully chosen for one's self" ((13), p. 102). In the case of pain management this would include the prerogative of the person in pain to participate as fully as possible in choosing his or her mode of pain management. Such an accent on respecting freedom could have, as indicated above, two roots. The first, respect of freedom as a condition for a moral community, which conveys negative rights (i.e., not to be lied to, not to be subject to coercion, etc.) and is the hard core of morality. One cannot disagree with freedom as a constraint upon action and still understand the moral community as one not based on force. It is concern for freedom as a value that conveys positive rights as a means of achieving that value (e.g., establishing institutional procedures that maximize the participation of patients/clients) and is a part of the soft core of morality. It involves a central moral value, but is not a necessary condition for the moral community as one not based on force. In addition, special obligations develop positive rights in institutions supported through public funds. The public may, for example, wish to give greater weight to individuals participating in the management of their own pains than to the ease of institutional operations. A good example of the move from paternalistic to non-paternalistic approaches to pain management is the successful change in the level of self-determination now accorded women in childbirth.

SOME PARTICULAR ETHICAL CONCERNS IN PAIN MANAGEMENT

It is over the control of elements of pain management that much contention arises. Much of the vexation in fact focuses on rather everyday treatment issues. For example, Fagerhaugh and Strauss record the following patient remarks:

> I don't get it. One nurse says don't hold off asking for pain shots. Another says hold out.
>
> Some nurses offer pain shots. Others give the shot only when I ask for it.
>
> Some nurses are regular time nuts, giving the shots to the minute. Others are not so exacting.
>
> When I complain of pain some nurses try to find out more about the pains. Others say, let me check the last time you had a shot.
>
> Some nurses plan the drug so it won't be so painful to get up and walk around. Others just come in and command: "It's time for you to walk now" ((9), p. 68).

These remarks reflect the varying opportunities afforded to patients to determine their lifestyles in hospitals, in particular to co-determine the management of their own pains. The problems are complex and involve not only issues of staff recalcitrance, institutional needs, varying levels of knowledge, but also the fact that many patients are not inclined to assume co-responsibility for managing their pains. Also, in a society where access to most addictive substances is greatly restricted (special drugs such as tobacco and alcohol excepted), there is likely to be a feeling on the part of some in society that co-participation of therapist and patient in the control of pain, including levels of pain medication, is in some sense illicit. Indeed, in a society that no longer has generally accepted moral principles to forbid the suicide of competent terminally ill patients, there still remain feelings of ill ease in allowing a patient dying in severe pain to decide not only to refuse all further treatment, but to accelerate death as well ((9), pp. 163-166). We are still far from having drawn the conclusions implicit in fashioning a secular, pluralist, and tolerant society where different views of risks and benefits in pain management are likely to exist - namely, that free individuals should, as far as is compatible with the duty of forbearance against violating the rights of others, be allowed to determine the character of their own lives and deaths. In the case of pain management, this will involve negotiations between pain managers and those in pain, restrained at least by duties of full free and informed consent.

Concern with free and informed consent will as well have an impact upon what use of placebos in research or practice will be justifiable - namely, only that deception in the use of placebos to which consent is given (explicit consent) or which is in some sense expected or considered by the person deceived to be of no moment (implicit consent). One might think, for example, of the consent to deception that occurs in poker, or in an agreement to be a physician or patient in a double-blind clinical trial. Also stating "this should help you with your pain" when giving a placebo might not be deceptive, if one has good evidence that there will be an analgesic effect and that the person in pain has no interest in knowing the mechanism by which the analgesic effect is achieved. However, one could not lie about the nature of the material given, nor refuse to give information about the nature of the material when asked. Stating that the placebo is morphine or some other directly effective drug, when it is not, would involve unjustified deception on the grounds of a failure to respect the individual as a person (unless, for example, the person has agreed to a possible deception as a part of a double-blind study). The fault would not lie simply in one withholding a more efficacious therapy, but in not regarding individuals as free persons ((18), pp. 13-14). In fact one could only use a placebo when one was sure that the patient did not wish to have full information. The same considerations will count against the use of coercion in bringing patients into experimental protocols for pain management ((32), p. 250). Given the desperation of many suffering from pain, they may be individuals easily deceived or coerced. How these issues will be resolved in concreto will depend on how the participants view the therapist (pain management consultant)/patient (client) relationship.

This last point, however, brings the reflections concerning paternalism full circle. Those who care for the suffering should be good counselors of finitude. To those who are competent they should give as complete and accurate information as possible, including the therapist's experience with the consequences of various choices among modes of pain management. Such counseling may be directive but may not be coercive. On the other hand, therapists are also free individuals and may be unwilling to use certain modes of pain management. However, with regard to incompetents, therapists have an opportunity to act paternalistically and to choose as best they can in the best interests of the patient. There is no free choice to which to appeal. In such circumstances one may appeal to the wishes of the immediate family with whom the incompetent lives, as likely good judges of those interests, because it is in terms of that social unit that the life of the incompetent is defined. Special limitations arise, however, in the case of a previously competent individual whose past competent wishes may be known, or in the case of an individual who will become competent and whose likely wishes should be given weight.

CONCLUSION

As these reflections suggest, pain management raises numerous value issues. This should be expected. Pain and suffering embrace a large part of our universe of values. The ethical questions raised by pain management can procrusteanly, however, be put into two major categories. The first is procedural. It arises, for example, in concerns for free and informed consent. It involves the ways in which free individuals may agree on joint projects, in this case pain management. The second involves particular hierarchies of values in which the goods of adequate pain control are to be balanced against risks such as permanent physical damage, disruption of institutional operation, accelerated tolerance to analgesic agents, and addiction. Given the likely lack of agreement regarding such hierarchies, this second set of problems argues for creating latitude especially in public institutions for widely differing choices in pain management. Thus, the ethical dilemmas of pain management reflect the general problems of moral conduct: How to allow free agents to create peacefully their own ways of living and dying.

REFERENCES

(1) Annas, G.J. 1975. The Rights of Hospital Patients. New York: Avon.

(2) Bakan, D. 1976. Pain - The existential symptom. In Philosophical Dimensions of the Neuro-Medical Sciences, eds. S.F. Spicker and H.T. Englehardt, Jr., pp. 197-207. Dordrecht, Holland: D. Reidel.

(3) Casey, K.L., and Melzack, R. 1967. Neural mechanisms of pain: A conceptual model. In New Concepts in Pain and Its Clinical Management, pp. 13-31. Philadelphia: F.A. Davis.

(4) Dworkin, G. 1972. Paternalism. Monist (La Salle, IL) 56: 64-84.

(5) Ellin, J. 1978. Comments on 'paternalism and health care.' In Contemporary Issues in Biomedical Ethics, eds. J.W. Davis, B. Hoffmaster and S. Shorten, pp. 245-254. Clifton, NJ: Humana.

(6) Engelhardt, H.T., Jr. 1975. John Hughlings Jackson and the mind-body relation. Bulletin of the History of Medicine (Baltimore) 49: 137-151.

(7) Engelhardt, H.T., Jr. 1976. Ideology and etiology. J. Med. Philos. (Chicago) 1: 256-268.

(8) Engelhardt, H.T., Jr. 1976. The conceptual roots of the neural sciences. Book Review of The Self and Its Brain by K. Popper and J. Eccles. J. Nerv. Ment. Dis. (Baltimore) 169: 257-262.

(9) Fagerhaugh, S.Y., and Strauss, A. 1977. Politics of Pain Management. Menlo Park, CA: Addison-Wesley.

(10) Fordyce, W.E. 1974. Treating chronic pain by contingency management. In Advances in Neurology, ed. J.J. Bonica, vol. 4, pp. 583-589. New York: Raven.

(11) Fordyce, W.E. 1978. Learning processes in pain. In The Psychology of Pain, ed. R.A. Sternbach, pp. 49-72. New York: Raven.

(12) Foucault, M. 1973. The Birth of the Clinic: An Archaeology of Medical Perception. Tr. A.M. Sheridan Smith. New York: Random House.

(13) Fried, C. 1974. Medical Experimentation. New York: American Elsevier.

(14) Graber, G.C. 1978. On paternalism and health care. In Contemporary Issues in Biomedical Ethics, eds. J.W. Davis, B. Hoffmaster and S. Shorten, pp. 223-244. Clifton, NJ: Humana.

(15) Illich, I. 1976. Medical Nemesis. New York: Pantheon.

(16) Jackson, J.H. 1915. On the nature of the duality of the brain. Brain (London) 38: 80-103.

(17) Jackson, J.H. 1958. Selected Writings of John Hughlings Jackson, ed. J. Taylor. London: Staples Press.

(18) LeRoy, P.L. 1977. Overview: In search of the answer to chronic pain. In Current Concepts in the Management of Chronic Pain, ed. P.L. Leroy, pp. 1-17. New York: Stratton.

(19) Linnaeus, C. 1763. Genera morborum, in auditorium usum. Upsallae: C.E. Steinert.

(20) Melzack, R., and Casey, K.L. 1968. Sensory, motivational, and central control determinants of pain: A new conceptual model. In The Skin Senses, ed. D. Kenshalo, pp. 423-439. Springfield, IL: C.C. Thomas.

(21) National Commission for the Protection of Human Subjects of Biomedical and Behavioral Research. 1978. The Belmont Report: Ethical Principles and Guidelines for the Protection of Human Subjects of Research with appendices in two volumes. Bethesda, Md.: DHEW. DHEW Publication no. s (OS) 78-0012, 78-0013, 78-0014.

(22) Parsons, T. 1951. The Social System. New York: Free Press.

(23) Parsons, T. 1957. The mental hospital as a type of organization. In The Patient and the Mental Hospital, eds. M. Greenblatt et al., pp. 108-129. Glencoe, IL: Free Press.

(24) Parsons, T. 1958. Definitions of health and illness in the light of American values and social structure. In Patients, Physicians and Illness, ed. E.G. Jaco, pp. 165-187. Glencoe, IL: Free Press.

(25) Parsons, T. 1958. Illness, therapy and the modern urban American family. In Patients, Physicians and Illness, ed. E.G. Jaco, pp. 234-245. Glencoe, IL: Free Press.

(26) Pilowsky, I. 1969. Abnormal illness behavior. Brit. J. Med. Psych. (London) 42: 347-351.

(27) Pitcher, G. 1976. Pain and unpleasantness. In Philosophical Dimensions of the Neuro-medical Sciences, eds. S.F. Spicker and H.T. Engelhardt, Jr., pp. 181-196. Dordrecht, Holland: D. Reidel.

(28) Sauvages de la Croix, Francois Boissier de. 1768. Nosologia methodica sistens morborum classes juxta sydenhami mentem et botanicorum ordinem. 5 vols. Amsterdam: Fratrum de Tournes.

(29) Seneca. Letter LXX. Suicide.

(30) Siegler, M., and Osmond, H. 1973. The 'sick role' revisited. Hastings Center Studies 1: 41-58.

(31) Sternbach, R.A. 1974. Varieties of pain games. In Advances in Neurology, ed. J.J. Bonica, vol. 4, pp. 423-432. New York: Raven.

(32) Sternbach, R.A. 1978. Clinical aspects of pain. In The Psychology of Pain, ed. R.A. Sternbach, pp. 241-264. New York: Raven.

(33) Veatch, R.M. 1974. Drugs and competing drug ethics. Hastings Center Studies 2: 86-90.

(34) Wulff, H. 1976. Rational Diagnosis and Treatment. Oxford: Blackwell Scientific.

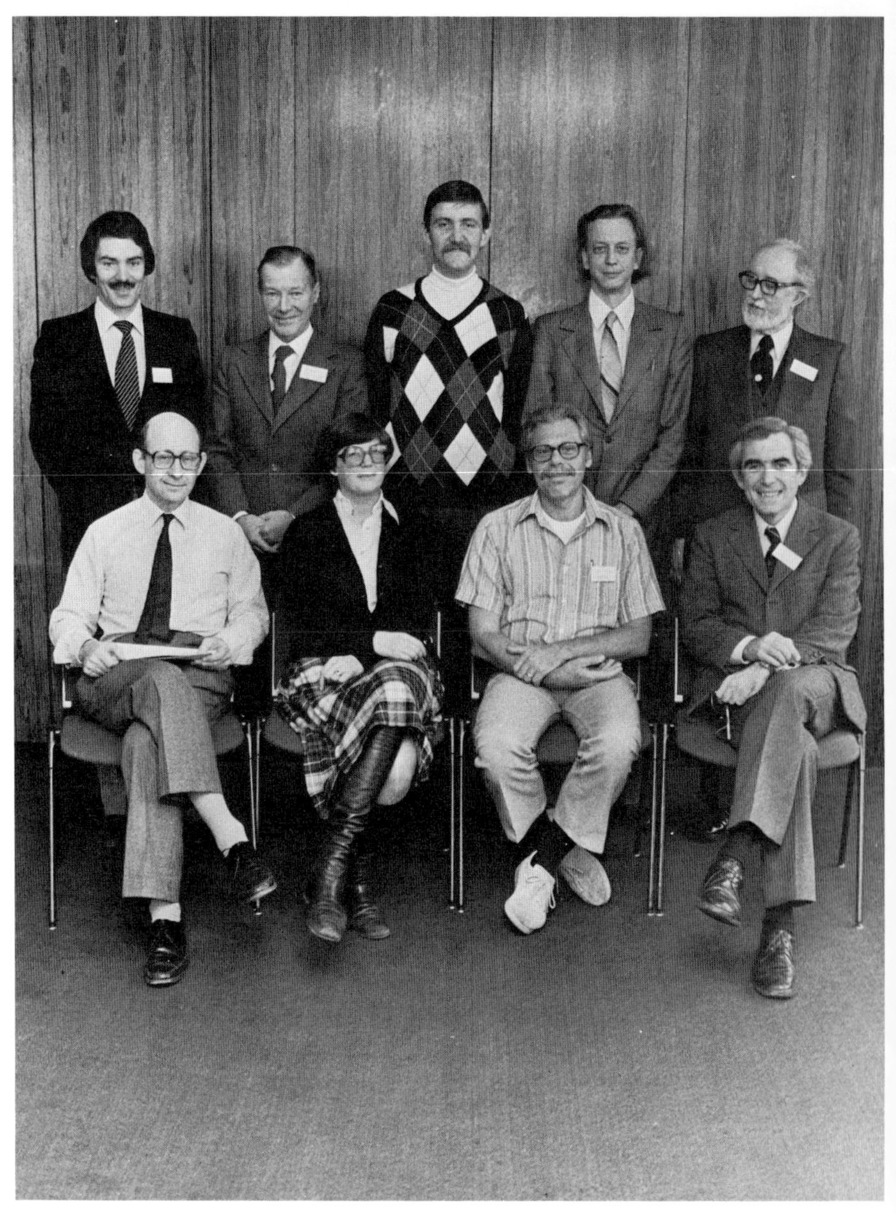

Group on <u>The Principles of Pain Management</u>: Seated, left to right: Harold Merskey, Margareta Eriksson, Dick Sternbach, Issy Pilowsky. Standing: Volker Sturm, Albrecht Struppler, Bengt Sjölund, Tris Engelhardt, Jr., Ray Houde.

Pain and Society, eds. H.W. Kosterlitz and L.Y. Terenius, pp. 483-500.
Dahlem Konferenzen 1980. Weinheim: Verlag Chemie GmbH.

The Principles of Pain Management Group Report

H. Merskey, Rapporteur
H. T. Engelhardt, Jr., M. B. E. Eriksson, R. W. Houde,
K. Mizumura, I. Pilowsky, B. H. Sjölund, R. A. Sternbach,
A. Struppler, V. Sturm

Q: "What is a necessary condition of the experience of pain"?

A: "Consciousness."

(An exchange during group discussion)

It is not possible to manage pain in a theoretical vacuum. Our concepts of the nature of pain, of who may be a patient with pain, and of what factors may cause pain all influence our ideas of treatment and management. In the subsequent discussion it will appear that ideas about the treatment of pain also affect our concepts regarding pain and patients. Meanwhile, for the purposes of this group, it has been agreed that it is necessary to explore the prior concepts and questions related to pain before proceeding to consider management.

There are many subsidiary or background questions which are related to these statements. Some of them are as follows: what are the types of bias in our work due to differences in the samples of patients with pain? In other words, what types of patients are different people managing? To what extent should we try to evaluate the psychological aspects in the initial management of patients? What are the implications of different terms, e.g., acute and chronic pain? Can there be an objective measure of pain? Is the social aspect an invariable concomitant of pain and how can it be assessed? How can we link our knowledge of physical and psychological mechanisms with our methods of treatment? How does our way of thinking about science affect our approach to pain?

The foregoing questions involve consideration both of factual data and of concepts. A number of them also relate to our ideas of the facts and theories and problems of medicine. More direct questions about treatment include: Are drugs the answer? Will they encourage or cause "pain behavior"? What is the place of stimulation techniques? What are the proper limits of destructive surgery and phenol blocks? Is an eclectic approach the best one? Should there be pain clinics? Can anything be done for prevention and for prediction of high risk cases? Can drug dependence be justified and is some dependence no more for pain than spectacles are for myopia? Should we consider an economic factor in medicine and who should control the system for pain management? Should it be the patient or the physician? What values are relevant? What arrangements should generate the system and values which will be most satisfactory or nearest to the ideal?

The group believes all these questions can be grouped into three major categories as in the following table.

TABLE 1 - Classes of questions about pain.

PATIENTS	CONCEPTS	TREATMENTS
Who are they?	What are they? a) phenomenological b) methods of explanation c) expectations based on social roles	What are they and how do we assess them?

The categories are not isolated from each other. Every question in one category has a bearing on another category. The figure below sets this out diagrammatically for heuristic purposes, showing ways in which one can isolate different basic dimensions of pain research and therapy.

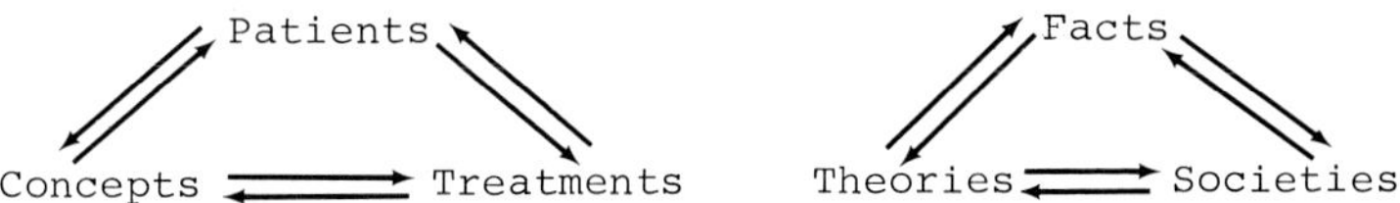

FIG. 1 - Relationship among patients, concepts, and treatment.

The relationships in the diagram are two-way. If the scheme provided is sound, we should be able to develop a tolerable framework in which to study pain and its treatment. In the course of the sessions it became clear that ideas about concepts were discussed extensively first in the context of the nature of the patients encountered and then as a response to problems found with treatment and management. These two themes are therefore reviewed in the next two sections.

WHO ARE THE PATIENTS?

The answer to this question depends upon location of the physician, selection processes, whether the pain is acute or chronic, the characteristics of the therapist, and the nature of what he has to offer. This applies to a pain clinic or a general practitioner as much as to an orthopedic surgeon or a dentist. In general practice patients only report a tiny proportion of their symptoms to their general practitioner. Findings in this field immediately call into question the representative nature of any sample from a hospital, a clinic, or an individual physician.

Some types of setting in which patients have been described can be listed as follows.

- Different sorts of pain and headache clinics
- Psychiatric hospitals and departments
- Neurological and neurosurgical services
- Dental and other types of service for facial pain
- Cancer treatment centers

- Rheumatology departments
- Anesthesiology departments

Centers try hard to label patients. Diagnostic labels can, on the one hand, usefully direct our attention to some important views, or, on the other, divert us from other important matters. For example, referring to a patient as "psychiatric, dental, organic" and so forth may lead us to see him or her as a case, not as a person with his or her own special desires, interests, and wishes. It may also lead us to fail to attend to all the relevant therapeutic approaches. As a result we must examine the ways in which classifications direct research, therapy, and the ways in which we are willing to acknowledge patients as collaborators in their care. Diagnostic labels not only describe reality, but evaluate reality, and create social roles for patients.

Certain trends are evident from the different settings. Patients selected for psychiatric illness and pain in the absence of physical lesions have many neurotic features (hysterical, anxious, exogenous depression, and occasionally other diagnoses). Such patients without lesions whose pain is of short duration may show comparatively more evidence of anxiety and depression than of hysterical features, while those with continuing psychiatric illness manifest more emotional changes later in the illness. Patients with neurological lesions show relatively more evidence of anxiety and depression. On psychological tests facial pain patients, low back pain patients, and patients from pain clinics tend to show neurotic trends including some hysterical features. Furthermore, there is a relationship between complaint behavior and personality variables like neuroticism, introversion, and extraversion. This relationship is affected by cultural variables but no ethnic differences have been proved in respect to the experience of pain. Amongst the various findings, the relationship between pain and depression excited particular attention, together with a need for more information on the latter theme.

In reports on psychiatric patients, the commonest type of pain is headache and this is the case in general practice. Reports from N. American pain clinics, where headache is usually referred to headache clinics, emphasize low back pain as the commonest type. It follows that reports on populations of patients with pain should always indicate the country, place of origin, type of medical practice from which they come, the sites of pain in the patients studied, and the principal physical and psychiatric diagnoses and supporting evidence for them.

The frequency of pain in overall patient populations is also a matter of interest and has been the subject of a variety of reports. In time perhaps the International Association for the Study of Pain (IASP) might consider attempting to generate some standardized comparative studies in different samples and in different patient populations. The epidemiology of pain, as a complaint, is virtually untouched as a field of study, except for some studies of migraine and headache, and yet such enquiries meet very little resistance in populations under survey. The status of the patients in regard to how many may be entitled to compensation also requires definition. The differences in experiences in early life between patients with pain related to lesions and those without lesions have hardly been touched upon in any studies and are a topic of enquiry which is theoretically very important. At present that topic is the subject of speculations but almost no controlled evidence.

Classificatory work, which goes beyond pain terms and groups and describes syndromes associated with pain, has been begun and more is required. Illness classifications based on aspects of pain have figured in the evolution of systematic classifications (cf. Engelhardt, this volume). A classificatory system for pain which provides specific descriptions for pain syndromes is feasible, as demonstrated by the work of Bonica, and ought to be more widely instituted. In order to encompass the various purposes of therapy and research, a multi-dimensional system of classification is required.

This review of knowledge about "Who are the patients?" concludes that if answers to this question are sought we should obtain much more sound information about the relationship among pain, organic lesions, human personality, psychiatric illness, and social relationships. This is in addition to any basic epidemiological information about the true incidence and prevalence rates of chronic painful illness, which except perhaps for headache and one or two categories in the musculoskeletal systems, is also seriously lacking.

Further in this section the group expressed distinct concern about the need for all patients to have an adequate basic physical assessment as well as psychological and social evaluation. Although this statement ought to be axiomatic, our experience was such that it was felt necessary to emphasize this need as well as the need to have an open sympathetic discussion with the patient in the light of the results of the enquiries into his or her complaint and condition.

The Nature of the Data

Phenomenological aspects of pain include what we mean by pain, how it is described, and other clinical features by which it may be defined. The IASP (1979) has published a list of Pain Terms with definitions. The aim of this list is to promote consistency in the use of terms so that work from different places may be more readily compared. The specific definition of the word pain as "an unpleasant sensory and emotional experience which we associate with tissue damage and describe in terms of tissue damage" serves an additional function. It emphasizes the necessity to view pain as a subjective experience described in the language of psychology. As such it is distinct from the very important events in sensory receptors, nerves, and the spinal cord and higher parts of the nervous system which occur as a result of noxious stimulation. Those events have to be described in their own terms, relevant to physical measurements. One philosophical viewpoint about this situation is that it represents a parallelism of properties.

The fundamental events have concomitant psychological properties and physical ones. This question is not simply a metaphysical topic but influences the ways in which physiological data are understood and clinical practice conducted.

TREATMENTS

General Aspects

It is largely accepted that pain does not have a one-to-one relationship with intensity of noxious stimulation. The influence of emotional states, mood changes, arousal, and the significance of the situation in which a lesion occurs have all been promoted as factors which influence the occurrence or severity of pain. The social context is further held to influence the expression of ideas, feelings, or reports by individuals in regard to pain which they may experience, and all these considerations bear upon the forms of treatment to be employed.

A simple position can be taken based on two propositions. Some pain is a consequence of noxious stimulation or other organic or pathophysiological disturbance. Some pain, by contrast, results from emotional causes and no direct physical agent can be detected. The definitions and approaches to phenomenology which have been presented in the last section are shaped by this theoretical position. A third proposition which it entails is that the subjective experience may be determined to a varying extent by these two groups of causes. Parenthetically we can note that few workers currently feel that it is usually possible or suitable to try and dissect out which bit of the pain experience is emotionally determined and which is organically induced. However, all agree that assessment of the relative importance of organic and psychological causes is essential in each case. Some group members emphasize that at times pain can be recognized as wholly due to organic causes, others disagree. It can also be remarked that some differences are described or anticipated in the subjective reports of individuals who have pain for these different reasons.

One of the immediate therapeutic consequences of the foregoing principal assumptions is that appropriate standard physical and psychiatric treatments would be instituted for a complaint of pain. Part of the reason for the emergence of other methods of explanation and treatment is the failure of these routine approaches in many cases.

Another point of view is that even though emotional changes and causes are important, there may always be a substratum of physical change occurring outside the brain so that a person with an emotional difficulty may emphasize or experience minor sensory changes more than usual. In that case what would ordinarily be a transient mild ache is felt as a troublesome pain. The argument is that we select, unconsciously, some pain or related sensation from our repertoire of experiences and it then develops obtrusive unpleasant characteristics.

The opinion that pain may result from thought processes is supported by anecdotal evidence of such happenings, by the occurrence of pain which can be demonstrated to have symbolic functions, especially conversion reactions and the couvade syndrome, and by the frequent evidence of hysterical characteristics with chronic pain without lesions. That opinion is also implicit in the generally accepted view that pain may be a conversion symptom and in some of the principles of cognitive therapy (see below). It gains some extra strength from the view that alternative mechanisms (especially a tension-pain theory) have failed to provide adequate evidence when tested. The view that pain has not been shown to arise from thought processes may be supported on the basis that the direct evidence so far presented is insufficient and does not carry conviction.

Also, examples of pain without a physical basis occurring in dreams have not been reported and it is hard for anyone to develop a conscious experience of pain deliberately by processes of imagination.

Some less controversial general problems were also emphasized. Emergency measures are rarely needed for the treatment of chronic pain. It follows that it is usually desirable to use the least invasive or toxic treatment possible. However, there are instances of severe pain illness, where it is a mistake to delay, on principle alone, proceeding to invasive measures. Even so the latter should not be introduced without adequate attention to the emotional and social situation of the patient.

The possibility of an organic diagnosis being missed or a relevant psychiatric diagnosis being ignored leads to emphasis on the need for adequate interdisciplinary consultation. The possible institution of damaging treatment based on a wrong diagnosis or indications reinforces the need for appropriate education of medical practitioners so that they can recognize the best way to manage the patient. A multidisciplinary clinic sometimes provides a safety net to make up for such deficiencies in education or practice.

Psychological Treatments

Consideration of the psychodynamics of pain has been part of the psychoanalytic contribution to the understanding of pain. Individual responses have often been reported in the treatment of pain by analytically oriented psychotherapy. Speculations about pain and guilt and about pain and masochism derive from this source, as also do ideas about the importance of family background and marital conflict in promoting pain. However, treatment for chronic pain by techniques related to these ideas has had only limited success.

One of the new approaches is to formulate phenomena related to pain in terms of behavior. Statements about pain and actions such as resting, or complaining or refusing to rest after exertion are labelled as "pain behavior." Treatment is then directed according to an operational hypothesis towards reducing "pain behaviors" (extinction) and encouraging behavior which is usually or partly incompatible with pain (reinforcement). This approach does not necessarily deny but does diminish attention to the subjective experience of the individual. There was a strong feeling in the group that it would be more satisfactory to speak of "pain-related behavior."

Another approach whose theoretical principles are largely new is found in cognitive therapy. This is based on the hypothesis that the patient has faulty ideas which lead him to construe his environment wrongly and experience it in ways which are mistaken. If his view of himself in relation to his environment changes so may his experiences, including his mood. This implies that ideas which result from false "cognitions" may be altered by providing better cognitions. A second object of cognitive therapy has to do with teaching patients to identify their reactions to stress and adopt better "coping skills" or strategies for relieving pain such as "distancing" from the pain, gaining awareness of possibilities of control over it, using relaxation, concentration, or distraction, deliberately cultivating alternative imagery to reduce pain and giving self-instructions like "calm-down," "concentrate on the present," etc. Like behavior therapy for pain, cognitive therapy has operant characteristics.

Cognitive therapy has been widely investigated so far in the laboratory, but there have been few clinical reports. However, these include at least two controlled studies with positive results. The conceptual standpoint of cognitive therapy clearly requires the view that pain may be reduced by altering thought processes. The evaluation of its usefulness has scarcely begun and much more controlled evidence is needed.

During the review of psychological therapies a consensus readily emerged that the scientific evidence for the usefulness of all the treatments under consideration is poor. The good example of research into psychotherapy was cited by comparison and the following requirements were noted to be needed:

systematic evidence of the characteristics of the patients treated, controls, investigation of single modalities, good outcome measures which should include both the doctor's view and the patient's view and long-term follow-up studies. This is not intended to be an exhaustive list. It applies as well to somatic therapies.

Some other conclusions noted are as follows: the revisions of theory which are being undertaken are a response to failures with a residual group of patients. Many others do respond to available treatments and also some of our expectations may be too high. Those treatments seem to work best which possess or require high activity, high visibility, high contact, and high apparent relevance. The adherence of the patient to the program has to be obtained and this is facilitated if the patient's pain is taken seriously. Whilst the latter precept is axiomatic in terms of the human consideration which should imbue the doctor-patient relationship, it is also essential to the success of treatment. It leads on to the observation that management is not the same as treatment.

Somatic therapies

Like the psychological therapies, all somatic therapies involve the doctor-patient relationship. They are often misused but definitely have a place. It was not possible for the review of somatic therapies to be exhaustive for all treatment or even adequately detailed about several. However, most standpoints were agreed to quite readily.

Pharmacological Methods

Drug therapy is undoubtedly useful. There is a need for better analgesics. No drug can be expected to have only one effect, hence long-term administration of any medication is likely to lead to unwanted somatic changes. However, existing analgesics are subject to disadvantageous side effects, particularly the narcotics to which tolerance develops, whilst other drugs are less effective and also have hazards.

Narcotics are potent but on chronic administration are liable to cause dependence with side effects. They are therefore usually reserved, in long-term use, for patients with malignant diseases. In recent years it has been emphasized that they must be used as part of the comprehensive treatment of cancer patients. For pre-terminal patients with pain it is considered proper to use large doses of opiates sufficient to control pain adequately.

There are strong clinical impressions that tricyclic antidepressants and monoamine oxidase inhibitors relieve some patients in pain. There are also a few controlled trials to this effect in patients with pain and depression combined. More trials are needed. Antidepressants are generally not thought to be effective for pain in the absence of depression. Overall there is a need for more controlled studies with antidepressants using adequate methods of recording and assessing pain, depression, the type of depression, and the outcome.

Local anesthetic nerve blocks have a variety of uses. These were not discussed in detail. There is a consensus that repeated temporary blocks are preferable to neurolytic blocks or surgical section of nerves which appears to cause denervation hypersensitivity or other pain-generating mechanisms.

Destructive Measures

These were not reviewed in detail. The general current view was stated that for pain due to neoplasms it is best for any such treatment to be given relatively early. In chronic pain without neoplasms there is little or no place for destructive surgery because it is not sufficiently effective to justify the risk of complications which include additional pain of the deafferentation type. One exception occurs in the treatment of trigeminal neuralgia. If carbamazepine and transcutaneous electrical nerve stimulation (TENS) are ineffective, thermocoagulation of the Gasserian ganglion can be successful. In cancer patients suffering from cervical, neck, and facial pain, thalamotomy may be indicated. Cancer pain originating from lower sites may be treated by percutaneous or open chordotomy.

Electrical Stimulation Techniques

These are held to operate by activation of control systems. TENS is a benign procedure. A combined approach using acupuncture-like stimulation and conventional TENS has a 50% rate of effectiveness at a two-year follow-up provided that the patients have lesions and provided that the lesions do not affect the viscera. Less selected groups with conventional TENS alone show less improvment after 12 months (Sjölund and Eriksson, this volume).

Stimulation by implanted devices should be considered only when TENS has proved to be ineffective. From the present clinical experience as reported in retrospective studies this mainly applies to those patients with pain due to organic lesions, but of nonvisceral origin, the aim being to reach presumed control systems that are not accessible to a sufficient degree by stimulation of peripheral nerves.

Two sets of procedures are available at present, dorsal column stimulation (DCS) and stimulation of deep brain structures (DBS). It appears that dorsal column stimulation should be considered for lesions in the distal neuraxis, e.g., in the periphery, the nerves, the roots, and possibly the spinal cord, whereas DBS may be used only after DCS has failed or if the lesion is in more proximal parts of the neuraxis.

Interestingly, "deafferentation pain" seems to respond better to DBS in the ventral part of the ventroposterolateral thalamic nucleus whereas pain due to excessive noxious stimulation appears to benefit from DBS in periventricular and periaqueductal areas. Implanted electrodes may rarely give rise to gliosis, infection, and other undesirable consequences. For these reasons prospective controlled studies of these methods should precede their more general use.

New Therapies

It was evident during the review of different therapies that many of the new ones were first used with much enthusiasm and later found to be disappointing.

Figure 2, which is a popular curve, illustrates the way in which a reasonable treatment may come into use on the basis of a preliminary investigation and achieve recognition which quickly becomes excessive. Subsequent disappointment may then lead to either the disuse of a worthwhile measure or to its correct employment. Examples were given of surgical techniques, new drugs, and behavioral therapies.

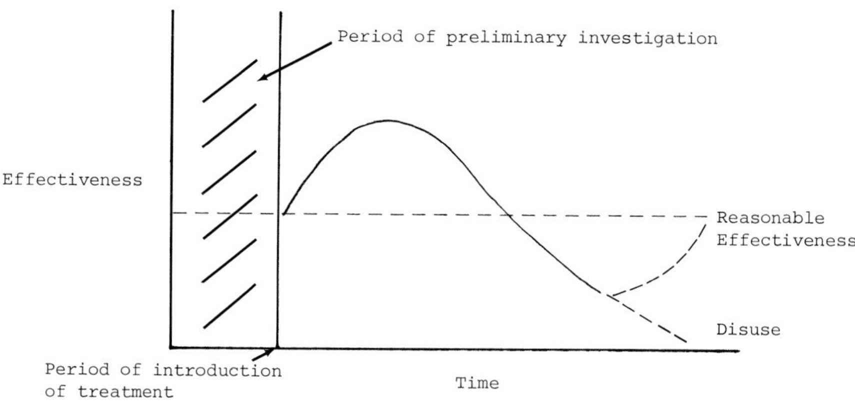

FIG. 2 - A Popular Enthusiasm Curve

The tendency can be moderated if there is proper experimental research, consisting of basic research on animals, if appropriate, and of controlled clinical trials with regular public reviews of findings. Therapists should also be adequately advised of correct indications and encouraged to produce careful outcome studies with reports of findings at successive stages of follow-up.

Multidisciplinary "pain clinics" or centers may avoid the errors of uncritical application of new therapies by adhering to the above practices.

Pain Clinics

The recent rapid growth of multidisciplinary pain clinics has the advantage of providing specialty skills and colloboration, and not merely consultation, among therapists. Two disadvantages, however, are that the centers may substitute for a general education of the medical practitioner in the proper management of patients with pain and the patient may be "forgotten or lost" in the administrative maze of the institution. We think that the "clinic" itself is not always required. The essential need is for a regular formal commitment to collaborative multidisciplinary meetings with the patient as a focus.

SOCIAL ASPECTS

Social influences on pain have been mentioned in passing but require more consideration (cf. Pilowsky, this volume). The notion of illness behavior provides another way of formulating the situation concerning chronic pain and relates well to sociological concepts. Chronic pain is identified as a form of illness behavior in which there is often a discrepancy between the somatic findings and the patient's complaints and behavior. This discrepancy results in a disagreement between doctor and patient. It may result in rejection or partial rejection of the individual's status as a sick person. There are social factors like low socioeconomic status which predispose the patient to require a sick role and to suffer in some ways, if it is not accorded to him. It is necessary to understand the benefit of the sick role and its advantages for many patients with chronic pain.

Chronic pain often involves a socially unacceptable claim to the sick role as it is most often associated with hypochondriacal and hysterical patterns which can be notoriously unresponsive to existing psychiatric treatments. On the whole we are better at recognizing some of the causal factors than at changing them. This is perhaps even more the case with regard to the intrapersonal factors which promote chronic pain, than with regard to the social ones. The ways in which the sick role can be relinquished therefore need particular study. Whatever the exact position may be in these matters, concepts related to the sick role offer a potentially useful universe of discourse within which to consider social and cultural aspects of pain. It may be developed by attention to marital, family, and social data in the individual patient and some hold that these aspects must be evaluated in all chronic pain patients.

It was noted that there are ethnic and social class associations with the complaint of pain or with the way in which it is expressed. This may vary from group to group and within groups in different circumstances. Evidence which suggests a difference between ethnic groups in the liability to feel pain is contradicted by other studies or is open to other interpretations. There is, however, strong evidence that the expression of pain, the way in which it is or is not accepted, and the way in which it influences behavior all vary considerably according to the traditions and expectations of different groups. There has been little if any direct application of these principles to the management of chronic pain, although it can be presumed that they are applied, at least sometimes, by physicians who understand the relevant cultural situations.

REFERENCES

(1) Andersson, S.A. 1979. Pain control by sensory stimulation In Advances in Pain Research and Therapy, eds. J.J. Bonica et al., vol. 3, pp. 569-585. New York: Raven Press.

(2) International Association for the Study of Pain. 1979. Pain terms: A list with definitions and notes on usage. Pain 6: 249-252.

(3) Long, D.M.; Campbell, J.N.; and Gucer, G. 1979. Transcutaneous electrical stimulation for relief of chronic pain. In Advances in Pain Research and Therapy, eds. J.J. Bonica et al., vol. 3, pp. 593-599. New York: Raven Press.

(4) Merskey, H. 1979. The contribution of the psychiatrist to the treatment of pain. In Pain, ed. J.J. Bonica. Proc. Ass. Res. Nerv. Ment. Dis. New York: Raven Press.

(5) Meyerson, B.A.; Boethius, J.; and Carlsson, A.M. 1979. Alleviation of malignant pain by electrical stimulation in the periventricular-periaqueductal region: Pain relief as related to stimulation sites. In Advances in Pain Research and Therapy, eds. J.J. Bonica et al., vol. 3, pp. 525-533. New York: Raven Press.

(6) Sternbach, R.A. 1978. The Psychology of Pain. New York: Academic Press.

List of Participants

AKIL, H.
Mental Health Research Institute
University of Michigan
Ann Arbor, MI 48109, USA

Field of research: Biochemistry and physiology of endorphins

ALBE-FESSARD, D.G.
Laboratoire de Physiologie des Centres Nerveux
Université P. et M. Curie
75230 Paris, France

Field of research: Central reception of pain messages, animal models for pain diseases

BASBAUM, A.I.
Department of Anatomy
University of California
San Francisco, CA 94143, USA

Field of research: Neuroanatomy of pain and pain modulation, synaptic relationships of peptides and monoamines in the spinal dorsal horn

BESSON, J.-M.R.
Unité de Recherches de Neurophysiologie Pharmacologique, INSERM (U. 161)
74014 Paris, France

Field of research: Physiology and neuropharmacology of pain

BOND, M.R.
University Department of Psychological Medicine, Southern General Hospital
Glasgow G51 4TF, Scotland

Field of research: Psychological and psychiatric studies of chronic painful disorders (benign and malignant)

BRINKHUS, H.
II. Physiologisches Institut
Universität Heidelberg
6900 Heidelberg, F.R. Germany

Field of research: Neuronal correlations with nocifensive behavior (thalamus)

CARLI, G.
Istituto di Fisiologia Umana
53100 Siena, Italy

Field of research: Pain and animal hypnosis, somatosensory system, position neurons

CARSTENS, E.
II. Physiologisches Institut
Universität Heidelberg
6900 Heidelberg, F.R. Germany

Field of research: Neurophysiology and neuropharmacology of pain mechanisms

CASEY, K.L.
Department of Physiology
University of Michigan Medical School
Ann Arbor, MI 48109, USA

Field of research: Central nervous system, neurophysiology of pain

CERVERO, F.
Department of Physiology
University of Edinburgh Medical School
Edinburgh EH8 9AG, Scotland

Field of research: Neurophysiology of sensory systems

CHAPMAN, C.R.
Department of Anesthesiology RN-10
University of Washington
Seattle, WA 98195, USA

Field of research: Perception of pain in man, measurement of human pain in the laboratory

CRAIG, K.D.
Department of Psychology
University of British Columbia
Vancouver, B.C. V6T 1W5, Canada

Field of research: Clinical psychology, sociocultural determinants of pain experience and behavior

DUM, J.E.
Abteilung Neuropharmakologie
Max-Planck-Institut für
Psychiatrie
8000 Munich 40, F.R. Germany

Field of research: Neuropharmacology, opiates, behavioral methods

ENGELHARDT, H.T., Jr.
Kennedy Institute of Ethics
Georgetown University
Washington, D.C. 20057, USA

Field of research: Philosophy and history of medicine

ERIKSSON, M.B.E.
Department of Clinical Neurophysiology, University Hospital
221 85 Lund, Sweden

Field of research: Clinical and experimental work on management of pain and mechanisms of pain control by stimulation techniques

FINER, B.L.
Samariterhemmet, Box 609
751 25 Uppsala 1, Sweden

Field of research: Hypnosis and pain

FISHMAN, J.
The Rockefeller University
New York, NY 10021, USA

Field of research: Opiates, endocrinology, steroid hormones

HANDWERKER, H.O.
II. Physiologisches Institut
Universität Heidelberg
6900 Heidelberg, F.R. Germany

Field of research: Physiology of nociception

HERZ, A.
Abteilung Neuropharmakologie
Max-Planck-Institut für
Psychiatrie
8000 Munich 40, F.R. Germany

Field of research: Opiate research, endorphins, pain, drug dependence

HÖLLT, V.
Max-Planck Institut für
Psychiatrie
8000 Munich 40, F.R. Germany

Field of research: Opioid peptides

HOUDE, R.W.
Memorial Sloan-Kettering Cancer
Center
New York, NY 10021, USA

Field of research: Clinical evaluation of analgesic drugs and management of pain due to cancer

IGGO, A.
Department of Veterinary Physiology
University of Edinburgh
Royal (Dick) School of Veterinary
Studies
Summerhall, Edinburgh EH9 1QH, Scotla

Field of research: Neurophysiology

KNIFFKI, K.-D.
Physiologisches Institut
Universität Kiel
2300 Kiel, F.R. Germany

Field of research: Muscle pain and its central aspects

KOSTERLITZ, H.W.
University of Aberdeen
Unit for Research on Addictive Drugs
Marischal College
Aberdeen AB9 1AS, Scotland

Field of research: Opioid peptides and their receptors

MELZACK, R.
Department of Psychology
McGill University
Montreal, Quebec H3A 1B1, Canada

Field of research: Sensory and psychological modulation of clinical pain, neurochemical mechanisms of analgesia

MERSKEY, H.
London Psychiatric Hospital
London, Ontario N6A 4H1, Canada

Field of research: Pain

MIZUMURA, K.
Physiologisches Institut
Universität Kiel
2300 Kiel, F.R. Germany

Field of research: Thalamic neurons which respond to noxious stimulations (algesic substances and strong mechanical stimulation) in the muscle of cats

NATHAN, P.W.
Medical Research Council
National Hospital for Nervous Diseases, London WC1N 3BG, England

Field of research: Pain: mainly anatomy of pathways in human CNS and effects of substances related to the sympathatic nervous system on painful states with hypersensitivity

PILOWSKY, I.
Department of Psychiatry
University of Adelaide
Adelaide, S.A. 5001, Australia

Field of research: Psychosocial aspects of chronic pain diagnosis and treatment of abnormal illness behavior

PROCACCI, P.
Centro di Algologia, Clinica Medica
Università di Firenze
50134 Florence, Italy

Field of research: Visceral pain, referred pain, transcutaneous electrical stimulation, history of medicine

REEH, P.
Institut für Physiologie und Biokybernetik
Universität Erlangen
8520 Erlangen, F.R. Germany

Field of research: Objective pain measurement in man (tooth pulp evoked potentials)

SCHMIDT, R.F.
Physiologisches Institut
Universität Kiel
2300 Kiel, F.R. Germany

Field of research: Neurophysiology of muscle pain

SJÖLUND, B.H.
Department of Neurosurgery
University Hospital
221 85 Lund, Sweden

Field of research: Stimulation-produced analgesia, mechanisms of action and clinical application

STERNBACH, R.A.
Pain Treatment Center
Scripps Clinic and Research Foundation
La Jolla, CA 92037, USA

Field of research: Pain

STRUPPLER, A.
Neurologische Klinik
Technische Universität
8000 Munich 80, F.R. Germany

Field of research: Studies in experimental pain in man, mechanisms of action

STURM, V.
Abteilung Neurochirurgie
Universität Heidelberg
6900 Heidelberg, F.R. Germany

Field of research: Thalamic electrostimulation in chronic pain syndromes

TAKAGI, H.
Department of Pharmacology
Kyoto University
Kyoto 606, Japan

Field of research: Mechanism of action of opiates and opioid peptides

TERENIUS, L.Y.
Department of Pharmacology
Uppsala University
Box 573, 751 23 Uppsala, Sweden

Field of research: Opioids, pain

TU, W.
Department of History
Berkeley, CA 94720, USA

Field of research: Confucianism, Chinese intellectual history, philosophies of East Asia, Asian and comparative thought

WALL, P.D.
Cerebral Functions Group
Department of Anatomy
University College
London WC1E 6BT, England

Field of research: Pain mechanisms

WILLIS, W.D.
Marine Biomedical Institute
University of Texas Medical Branch
Galveston, TX 77550, USA

Field of research: Pain mechanisms in monkey spinal cord and thalamus

WOLFF, B.B.
Pain Study Group
New York University Medical Center
New York, NY 10016, USA

Field of research: Behavioral mechanisms of human pain, human pain measurement, human analgesic assays, pain control and management

ZIEGLGÄNSBERGER, W.
Max-Planck-Institut für Psychiatrie
8000 Munich 40, F.R. Germany

Field of research: Narcotic analgesics, pain mechanisms, neuropeptides

ZIMMERMANN, M.
II. Physiologisches Institut
Universität Heidelberg
6900 Heidelberg, F.R. Germany

Field of research: Peripheral and central neurophysiology of pain, development of cutaneous receptors in regenerating nerves

Subject Index

Author Index

Dahlem Workshop Reports

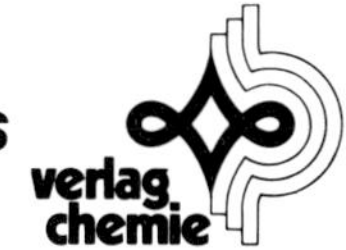

Life Sciences Research Report 6

Function and Formation of Neural Systems

Dahlem Workshop Report on
"Function and Formation of Neural Systems"
held in Berlin between the 7–11 March, 1977.

Editor: Gunther S. Stent, University of California, Berkeley.

Only recently has it been possible to take recordings from single nerve cells, to map their fine structure and their connections, and to test models of nerve cell network functions on computers. New research in "neuroethology" has discovered some nerve cell wiring diagrams and can account for behavioral acts of animals in terms of identified circuits.

This Dahlem Workshop brought together an international group of scientists active in such studies of the nervous system. They compared results obtained from widely different animals – from worms to snails and flies through fish and frogs to cats, monkeys, and man. Their report shows to which extent some general principles of the organization and development of the nervous system have emerged.

1977. 365 pages, with 6 figures and 1 table.
Softcover. ISBN 0-89573-090-1

Fields of interest:
Physiolgy, Neurology, Molecular Biology, Biophysics, Anatomy, Zoology, Ethology, Cybernetics, Psychology.

Dahlem Workshop Reports

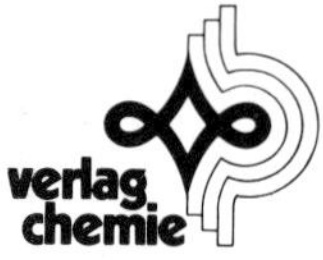

Life Sciences Research Report 10

Abnormal Fetal Growth: Biological Bases and Consequences

Dahlem Workshop Report on
"Abnormal Fetal Growth: Biological Bases and Consequences"
held in Berlin between the 20–24 February, 1978.

Editor: Fred Naftolin, Royal Victoria Hospital, Montreal.

Interest in *normal* and *abnormal* fetal growth has intensified due to progress in two major areas of importance:
– our growing understanding of normal and disordered cell biology makes the developing fetus an ideal model for theoretical and applied studies, and
– the availability of physical measurements of the developing fetus in the clinical situation has given immediate relevance to the early detection, understanding and treatment of abnormal growth.

The contributors have attempted to focus a multidisciplinary approach on the opportunities and challenges presented by this problem. The reader will find the views of Embryologists, Cell Biologists, Perinatologists and others represented here. This mixture of backgrounds brings a flavor and critical approach to the problem of Abnormal Fetal Growth which is not generally available. The result is a definition of the problem and many clues to its observation and solution.

1978. 291 pages, with 15 figures and 15 tables.
Softcover. ISBN 0-89573-094-4

Fields of interest:
Pharmacy, Biochemistry, Genetics, Physiology, Pathology.